THE PERI DIET

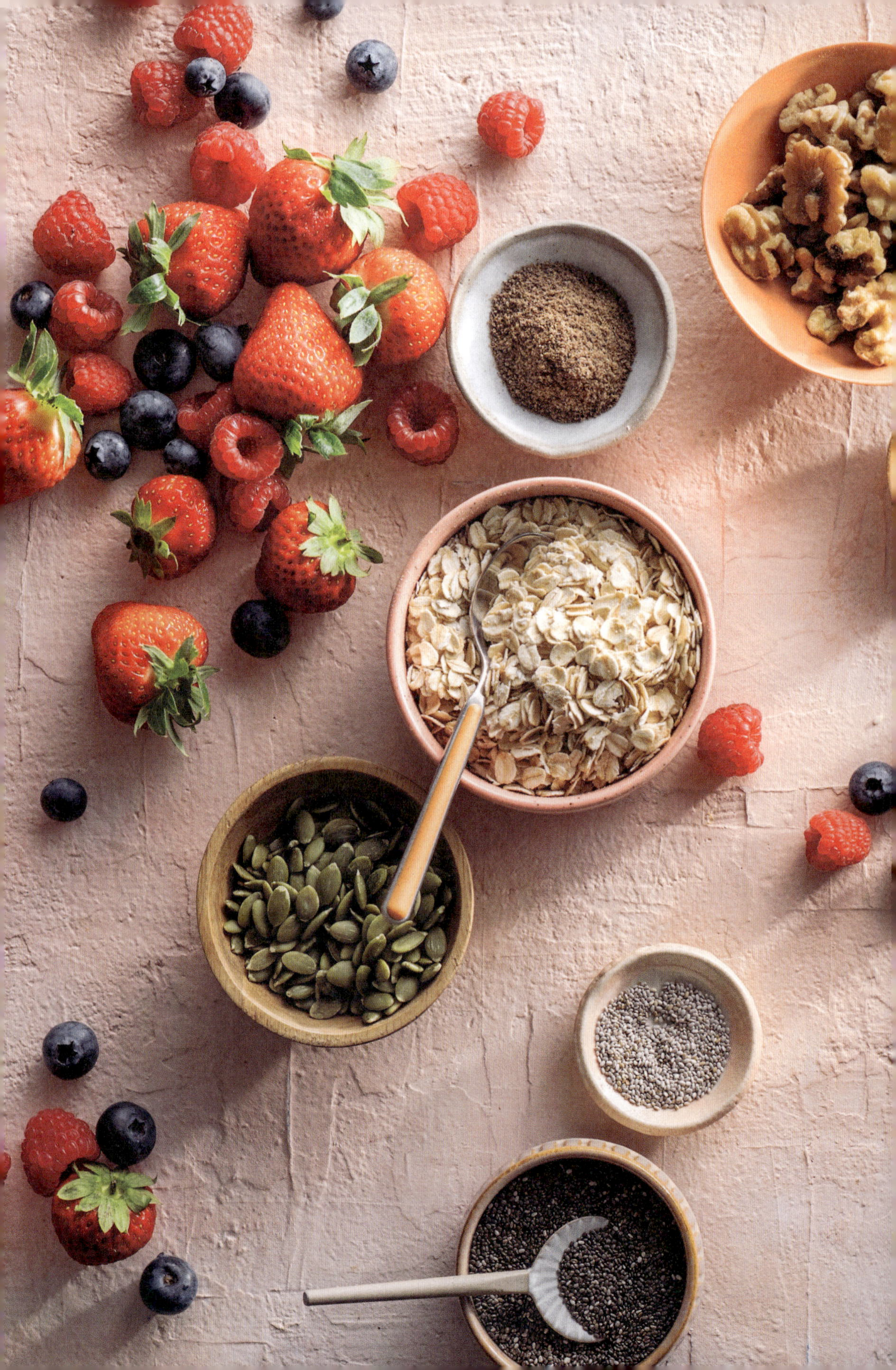

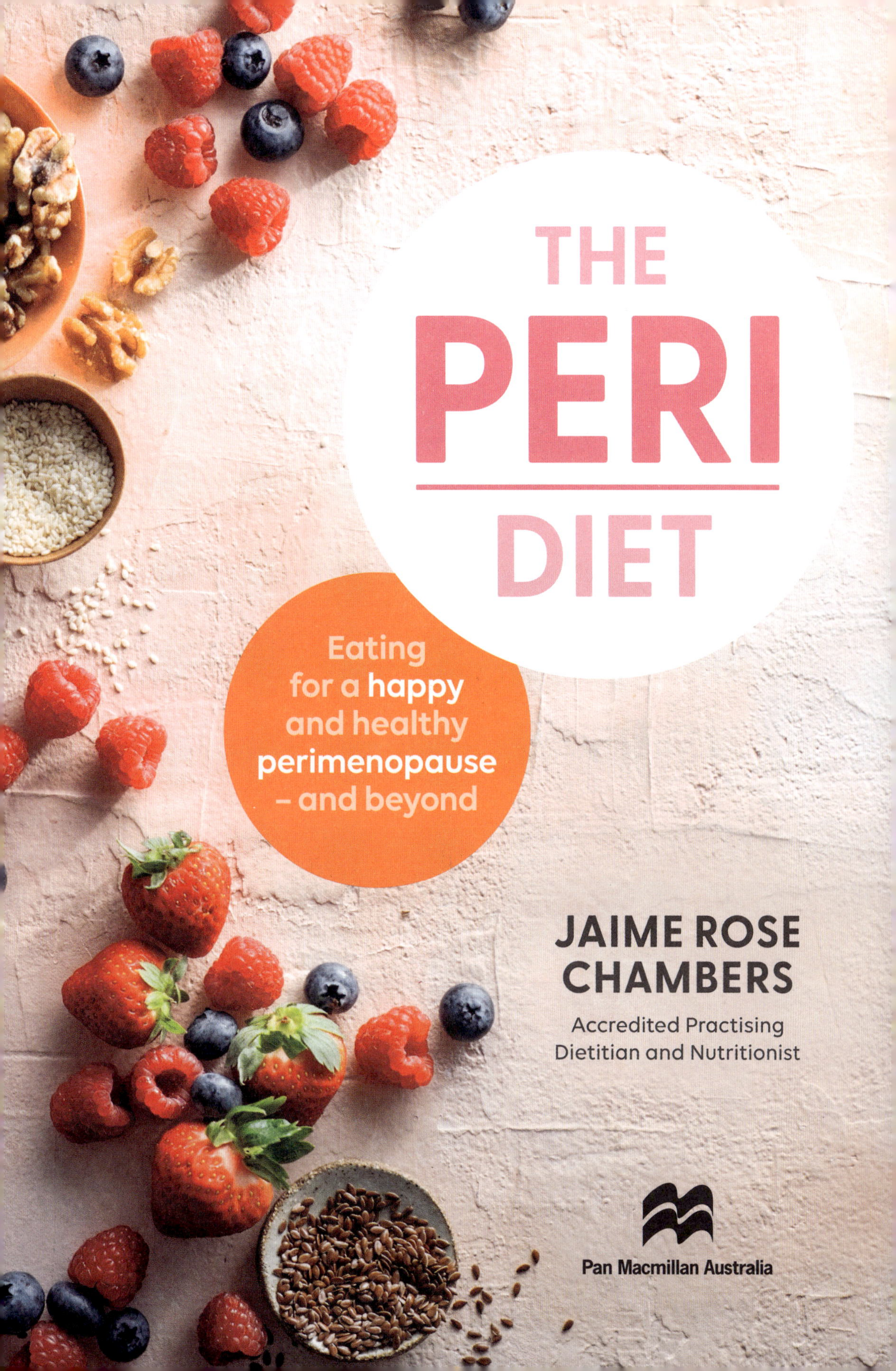

THE PERI DIET

Eating for a **happy** and healthy **perimenopause** – and beyond

JAIME ROSE CHAMBERS

Accredited Practising Dietitian and Nutritionist

Pan Macmillan Australia

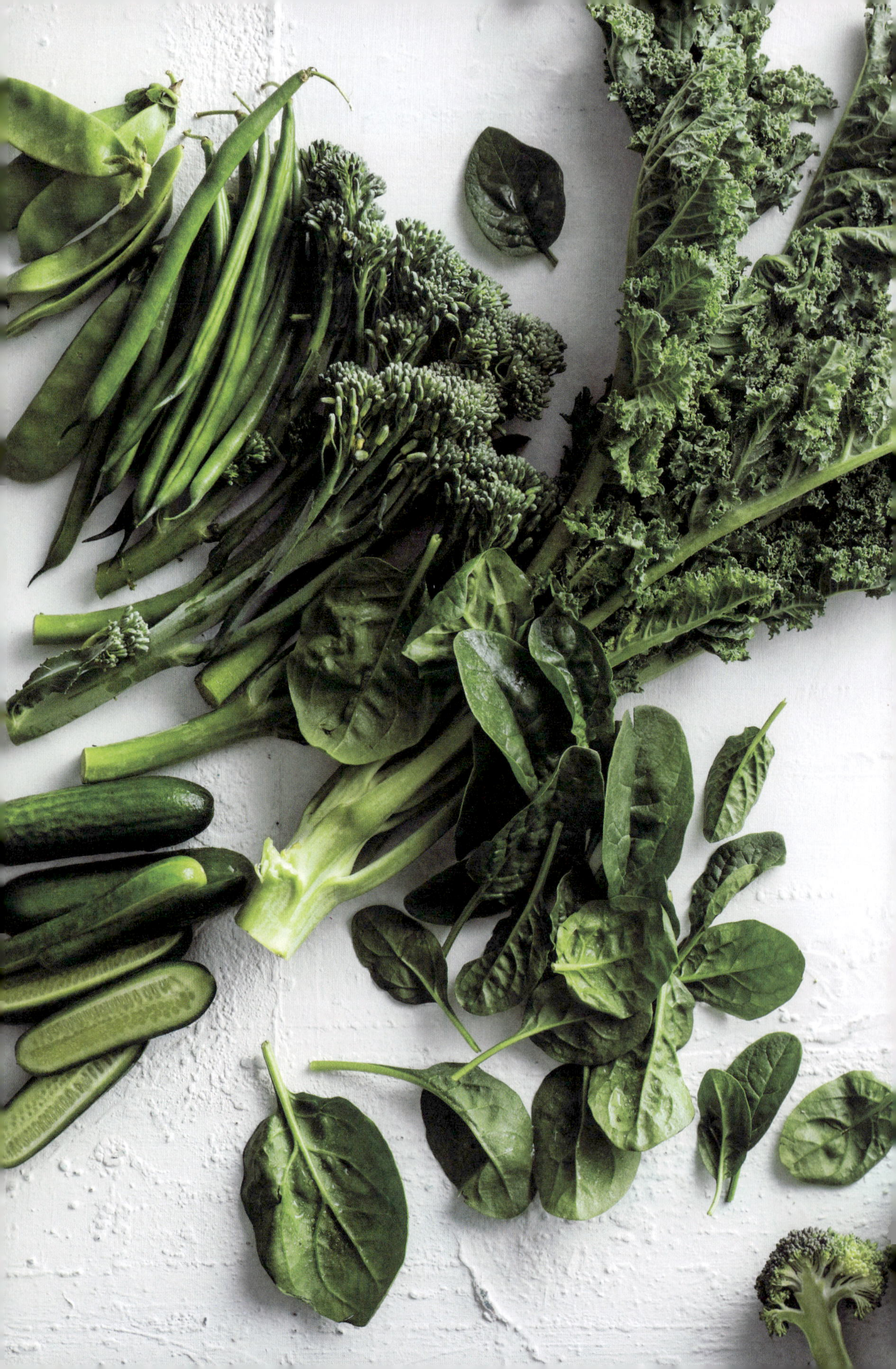

Contents

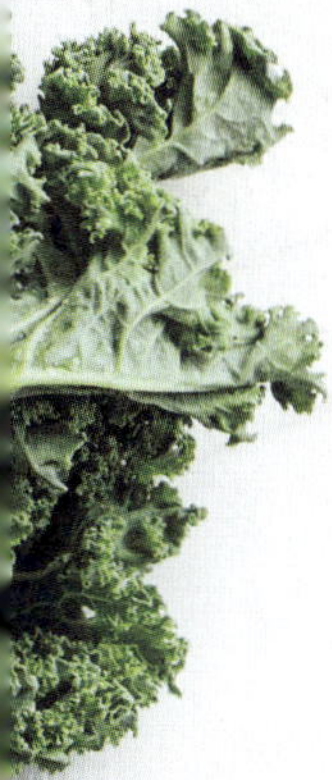

RECIPES

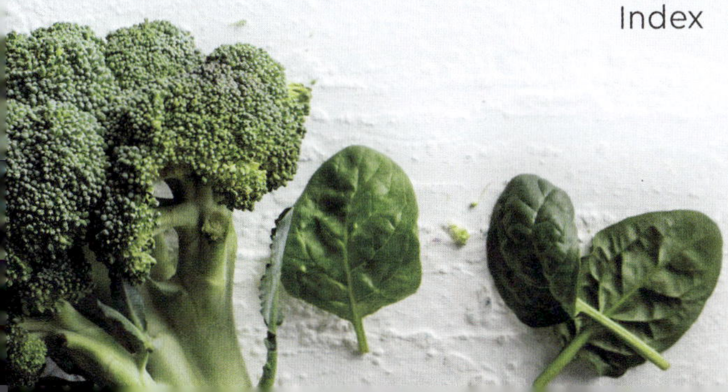

Introduction

Welcome to The Peri Diet. As I write this, I'm 42 years old and over the past couple of years, I've started noticing small changes in my body. For one thing, my overall shape has altered following the births of my children. Also, my periods are now often longer or shorter, heavier or lighter, than usual. Likewise, my hormonal symptoms are a little different. Not by much – but it's enough that I know I'm in that 'peri zone'.

Being in my early forties, I'm certainly within the age range for perimenopause. This is the phase that occurs before menopause, which is the point at which a woman's ovaries run out of eggs and her reproductive hormones fall. The average age for menopause in Australia is 51 and we can spend years in the transitional phase leading up to it. So learning what to expect from peri and how to feel our best during this time of change is incredibly important – not only because it can help to minimise disruptive symptoms but also because it can set us up for long-term health in the years that follow.

I'm fortunate that my job as a dietitian and nutritionist has armed me with a lot of knowledge about the challenges of perimenopause. I've done plenty of research, of course, but I've also amassed 15 years of hands-on experience by managing so many peri and menopausal patients over that time. Thanks to this, I have a sense of confidence about facing this significant life transition myself. Of course, I may not always feel this way, but right now, when I monitor my body and notice the changes that are happening, I'm able to be more objective about them. Most importantly, I've not been completely caught off-guard the way many women are. Right now, I'm gearing myself up physically and mentally so I'm in the best position to manage and minimise unwelcome symptoms such as hot flushes, mood changes and sleep disruption, and get through the other end successfully. That's what I hope for you, too, and exactly why I wrote this book!

Talking about peri

A woman is deemed to be officially in menopause once she has gone 12 months without a period. Historically, menopause itself has been given most of the medical (and media) attention – still not enough, quite frankly – but it isn't the most significant time of this lifestage. It is perimenopause, the lead-up to those 12 period-free months, when most of the action happens.

Up until relatively recently, medical professionals didn't consider perimenopause a phase worth discussing. It was seldom acknowledged and it certainly wasn't linked with the many symptoms women were experiencing. Doctors may have talked to their patients about 'the change' of menopause, but the transitional time leading up to it wasn't widely discussed, and consequently, women didn't anticipate the many associated symptoms. Thankfully, this is changing. There seems to be an outpouring of information about perimenopause now, which is brilliant for all of us who are currently experiencing it (or will in the future). On social media especially, I've noticed that women are talking about it a lot, and they're talking loudly! And so they should.

Because peri can be bloody hard. For most women, it is more difficult than menopause, plus it can last for as long as 10 years. While some women may be lucky enough to sail through it and barely notice changes, some will experience symptoms so distressing that their relationships, career and mental wellbeing are significantly impacted.

I've heard plenty of stories about perimenopausal women being put on antidepressants and anti-anxiety meds because their GPs didn't realise that perimenopause could be at the root of their challenges. I've also known women who were terrified they were developing Alzheimer's because they were suddenly forgetting things and finding it increasingly difficult to do their job well. Recently, a woman in her late forties told me about going to her GP to discuss options for managing what she knew to be peri-related symptoms. Her GP had never heard of perimenopause and brushed it off completely. Unfortunately, this isn't the first time I've heard this. That's why, if you want the most up-to-date information and guidance for this hugely transformative stage of life, it's vital to find a medical practitioner who specialises in women's health and perimenopause. Your GP may be wonderful in other areas, but if they don't have enough (or any) experience with perimenopause, they're unlikely to be able to give you the support you need at this time.

Peri puzzle pieces

One factor that plays a role in your experience of perimenopause is your genetics – specifically how your mother experienced this phase of life. If you're able to, ask her what she remembers about it, and what her symptoms were. Research suggests that your experience is likely to be similar. Your menstrual history and overall health may also influence your experience of perimenopause.

There are excellent books, online resources and podcasts available that discuss the finer details of peri, and the range of pharmaceutical, psychological and alternative therapies that can help manage symptoms. I'll leave those puzzle pieces to the professionals who specialise in those areas, and I urge you to seek support from as many experts as you need to. For this book, I'll stick to my area of expertise, which is nutrition.

The role of diet

Diet is a very important piece of the perimenopause puzzle. While our food choices won't single-handedly eliminate all the symptoms or even prevent hormonal weight gain, many women do notice significant improvements when they adjust their eating patterns. It's impossible to predict the factors that will move the needle for you, but your current baseline diet might give you a clue. If you're already eating in a way that aligns with the recommended eating patterns for perimenopausal women, you might not notice much of a change by tweaking your diet. But if your current diet looks nothing like the recipes in this book, your symptoms may significantly improve when you start eating this way.

I've written this book to be a support pillar for you during peri. The info here will help you to make easy nutritional changes, so you can enjoy a better peri experience. I'll steer you away from foods that may be exacerbating symptoms while guiding you towards ingredients that may minimise or even eliminate some of those gnarly symptoms. And you won't have to cook your own meal and eat it in the corner! These are family recipes full of great flavours and crowd-pleasing textures.

This phase of life comes with a lot of unpredictability and many challenges. We may not be able to control what's around the corner, but we can grab that grocery cart by the horns and fill it with food that optimises our chances of feeling our best.

Bon appetit! Here's to ageing gracefully and deliciously.

Jaime

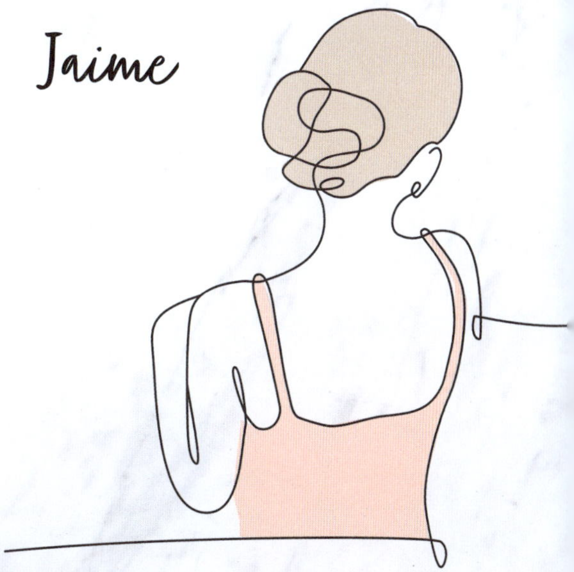

Chapter 1

Symptoms of peri

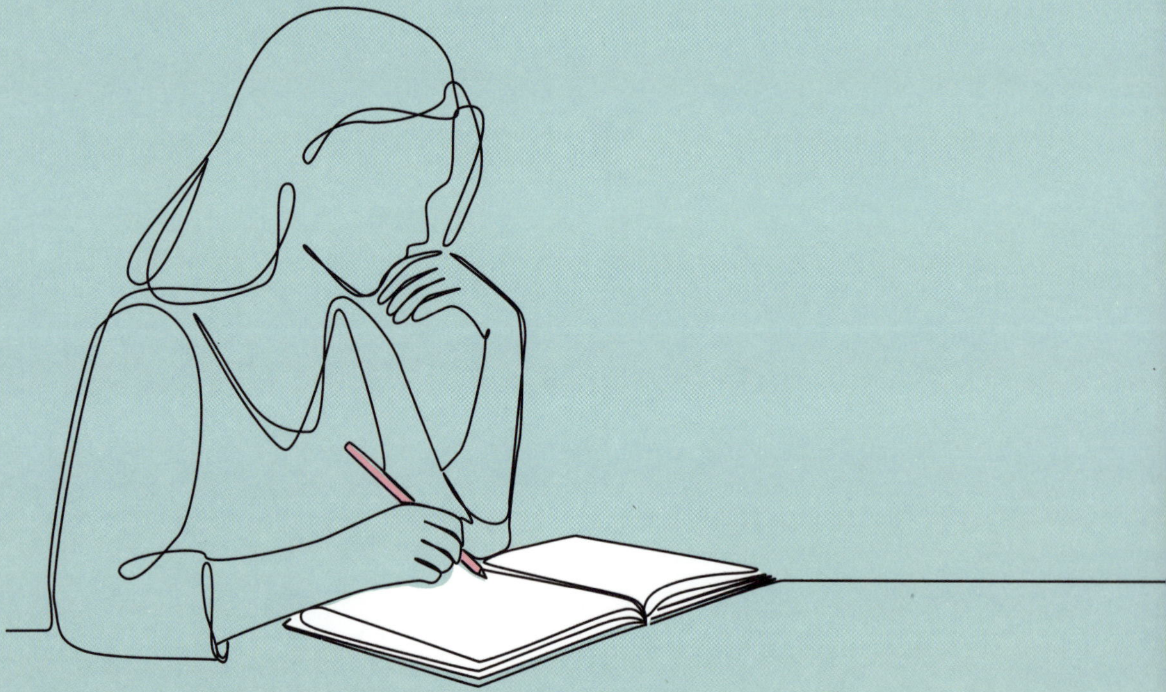

Menopause occurs when a woman has gone 12 consecutive months without a period. From that point, she is 'postmenopausal'. Essentially, menopause is the opposite of puberty – what one researcher calls 'the undoing of puberty'. And, like puberty, it's a natural part of the ageing process.

People don't always believe me when I tell them this mind-blowing fact, but I assure you that it's true: each baby girl is born with 1–2 million eggs inside of her. (Amazing, I know!) These immature eggs are in the follicles of her ovaries, and by the time she hits puberty that egg count has shrunk to between 200,000 and 400,000. When an egg isn't fertilised during ovulation (as most aren't), her menstrual period ensues, and the ovulation cycle begins again.

By 37, we have roughly 25,000 eggs left, and by the time we hit menopause (around age 51) we have fewer than 1,000 of those 1–2 million eggs left. Our egg supply runs out, and when our ovaries stop producing eggs, the hormones needed for reproduction (namely oestrogen and progesterone) fall, triggering many, many changes.

As I've said, the average age Western women go through menopause is 51, though it ranges from 45 to 55 years old. Since the average life expectancy for women (in industrialised countries) is between 80 and 85 years old, most of us will spend roughly half our adult lives in a postmenopausal state. But since Western medicine tends to 'treat' menopausal symptoms as they present, rather than focus on prevention, living longer doesn't necessarily mean we'll have a better quality of life. For that, symptoms need to be prevented in the first place.

We know that adopting healthy lifestyle habits, such eating well and exercising, early (ideally before peri but certainly during) is incredibly beneficial. Not only can it help to manage the symptoms of peri in the short term, it can also control risk factors and even prevent many future health problems.

Some women experience perimenopause symptoms as early as their 30s, but most of us enter this phase of life between 40 and 44. Each woman's experience is different: some barely notice a change and slide into menopause without breaking a sweat (quite literally), while others can struggle with a range of disruptive symptoms for up to 10 years. In fact, it's been suggested that peri symptoms drive as many as 90 per cent of women to seek support from their healthcare providers. Symptoms can impact many aspects of life – relationships with your partner, family and friends; work; physical and psychological health – making these often already demanding years even harder to navigate.

The reason symptoms are usually worse during perimenopause than during menopause is due to the dramatic fluctuations of hormone levels, namely of oestrogen and progesterone. Bodily systems, including the cardiovascular and central nervous systems, rely on many hormones to function normally. Oestrogen receptors throughout our body keep things ticking along, so when that oestrogen production begins to sputter out – as it does during peri – these systems aren't able to function as they normally would. This triggers the many symptoms associated with peri.

This decline in hormones isn't a linear process either; it's more of a rollercoaster, especially where oestrogen is concerned. There are big highs and lows of that hormone while progesterone falls at a steadier pace. These fluctuations in oestrogen mean that symptoms come in waves, change in severity and can really catch you off-guard.

Some peri symptoms such as hot flushes and night sweats are well known and quite common, but there are many others. Every woman is affected differently; we can also experience certain symptoms for a while, then have them change completely or ramp up or down. What can I say? Peri can be a mixed bag, full of surprises!

There's nothing worse than being blindsided by something you didn't see coming, so the best way to prepare and fortify yourself in the face of these changes is to know what could happen for you during this perfectly natural, but seismic, period of transition. So let's go through the symptoms now.

* Peri pause

The age a woman goes into menopause is often used as a health biomarker because epidemiological data indicates that every year later menopause occurs is associated with a 2 per cent decrease in mortality.

* Peri pause

Geographic location seems to impact the prevalence of hot flushes: 97 per cent of Turkish women experience them, followed by 83 per cent of Australian women, 76.5 per cent of European women and 58.8 per cent of North American women. Asian women experience the lowest occurrences of hot flushes at 45 per cent.

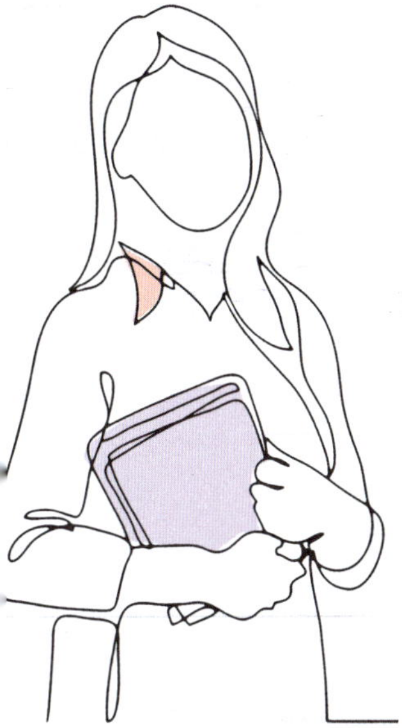

VASOMOTOR SYMPTOMS

Women in peri are as likely to experience vasomotor symptoms, such as hot flushes, as postmenopausal women – in fact, they can often be even worse in peri, since the hormone fluctuations are much greater during these years.

Hot flushes

Let's start with probably the most famous of the peri symptoms: the hot flush (or hot flash). A flushed face and neck, perhaps accompanied by beads of sweat on the forehead or upper lip, along with the tearing off of clothing and the fanning of the face are dead giveaways of a woman who's either peri or postmenopausal!

As many as 85 per cent of women experience hot flushes, which increase in frequency the closer you get to menopause. Research indicates that these hot flushes can persist for years – the average length of time falls somewhere between four and seven-and-a-half years. Whichever end of that spectrum you fall on, we can all agree that this is a long time to have to deal with such a visible and disruptive symptom. Despite this, studies suggest that only one in four women seeks medical advice for them.

Hot flushes mainly occur in the upper torso (head, neck and upper chest) and are triggered by small increases in core body temperature. When they happen, they usually last for 1–5 minutes, though some women can experience them for as long as an hour. Despite years of research, the exact mechanism of a hot flush is not fully known but it's thought to be directly related to the decline in oestrogen levels, since hot flushes are almost always completely resolved when a woman begins hormone replacement therapy (HRT).

What is known is that a hot flush is due to an abnormality in the hypothalamic thermoregulatory mechanisms – that's the part of the brain that governs our temperature. The drop in oestrogen affects this part of the brain and this causes a small increase in body temperature, which widens blood vessels, causing a surge of blood flow to areas of the body, which leads to that flush. Interestingly, the rate at which oestrogen declines may be more significant than the actual decrease in the hormone itself.

In terms of risk factors for hot flushes, there is likely a genetic component to whether a woman experiences this symptom, but a lot more research is needed in this area. So far, the only consistent risk factors associated with hot flushes are obesity, being of African descent, having a lower socioeconomic status, experiencing premenstrual symptoms, living a sedentary lifestyle and smoking. Triggers include alcohol, caffeine, spicy food, hot food and drink, stress and anxiety.

Changes to blood pressure

Hot flushes occur alongside changes in blood pressure. As blood vessels dilate, blood pressure drops. As they constrict, blood pressure rises. About 30–50 per cent of women develop hypertension (high blood pressure) before the age of 60 when menopause has well and truly set in. Hormonal changes, the vascular stiffness that comes with age and an increase in weight can all contribute to higher blood pressure.

Dizziness

When our blood pressure fluctuates, it can affect how blood moves through our body, causing us to feel dizzy.

Heart palpitations

A heart palpitation is an irregular heartbeat or a more intense heartbeat than you're used to. These occur because a drop in oestrogen levels can affect electrical activity in the heart.

SLEEP SYMPTOMS

The prevalence of sleep disturbances increases during peri. They can be one of the most debilitating symptoms, affecting quality of life, work productivity and relationships, as well as mental and overall health.

Night sweats

Night sweats come a close second to hot flushes in the most common symptom category, with as many as 80 per cent of women experiencing them. They're characterised by episodes of extreme heat and sweating during sleep, as well as increased heart rate and flushing of the face, neck and chest. In extreme cases, headaches and nausea can also accompany these night sweats. Ultimately, all of this leads to disrupted sleep. Much like hot flushes, night sweats are often worse during peri than they are during menopause.

Insomnia and night waking

Generally associated with vasomotor symptoms, night waking can be common in perimenopause. Changes in body temperature, which happen even when we're sleeping, can cause us to feel hot and uncomfortable and so we wake up, often several times a night, and may find it difficult to get back to sleep again. Having disturbed sleep over the long term can be very detrimental to our health and general functioning, leading to higher incidence of heart disease and mental disorders including depression and anxiety.

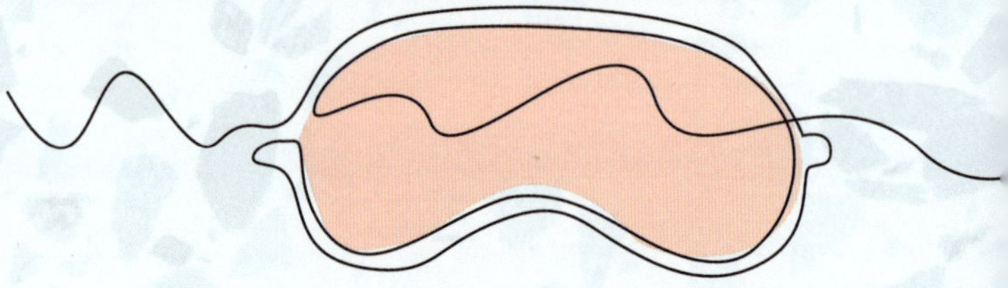

METABOLIC SYMPTOMS

Metabolism is the process of breaking down and accessing energy from our food and the way our body utilises that energy. The decline in oestrogen during peri leads directly to a decline in several processes that affect our metabolic rate. These include:

Decline in muscle mass

Peri can be a vulnerable period for the loss of muscle mass. It's believed this is because in peri, the oestrogen that usually protects the muscle is no longer available, which causes apoptosis (cell death), leading to a loss of skeletal muscle mass and strength. According to one study, women in late peri have a 10 per cent lower muscle mass than women in early peri.

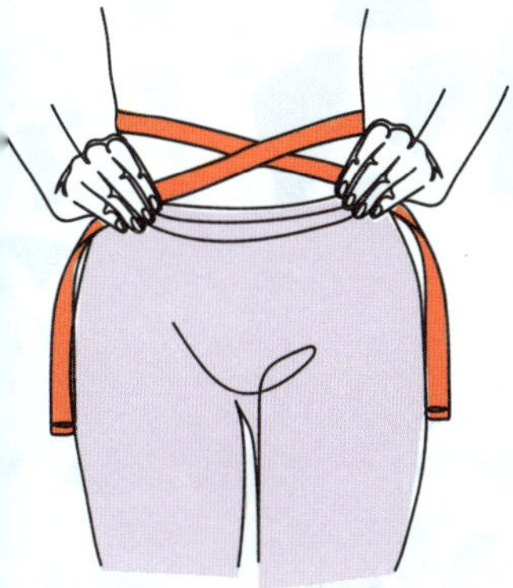

Weight gain and increased waist circumference

Fat mass and waist circumference increase the most during this phase of a woman's life – even more so than during menopause. The decline in oestrogen in perimenopause causes a change in the accumulation and distribution of fat, moving from the hips and thighs to the stomach. More of it gets deposited at a deeper level, around our organs. This visceral fat is the more 'dangerous' type of fat.

Fatty liver

There's also a rise in what is known as metabolic fatty liver disease in peri, which leads to that visceral fat (the fat that sits around our organs), plus changes to the proteins involved in managing the fat in the liver.

× Peri pause

WATCH YOUR WAIST CIRCUMFERENCE

The size of our waist is an important measurement during peri because this gives us an indication of internal fat deposits, which can coat our internal organs, affect their functioning and increase the risk of some chronic conditions. Generally, the greater your waist circumference, the greater your risk of those chronic conditions. To measure yours, place a measuring tape horizontally around your abdomen, in line with your navel (belly button).

INCREASED RISK	GREATLY INCREASED RISK
80 cm or more	88 cm or more

DIGESTIVE SYMPTOMS

Many women experience gastrointestinal symptoms during perimenopause, ranging from general discomfort to a change in bowel habits, bloating and pain. These have been associated with menstruation and periods of low oestrogen.

Constipation, diarrhoea, irritable bowel syndrome (IBS)

In the lead up to a period, bowel function will slow down for many women. Then, once their period arrives, it might speed up – resulting in loose stools. A similar pattern emerges during peri, too. Conditions such as IBS may come and go, along with symptoms such as constipation, diarrhoea (or both), wind, pain and bloating.

This happens because the brain's hypothalamus keeps our gut working properly, and when the oestrogen receptors in the hypothalamus are influenced by hormonal changes, this impacts gut function and digestion.

Another potential cause of gut-related issues can be diet-related. Feeling tired and either grabbing foods that give you an energy boost or not having the energy to put together a balanced meal means vital nutrients such as fibre may be sacrificed. Additionally, not drinking enough water or moving enough can also lead to changes in bowel habits.

Heartburn

According to one study, 42 per cent of women in perimenopause suffer from heartburn. Also known as reflux, or GORD (gastro-oesophageal reflux disease), this symptom occurs when highly acidic stomach contents head in the wrong direction and go into the oesophagus (the tube leading from the mouth to the stomach). It can feel like a horrible burning in the chest, and people can even mistake it for having a heart attack. It can also cause a burning sensation in the back of the throat and a bad taste in the mouth.

Not only does the drop in oestrogen change the amount of acid in the stomach, but the weight gain that often occurs in peri may also play a role. Causes include overeating, eating too quickly, eating whilst slouching or reclining after eating and having a hiatus or hiatal hernia, where the upper part of the stomach bulges up through the diaphragm putting pressure on the oesophagus. This is often picked up in a gastroscopy or endoscopy.

PSYCHOLOGICAL SYMPTOMS

> Around one in four women report mood changes in perimenopause.

Around one in four women report mood changes in perimenopause that can present like PMS (premenstrual syndrome). This can include feeling irritable and moody, low energy and difficulty concentrating.

Depression and mood changes

The most common psychological symptom of perimenopause is rapid mood change and irritability. This makes a lot of sense given that oestrogen binds to oestrogenic receptors in the brain, which interact with our serotonin and dopamine neurotransmitters. Serotonin is our 'happy hormone' and is responsible for boosting mood, memory and our stress response. By the time we've been through menopause there is a 50 per cent decrease in levels of serotonin.

There's also a decline in the production of endorphins – the hormones released in response to pain or stress because they're a natural painkiller. Endorphins are also associated with that happy high we get after exercising.

Hormone-related mood changes begin in puberty and continue for many women throughout their reproductive years as their mood fluctuates with their menstrual cycle. Many women report feeling cranky and irritable before their period; however during peri, women are two to five times more likely than premenopausal women to develop depression or depressive symptoms.

Brain fog and difficulty concentrating

The term brain fog refers to the way we might feel cloudy and unable to think clearly. It can look like not remembering why you walked into a room or why you're standing at the fridge. You might find yourself searching for your phone while it's in your hand or have difficulty remembering people's names. Brain fog can be very difficult, particularly if you have a very demanding job and/or countless family commitments to juggle.

Brain fog can become so severe that some women get tested for dementia. The cause, as always, is our declining oestrogen because it plays a big part in the functioning of our brain; this can also be exacerbated by disturbed sleep and stressors associated with this time of life.

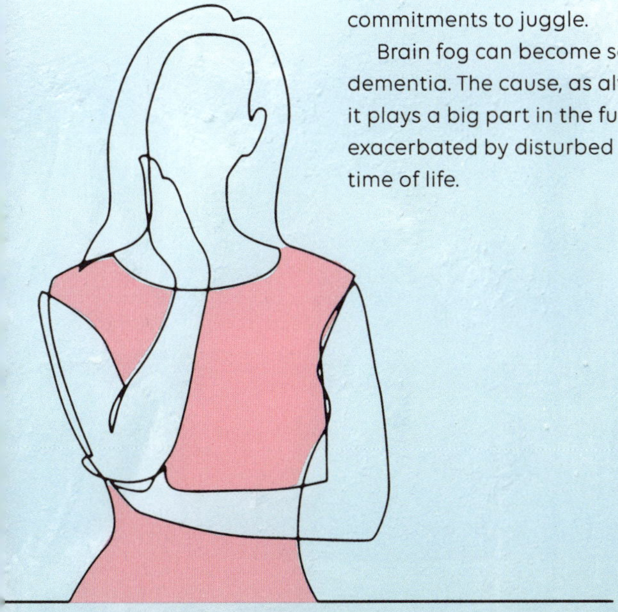

SEXUAL SYMPTOMS

Oestrogen promotes the health of the female reproductive system, including keeping the vagina moisturised, elastic and supplied with plenty of blood flow. The decline in oestrogen during peri can therefore cause vaginal dryness, and directly and indirectly affect sexual function and libido.

> If you experience any unusual bleeding, speak with your health care professional.

Vaginal dryness

Vaginal dryness due to lowered oestrogen is a common problem that often starts during peri and shows up in half of women by menopause. The lack of natural lubrication causes pain with penetration, making sex painful and decreasing a woman's desire for sex. Less lubrication can also increase the risk of urinary tract and yeast infections.

Changes in libido

Libido is our sexual drive and desire. It's widely accepted that sexual function gets worse (i.e. that desire goes down) as we approach menopause, with 40 to 55 per cent of women reporting low sexual desire. Other factors such as vaginal dryness, increased stress and feeling tired and irritable, as well as changes to our body and body image, can play into this lack of desire.

MENSTRUAL SYMPTOMS

During peri, some women find that the fluctuating hormones make their periods further apart, while others find it causes them to come closer together. Some women will have a very light bleed, whereas others can have a heavy bleed that lasts for a long time. (That being said, one of the positives of peri is that we're approaching a time when we'll no longer have to deal with bleeding every month!) Naturally, if you experience any unusual bleeding or other associated symptoms, speak to your health care professional.

ADDITIONAL SYMPTOMS

Other lesser-known symptoms of peri include:

Changes to taste and smell

This is a little-known symptom of peri believed to occur because oestrogen affects the pathways in the brain that control our taste and smell. This can happen in a similar way to when a woman is pregnant and suddenly craves something or loves a certain smell, but develops an aversion to other foods and odours.

Decline in bone mass

Peri (and particularly late peri) marks a time when an increase in bone resorption causes an acceleration in bone loss. We'll go into this in more depth on page 61.

Breast tenderness

Some women find that their breasts and nipples become very tender to the touch or ache when putting on a bra. Breasts can change shape and size during peri, and many women tell me that they're suddenly spilling out of their underwear. Hormones cause areas of the breast to swell and enlarge, and when these hormones drop off, they can cause the opposite effect, leaving breasts feeling smaller and deflated.

If breast tenderness is a concern for you, it might be worth looking into your caffeine intake (coffee, black tea, green tea, cola drinks, dark chocolate) since some studies have revealed that caffeine stimulates breast tissue and can make this area more sensitive.

Brittle nails

Nails can become brittle or soft and break more easily because they are made from a protein called keratin, which requires oestrogen for its production. As oestrogen levels decline, production of keratin goes down too, affecting the strength of the nail.

Dry and itchy skin

Falling oestrogen results in a loss of water and this causes the skin to thin and become dry, which tends to show up those wrinkles and crow's feet.

Bad breath and other oral issues

Oestrogen is involved with maintaining the structure and integrity of our bones and ligaments, including in our teeth and the mucous membranes in our mouth. Declining levels of oestrogen can result in reduced saliva production, which can lead to bad breath, as well as structural changes in the mouth that can cause a range of oral health concerns.

Limiting high-sugar and refined-sugar foods, including soda and fruit juices, can help prolong the health of your mouth. Be careful, too, when consuming so-called 'healthier' foods such as bliss balls and dried fruits since these are often very high in sugar and can get stuck in your teeth and cause tooth decay.

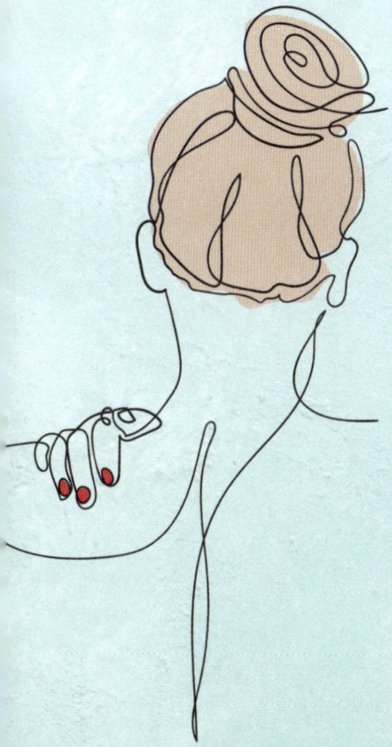

Tinnitus

A GP who specialises in perimenopause made an interesting observation about the connection between tinnitus and peri after many of her perimenopausal patients presented with constant ringing in the ears. Understandably, this symptom can be distressing and distract from everyday activities as well as disrupt sleep.

Joint and muscle pain

Oestrogen helps to lubricate our joints, so when those levels drop, muscle aches and pains often follow. It tends to be at its worst in the morning because this is when oestrogen levels are at their lowest.

Chapter 2

How to eat well during peri

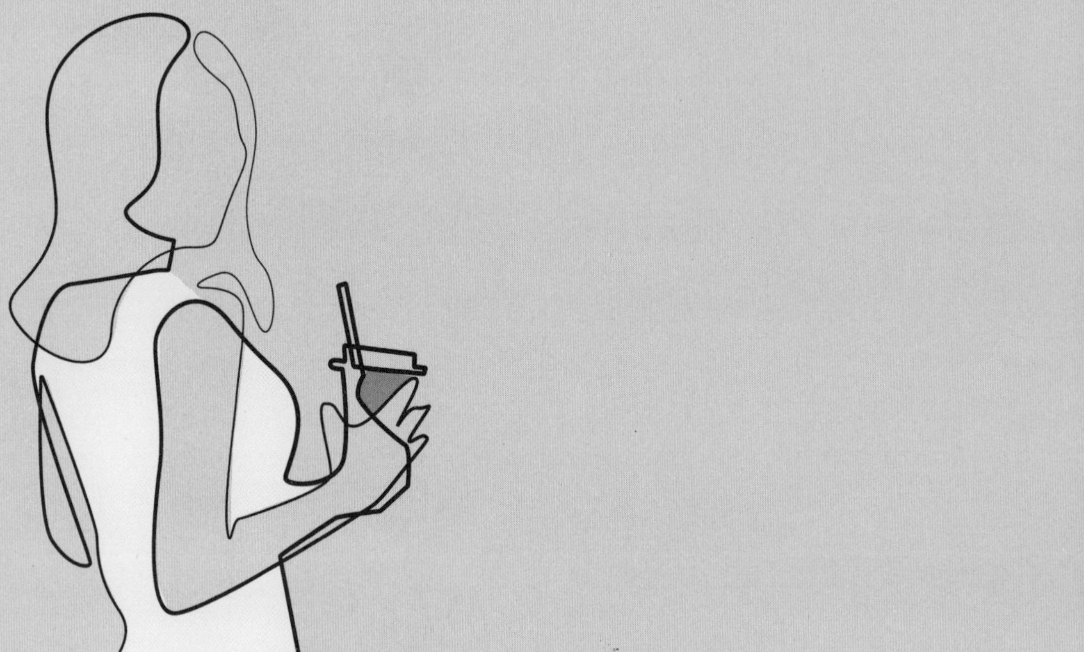

There's no specific diet plan you should be following diligently during perimenopause (though some diets may claim to be the 'one'). It's more a general way of eating that will best support your body and mind during this sometimes challenging time – and set you up for better health over the longer term.

My peri 'diet' is based on eating more of the foods and nutrients shown to have a positive impact on perimenopause and its symptoms, and limiting the foods known to trigger many of the symptoms we've just covered. It also encompasses foods that can protect against some of the common health issues that arise at this stage of life.

When it comes to perimenopause, so much is out of our control, but one thing we have control over is what we eat. Choosing food wisely can not only help to manage peri symptoms, it can also help to regulate weight and prevent – or at least minimise – the gain that often occurs during peri. A good diet can also protect the parts of the body, such as the heart, bones and brain, that are typically impacted by peri as well as the natural ageing process.

Taking care of yourself when you're busy and not feeling so good can be challenging. It can be hard to maintain consistency, especially while riding the ups and downs of your hormones and the various demands of life. The last thing we likely feel like doing when we're tired, hot, uncomfortable or moody is cooking an extravagant (or even basic!) meal. It can be tempting to grab takeaway or a ready-made meal, or even just eat cheese and bikkies with a glass of wine. But the problem with eating like this on a regular basis is that these meals tend to be higher in fat, salt and sugar than a proper meal made at home.

I know you already know all of this, and I'm not judging, believe me. I know how it is because I'm right there with you. That's why this book is dedicated to stacking the odds in our favour and making it more likely for us to eat in a way that best supports us during what can be a challenging few years.

In this book, I'm sharing some quick, easy throw-together meals, as well as great family recipes and snacks that can be batch-cooked on the days when we do have energy. If we can take advantage of those 'up days' by getting even one or two meals organised for the week ahead, we'll be so much more likely to consume meals full of vitamins, fibre and nutrients ready to go on those days we just CBF. (I'm sure you also know what that means!)

Building a good food foundation

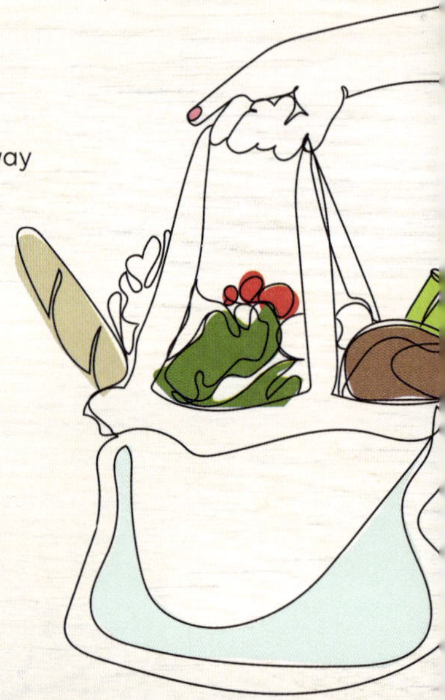

The first step to building a good food foundation for peri is finding a way of eating that suits your taste preferences and your lifestyle. The four eating patterns with the most research to back them up as being supportive to health – especially during peri – are the Mediterranean and Japanese diets, the DASH eating plan and a plant-focused diet.

Before we look at these foundation diets in detail, it's worth saying that how your body responds to changes in your diet varies. Some women find their symptoms are significantly improved, while others notice only mild changes. Like anything health-related, nutrition is very personal and results depend on a number of factors including:

Your baseline diet
What sort of diet do you have now? If you're starting from a balanced and nutritious baseline, you may not notice a significant change. If, however, your current diet doesn't include many or any of the peri-friendly foods we're about to discuss, you might notice a much bigger change in your symptoms.

Your baseline health status
Are you fairly healthy right now? Do you have any underlying health issues or conditions that might be impacted by peri?

Physical activity level
How active are you now? What kind of shape is your body in?

Genetics
This can play a big role in how your body responds to dietary changes.

Lifestyle
What are your stress levels like? Do you get enough sleep? Do you smoke? How long do you spend sitting down each day? How much do you drink?

Medications
Certain medications change the way our body responds to food.

Even if it improves your peri symptoms only mildly, following a healthy diet is still so important. It can improve your energy levels, maintain healthy bowel function and reduce the risk of chronic disease, just to name a few benefits.

THE MEDITERRANEAN DIET

The Mediterranean diet has been ranked the number-one diet in the world by health experts for several years now. To be clear, we're not talking about how we'd eat while on holiday in Rome – we're talking about the traditional diet and lifestyle habits followed by people living in the region (specifically the Greek island of Crete) many decades ago. The traditional Mediterranean diet encompasses not only food, but also a way of life in general. It features:

- a variety of colourful fresh vegetables and fruit, eaten daily
- healthy fats from extra-virgin olive oil, oily fish, avocado, nuts and seeds
- dairy, particularly fermented kinds like yoghurt
- legumes and eggs
- more seafood and less red and processed meat
- wholegrains
- spices and herbs
- seasonal, local produce; minimal processed foods
- moderate portion sizes
- alcohol in moderation
- enjoying meals with others
- getting enough rest
- daily movement.

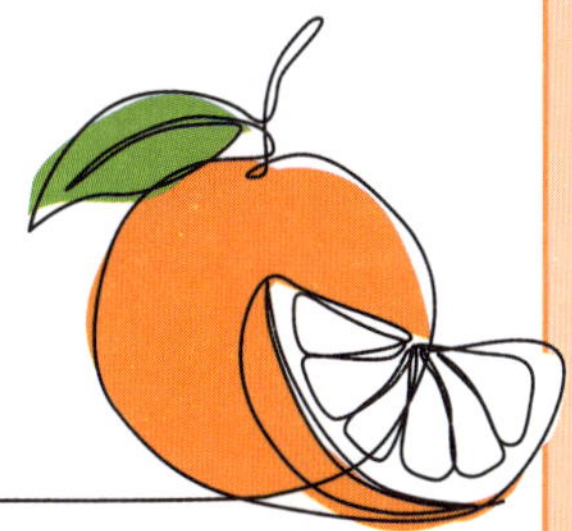

What the research says

The Mediterranean diet has been shown to lower the risk of developing a number of chronic diseases from heart disease, type 2 diabetes and bowel and breast cancers, to neurodegenerative diseases such as Parkinson's and Alzheimer's disease. Consequently, it's associated with a longer life span and healthy ageing.

In one study, a group of women following a Mediterranean style of eating (i.e. an anti-inflammatory diet rich in antioxidants) showed a slowing of cell reproduction and division, indicating a slowing down of the ageing process.

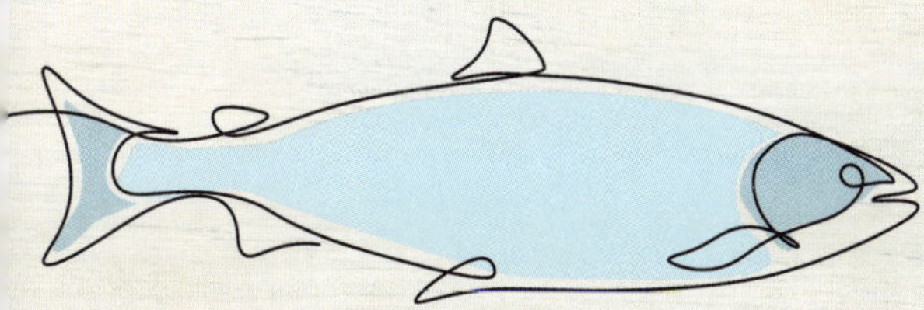

THE JAPANESE DIET

Recently, I read that Japan is possibly the 'poster child for how to "do" menopause'. It's true that Japanese women experience far fewer peri and menopausal symptoms than Western women: around 25 to 50 per cent versus 70 to 80 per cent. Japanese women generally experience less frequent hot flushes and night sweats, as well as less bone loss throughout peri. This difference is believed to be a result of diet. Like the Mediterranean diet, the traditional Japanese diet is low in animal products and high in plant-based foods, low in fat and high in fibre.

The traditional Japanese diet features a lot of soy-based ingredients such as tofu, plus seafood, fruit and vegetables, seaweed and fermented foods such as miso and natto.

Okinawa in Japan is one of the world's 'blue zones', which means its population has one of the highest life-expectancy rates in the world. Plant foods make up 90 per cent of the traditional diet, in which beans and vegetables, including purple sweet potato, play a starring role, and animal products only a very minor role. As a result, this eating pattern is anti-inflammatory and high in antioxidants, which have a protective effect on the body.

> The traditional Japanese diet is low in animal products and high in plant-based foods.

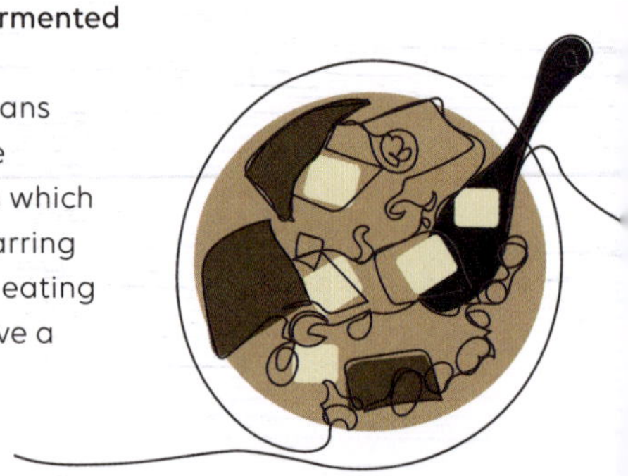

THE DASH EATING PLAN

DASH stands for 'Dietary Approaches to Stop Hypertension'. It's a flexible and balanced way of eating centred around meeting daily and weekly nutrition goals. There are no specific rules or restrictions – hence why it's referred to as a plan rather than a diet.

The DASH diet centres on vegetables, fruit and wholegrains, low- and no-fat dairy products, fish, poultry, beans, nuts and olive oil. It limits foods high in saturated fats, high-fat takeaway meals, full-fat dairy products, tropical oils like coconut and palm oils, sweetened drinks and sweets.

What the research says

Heart health is a big focus of the DASH plan, specifically the prevention or treatment of high blood pressure. It's also been shown to reduce cholesterol and diabetes. In a 2022 study of perimenopausal women who followed the DASH framework, subjects showed a significant improvement in diet quality and behaviours, as well as reduced body fat and waist circumference measurements.

This way of eating provides a lot of the minerals important for heart health such as potassium, magnesium and calcium, while also lowering sodium (salt). On top of that, it's also high in fibre and protein – which, as you'll soon learn, are both important when managing perimenopause.

A PLANT-FOCUSED DIET

This isn't a vegan diet – it's not even a vegetarian diet. It's simply a way of eating that features a strong focus on whole plant foods. There are no specific rules or guidelines to follow; it's just about eating a variety of different-coloured plant foods.

A plant-focused diet is based on eating fruits, vegetables, wholegrains, legumes, nuts and seeds for MOST of your meals and snacks, say at least 80 per cent. The remainder of the diet is made up with low-fat dairy, seafood, eggs and lean meat and chicken.

Overall, research shows that a plant-focused diet is associated with reduced perimenopausal symptoms.

Naturally, choosing to eat a vegetarian or vegan diet is great, too, as long as it's done correctly – and by that, I mean that it meets the nutritional guidelines. In my time in clinic, I've seen some less-than-ideal vegetarian and vegan diets. Often, people will have a diet full of ultra-processed food products, white breads and pasta and not a lot of whole plant foods yet think that this is 'healthy' just because they aren't eating meat.

Whether you choose to follow a plant-based, vegetarian or vegan diet, the key is to make sure whole plant foods make up about 80 per cent of the food you eat.

TO BUILD A PERI PROTOCOL TAILORED TO YOU, FOLLOW THESE TWO STEPS:

1 CHOOSE A FOUNDATION DIET

Review the four eating patterns above and choose one to be the 'foundational' framework of your protocol, which will be the way you'll eat 80–100 per cent of the time. Which of the patterns you choose will depend on the types of food you enjoy, as well as your individual requirements.

2 ADD PERI-SPECIFIC NUTRITION

On top of that solid foundation, you're going to start layering in foods shown to have positive impacts on peri symptoms and/or supporting a healthy weight throughout this journey. This is where you begin to weave in specific foods that match your nutrition goals and tackle any particular symptoms you'd like to address.

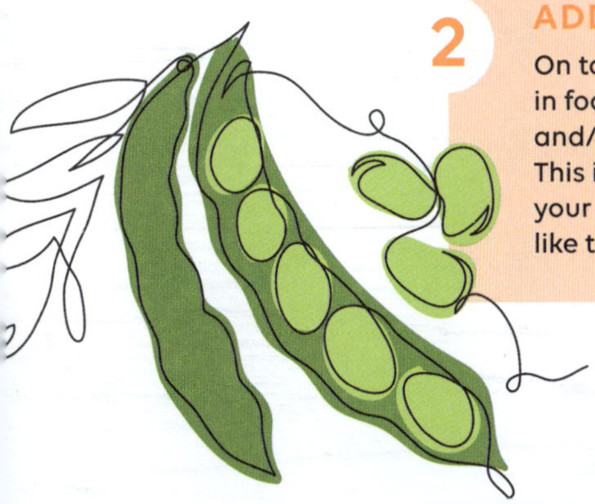

Top 10 peri nutrients

As I always say, we eat food, not nutrients! However, I think it's beneficial to underscore the importance of certain key nutrients during peri. That way, we can be aware of what our body needs and why – and which foods we can eat to ensure we are getting enough of the good stuff.

1 PROTEIN

Essential for building and maintaining muscle, protein is arguably the most important nutrient during peri. Higher protein intake during this time is associated with a higher lean muscle mass, lower frailty and better physical function. Research suggests that peri women can lessen or prevent weight gain and loss of lean tissue by prioritising protein. It is also associated with an overall improvement in symptoms. Protein's ability to support healthy weight management means that it also has long-term benefits, as it helps to reduce the risk of weight and metabolic-related diseases such as type 2 diabetes and cardiovascular disease. We'll go into detail about calculating your protein needs on page 31 and check out the protein counter on page 32.

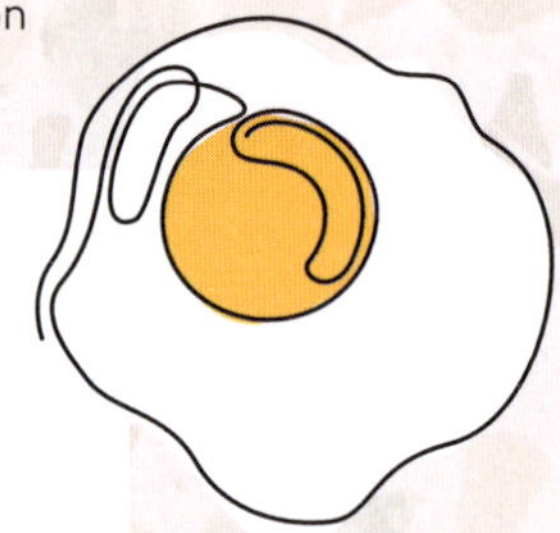

TOP SOURCES INCLUDE:

- lean meat
- poultry
- seafood
- dairy and eggs
- soy foods, such as tofu
- quinoa, nuts and seeds.

2 CALCIUM

Calcium builds and maintains bone; 99 per cent of the calcium in our body is stored there. It is an essential nutrient during peri because bone mass begins to decline at this time. In fact, it's estimated that five years into menopause, some women will lose as much as 10 to 20 per cent of their bone mass, leading to greater risk of osteoporosis.

TOP SOURCES INCLUDE:

- dairy products
- calcium-fortified plant milks
- tofu
- green leafy vegetables.

3 VITAMIN D

Vitamin D helps us to absorb calcium so it's also essential for bone health in addition to playing a strong role in immunity. The best source of vitamin D is sunshine; while it is found in some foods, it's often in low amounts and in a form that isn't easily used by our body. The Cancer Council has safe sun exposure guidelines on their website, but if you have a history of skin cancer or fair skin, or just want to avoid the sun, a vitamin D supplement may be necessary to maintain healthy levels.

4 LOW-GI CARBOHYDRATES

The glycaemic index (GI) is a food ranking system from 0 to 100 that measures how quickly a food raises blood sugar levels after eating. High-GI foods include anything made with a processed grain, such as white bread, pasta and rice, and anything containing refined sugars such as soft drinks and sweets. High-GI foods are rapidly digested, absorbed and metabolised, which can cause a spike in blood sugar and insulin levels (the hormone that removes sugar from our blood into our cells so we can use it as energy). This is particularly important for peri women, because declining oestrogen levels can cause our cells to become less responsive to insulin.

With low-GI carbohydrates, the sugar is released into the bloodstream more slowly, which means insulin has more time to do its job and our body has more time to manage the sugar in our blood. Eating low-GI foods is also beneficial during peri because not only do they keep us feeling fuller for longer, which is good for weight management, they're generally higher in nutrients, including B vitamins and fibre (see over the page). They can also help reduce the severity of hot flushes and insomnia.

TOP SOURCES INCLUDE:

- wholegrains e.g. oats, brown rice, whole wheat products
- starchy veg e.g. sweet potato, corn
- legumes
- quinoa
- apples and berries.

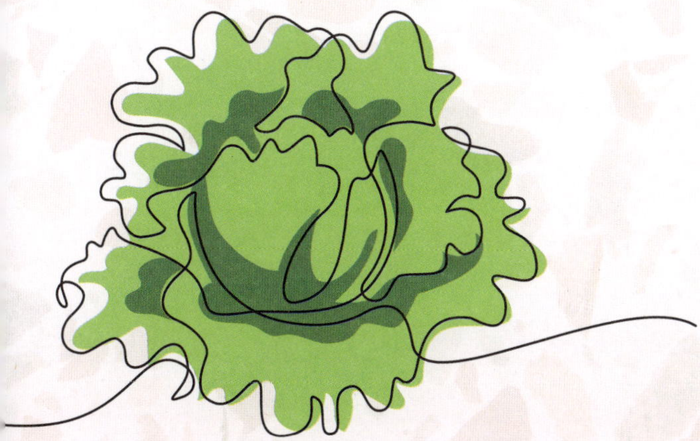

5 MAGNESIUM

Magnesium is essential for the maintenance of normal cell and organ function, energy production, blood sugar and insulin regulation, bone building and bone mineral density, muscle and nervous system function, brain function and mood stability. Studies show that maintaining optimum levels of magnesium can help to counteract the symptoms of perimenopause, particularly where bone density is concerned. It is also often taken as a supplement during peri to aid restful sleep.

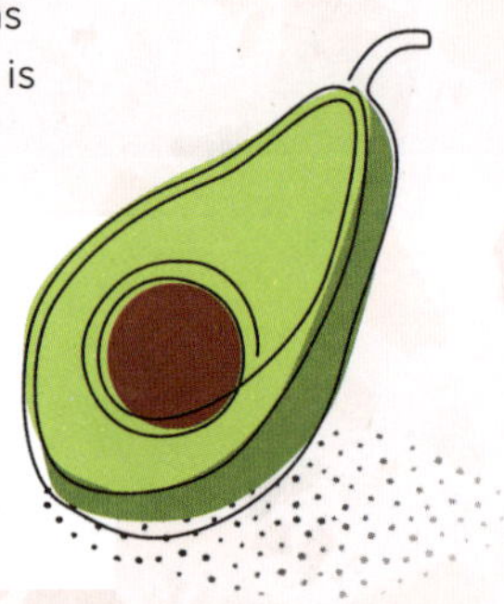

TOP SOURCES INCLUDE:

- pumpkin and chia seeds
- almonds and cashews
- avocado and spinach
- soy and cow's milks
- rolled oats
- wholegrains.

6 FIBRE

This nutrient feeds the beneficial bugs in our gut, which helps to support our digestion and immunity, as well as the production of anti-inflammatory chemicals in the gut and throughout our body. And since fibre helps us feel fuller for longer, it can help if your goal is weight management. It's also been linked with improved cholesterol and a lower risk of heart disease. Women need around 25 g of fibre each day. Eating a diet based mostly on whole plant foods (see page 23) is a great way to consume adequate fibre. Check out the fibre counter on page 50.

TOP SOURCES INCLUDE:

- fruit and vegetables
- wholegrains
- legumes
- nuts and seeds.

7 OMEGA-3 FATTY ACIDS

Omega-3 fatty acids are a type of unsaturated or 'healthy' fat found in abundance in oily fish; we'll explore them in more detail on page 44. They can help with many different symptoms of peri (mood changes, bone density, hot flushes and vaginal dryness), lower triglycerides (a type of 'bad' cholesterol) and support joint health.

TOP SOURCES INCLUDE:

- oily fish, such as salmon, trout, tuna and sardines
- flaxseeds and chia seeds
- walnuts.

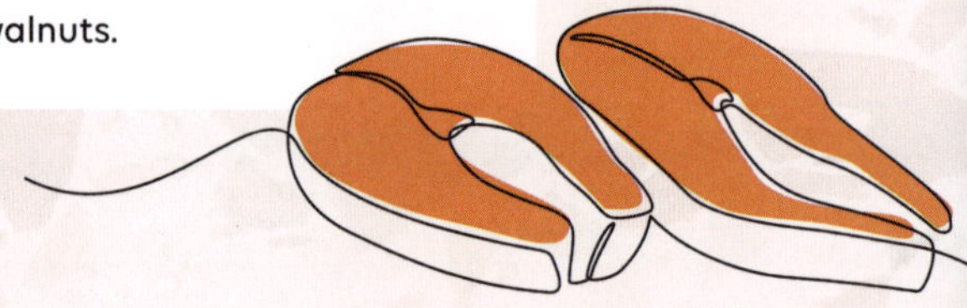

8 PHYTOESTROGENS

Phytoestrogens are found in plants, but they have similar chemical structure to oestrogen. They bind to oestrogen receptors, which are found throughout our body, and mimic what oestrogen does, albeit to a much milder degree. Because the decline of oestrogen in peri is one of the main causes of symptoms, eating foods rich in phytoestrogens can help to buffer this loss. There are two main types: isoflavones and lignans; we'll discuss them in detail on page 35.

TOP SOURCES INCLUDE:

- legumes, especially soy
- seeds, especially flaxseed
- wholegrains
- fruit and vegetables

9 IRON

Iron carries oxygen around the body and is also essential for energy production and immune function. When iron levels are low, we can feel incredibly tired, short of breath and dizzy. Women in their reproductive years are at the greatest risk of iron deficiency due to the blood loss from periods. A perk of menopause is that our iron needs from our diet drop and blood iron levels can increase once we're no longer having our period. Peri women, however, may experience longer and heavier periods of menstruation so it's important to keep an eye on iron levels during this time as dietary requirements may change. See page 67.

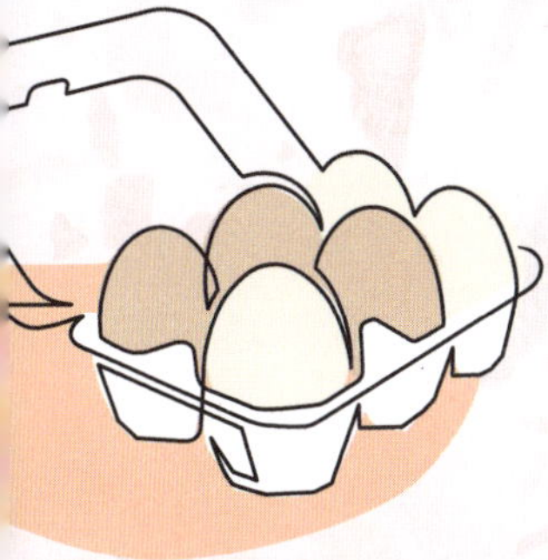

TOP SOURCES INCLUDE:

- red meat
- poultry and fish
- eggs
- legumes, including soy
- green leafy vegetables
- iron-fortified foods.

10 WATER

Water is an essential nutrient. As we age, the risk of dehydration increases because our body replenishes fluid at a slower rate thanks to those hormonal changes. The physical trigger for thirst is often less noticeable, too, so it's common to forget to drink. Dehydration causes headaches, feelings of sluggishness and constipation.

Chapter 3

Peri *power* foods

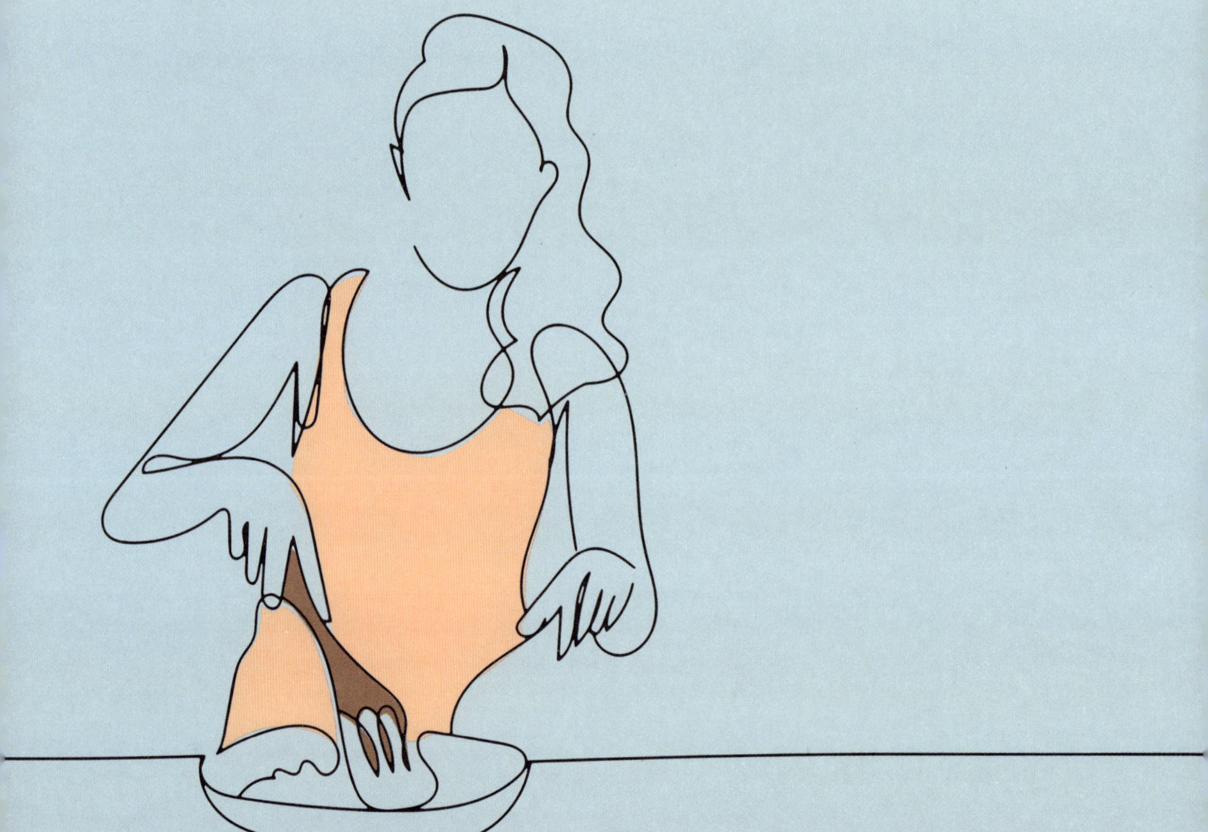

Peri power foods are specific foods and nutrients that have been shown in research to have a positive impact on peri symptoms, as well as supporting your health more broadly at this time. From protein to phytoestrogenic foods, fibre to oily fish, here are the key nutrients and ingredients to include in your diet during peri.

Protein is key

Protein is one of three major macronutrients that provide the body with energy – the other two being fat and carbohydrates – and it directly contributes to building and maintaining our muscles. As oestrogen falls during peri, muscle loss becomes a primary concern. From around the age of 40, muscle mass in women decreases by about 3 to 8 per cent per decade, and this increases to 10 to 15 per cent per decade by the time we're 60. To preserve or slow the decline in lean muscle, there are two things we must do:

1. **Eat enough protein to meet our increased requirements.**
2. **Stimulate our muscles with strength and resistance-based exercise.**

Loss of muscle doesn't just mean we lose strength; it's also regarded as one of the main causes of peri weight gain. Since muscles are an energy-burning furnace, the less we have, the less energy we are able to burn off. This means that whatever activity and eating pattern has kept your weight stable up to now can lead to weight gain.

PROTEIN HELPS US TO:

- build and maintain muscle
- maintain a healthy immune system
- regulate blood sugar levels
- change body composition to favour fat loss
- feel satisfied after a meal
- absorb dietary calcium, and therefore improve bone health
- create hormones
- recover from injury and heal wounds.

COMPLETE AND INCOMPLETE PROTEINS

The protein we eat is made up of a combination of amino acids, which are like a string of pearls. Once we've eaten protein, that string of amino acids gets prised apart into individual 'pearls', which are absorbed and used for many different functions. There are 20 amino acids in total and they are classified as either essential or non-essential. The 11 non-essential amino acids are produced by our body, but the remaining nine are not produced by us so we have to obtain them from our diet; these are known as essential amino acids.

When we describe a food as 'a complete protein', this means that all nine of the essential amino acids are available in that food. All animal-based protein sources are a complete protein and so are soy products and quinoa. Incomplete protein describes all other plant sources of protein, including legumes, nuts, seeds and some wholegrains.

> Animal-based proteins, soy products and quinoa are all complete sources of protein.

You don't need to have complete protein at every meal, but by eating a variety of foods over the day, you're likely to get a full range of complete proteins. If you're vegan, or following a plant-focused diet with not a lot of animal protein, you can eat complementary protein combinations to ensure you're getting complete protein. For example, if you eat a salad that includes wholegrains, nuts, seeds and legumes (including peanuts), that meal will give you all nine essential amino acids (i.e. a complete protein).

* Peri pause

SHOULD I USE PROTEIN POWDER?

Generally, it's not necessary because the average person should be able to get more than enough protein from a varied and balanced diet. However, protein powder can be a great tool if you're not going to be able to eat for a while after a training session, or if you find it difficult to meet protein requirements through diet alone, as can be common among vegan or vegetarian women. In my clinic, I often suggest adding protein powder to foods such as porridge made with water or plant milk, since they won't contain the amount of protein found in cow's milk or yoghurt.

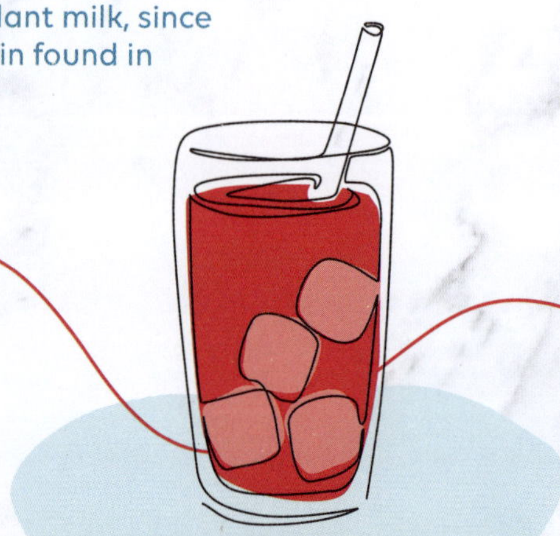

HOW MUCH PROTEIN DO I NEED?

There are the three main approaches to calculating how much protein you need. Each approach will provide roughly the same target.

1 PROTEIN PER MEAL

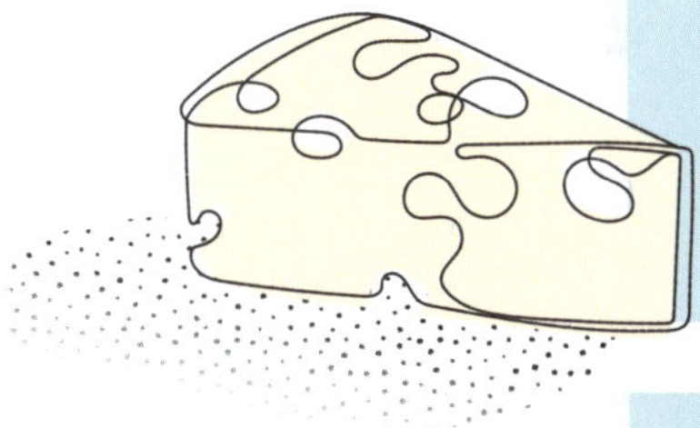

Aim for between 20 and 30 g protein in each main meal and 10 to 20 g in each snack. If, for example, you have three main meals and a snack each day, or two main meals and two snacks, this will average at around 100 g protein per day, which you can adjust based on your needs.

For example, 30 g at breakfast + 25 g at lunch + 12 g at afternoon tea + 35 g at dinner = 102 g protein

2 PROTEIN BASED ON BODY WEIGHT

General dietary recommendations for women are 0.8 g of protein per kilogram of body weight. This is to meet basic body functions; however if you've got higher needs (e.g. muscle loss in peri), the recommendation is to increase this to 1.2 g and if you're particularly active or are starting off with a lower muscle mass, this can go as high as 1.6 g of protein per kilogram of body weight.

Calculate 1.2 g of protein per kilogram of your current body weight. So, for example, if your current weight is 80 kilograms, calculate your protein needs using this formula: 1.2 g x 80 kg = 96 g protein per day

3 PROTEIN BASED ON PERCENTAGE OF ENERGY INTAKE

In Chapter 5, we'll be discussing various strategies to manage weight, and as part of that. I'll show you how to calculate your ideal energy intake, if that's something that interests you. From there, you can calculate the amount of protein you need. During peri, it's recommended that protein intake is higher – approximately 30 per cent of total energy. So, here's an example of what that might look like for a woman whose total energy intake should be 1,500 calories per day.

1,500 calories x 30 per cent = 450. Therefore, 450 calories of your daily intake should be protein.

There are 4 calories per gram of protein:
450 calories / 4 = 112.5 g protein per day

Protein counter

INGREDIENT	PROTEIN
Pork, raw (100 g)	33 g
Chicken, raw (100 g)	28 g
Beef, raw (100 g)	28 g
Lamb, raw (100 g)	25 g
Prawns (100 g)	24 g
Tempeh (100 g)	23 g
White fish, raw (100 g)	22 g
Oily fish, raw (100 g)	20 g
Tofu (100 g)	14 g
Cottage or ricotta cheese (½ cup)	18 g
Lentils, cooked (1 cup)	15 g
2 whole eggs	12 g

INGREDIENT	PROTEIN
Greek yoghurt (200 g)	10 g
Pulses e.g. chickpeas, cooked (1 cup)	9.5 g
Hard cheese e.g. cheddar (2 slices/40 g)	9 g
Edamame, podded (½ cup)	8.5 g
Cow's milk (1 cup/250 ml)	8 g
Baked beans (1 cup)	8 g
Soy milk (1 cup/250 ml)	7 g
Mixed nuts (30 g)	5 g
Quinoa, cooked (½ cup)	4.7 g
Peanut butter (1 tablespoon)	4 g

Distribute your protein needs

Since our body is only able to absorb a certain amount of protein at any one time, distributing your protein needs over the day is the best way to ensure you meet your target. The amount we can absorb at one time is not fully known and likely to be quite individual but it's believed to be around 25–35 grams. If you're exercising, to support muscle recovery it's recommended you have a serving of high-quality protein and carbohydrates within an hour of finishing your workout – this is especially true if you're strength-training. This is so your body can maintain its protein balance. There's no need to add an extra meal, snack or protein shake to achieve this as that will only increase your calorie intake. Instead, try timing breakfast after a morning workout, or dinner after a late afternoon session.

* Peri pause

IS IT POSSIBLE TO EAT TOO MUCH PROTEIN?

Yes! You need to be particularly careful if you have any renal or liver issues. Very high protein diets (i.e. more than 200 g protein per day) can put a strain on your organs and cause a loss of calcium. In this case, more is not necessarily better.

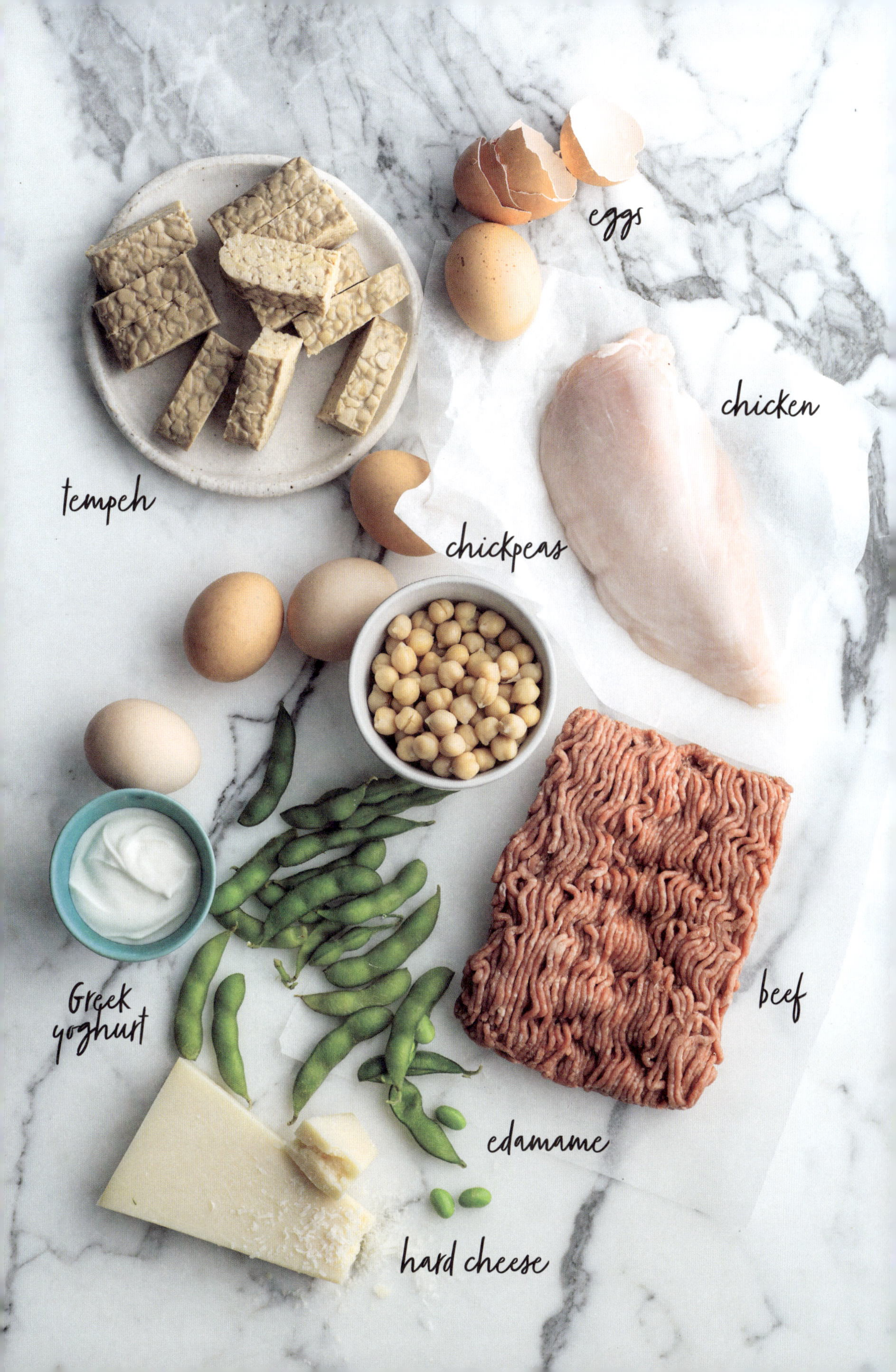
eggs
chicken
tempeh
chickpeas
beef
Greek yoghurt
edamame
hard cheese

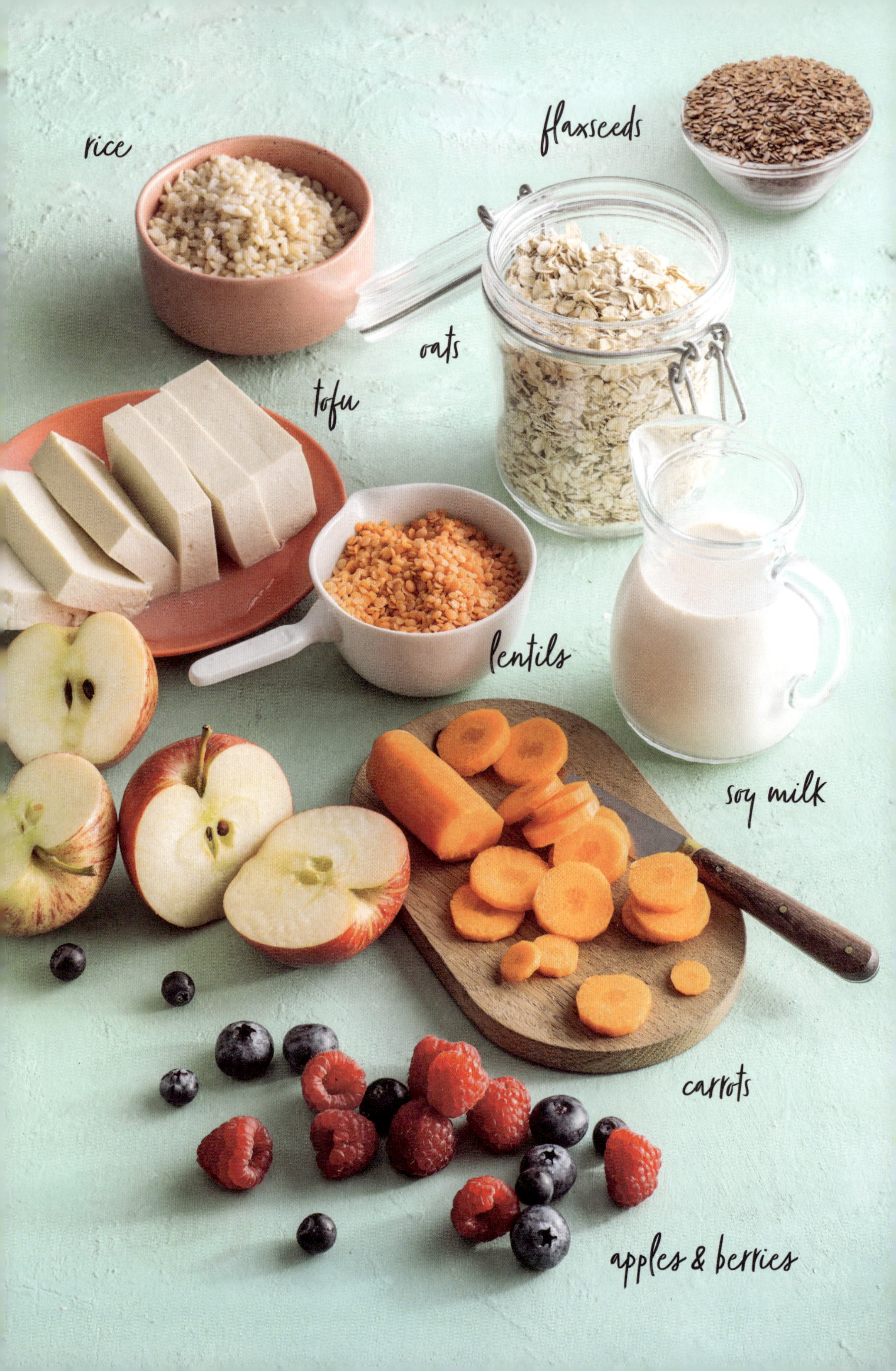
rice
flaxseeds
oats
tofu
lentils
soy milk
carrots
apples & berries

Phytoestrogenic foods

Found in a range of plant foods, phytoestrogens interact with oestrogen receptors in the body, though to a much milder extent than oestrogen itself. Eating a certain amount of phytoestrogenic foods consistently over time can help to tame some of the symptoms associated with peri by giving us an oestrogen-like boost when that hormone is low.

There are four groups of phytoestrogens:

- **Isoflavones/ isoflavonoids.** Soy is the richest source.
- **Lignans.** Mainly found in nuts, seeds, legumes, grains, vegetables and fruit. The best source is flaxseeds.
- **Coumestans.** Found in sprouted beans, alfalfa and spinach.
- **Stilbenes.** Found in red wine and peanuts.

In this section, I'll be focusing most of the attention on soy and flaxseeds because they contain significantly high amounts of phytoestrogens and have a lot of research backing up their benefits, especially in regards to perimenopause.

PHYTOESTROGEN-RICH FOODS INCLUDE:

- soy products
- flaxseeds
- alfafa
- mung beans
- berries and apples
- carrots
- oats
- barley
- rice
- pulses
- lentils.

SOY: SOURCES AND BENEFITS

Soy beans, also known as edamame, are a legume native to Asia. They feature prominently in the traditional Japanese diet (see page 22). Soy products can be made from whole soy beans or processed soy.

SOY PRODUCTS INCLUDE:

- tofu
- soy milk
- textured vegetable protein
- meat substitutes (e.g. soy burger)
- edamame pasta
- dry-roasted soy beans
- soy cheese
- soy yoghurt.

Fermented soy products (see page 52) include:

- miso
- natto
- tempeh.

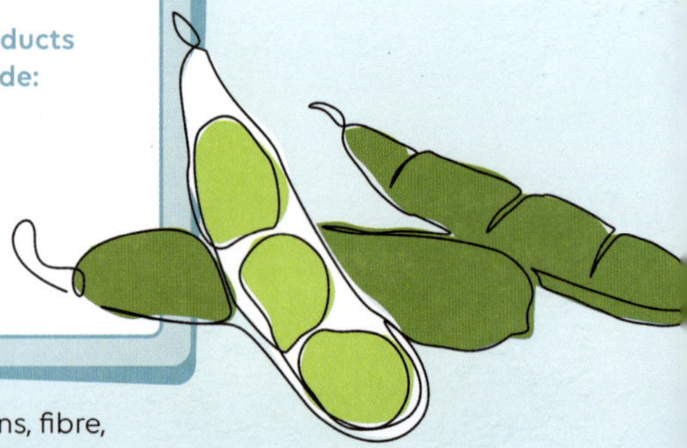

In general, these foods are nutritious and rich in B-vitamins, fibre, potassium and magnesium. Soy beans are also considered a complete protein (see opposite), which makes them an incredibly valuable source of protein for those following plant-based diets. Regular consumption of soy products as a high-quality protein source or in place of low-quality meat is likely to be beneficial.

Does soy increase breast cancer risk?

I can't talk about soy intake without discussing the purported link with breast cancer. The World Cancer Research Fund (WCRF) has recently reviewed all the available evidence on the link between foods high in isoflavones and breast cancer. It concluded that there's not enough evidence to prove this link exists. In fact, another study even found that breast cancer patients who increased their intake of soy-based foods following diagnosis lowered their risk of dying from the disease. Even so, more research in this area is needed, so there are currently no specific recommendations. As always, check with your health care professional for personalised advice.

What the research says

The link between soy and reduced peri symptoms was first noted in research when women in East Asian countries who ate soy products as a regular part of their diet reported lower rates of peri and menopausal symptoms. Some other interesting research reveals further benefits.

A recent study of postmenopausal women who were still experiencing menopause symptoms put the participants on a reduced-fat, vegan diet that included ½ cup of edamame each day. As a result, these women reported that their hot flushes decreased by up to 84 per cent, and they noted an overall improvement in their quality of life in psychosocial, physical and sexual domains.

In Japan, where isoflavone (the main phytoestrogen in soy foods) intake is an average of 31.7 mg per day, bone mineral density of women was shown to be significantly higher in the groups that ate the highest amount of soy products. However, the research isn't definitive on this and has shown some variability.

For health benefits, the recommended daily intake of isoflavones is 50 mg per day. In studies, the therapeutic dose of isoflavones ranged from 40 to 70 mg.

INGREDIENT	ISOFLAVONES	PROTEIN
Soy milk (1 cup/250 ml)	6 mg	7 g
Tofu, soft (100 g)	23 mg	9 g
Soybeans, mature, boiled (½ cup)	55 mg	15 g
Soy beans, dry-roasted (30 g)	40 mg	11 g
Edamame, boiled (½ cup)	16 mg	11 g
Soy cheese (30 g)	2 mg	4 g
Soy burger pattie (brand-dependent)	5 mg	14 g
Tempeh, cooked (100 g)	34 mg	15 g
Miso (30 g)	12 mg	3 g
Natto (30 g)	23 mg	5 g
Soy sauce (1 tablespoon)	0.02 mg	0 g

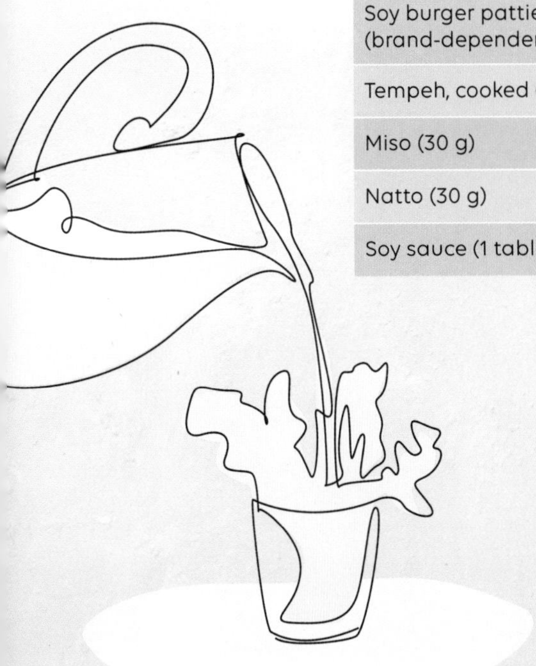

FLAXSEEDS: SOURCES AND BENEFITS

Flaxseeds (also known as linseeds) are a small brown seed from the flax plant. They contain the phytoestrogen lignans and are commonly found whole in muesli mixes and soy and linseed breads. Whole flaxseeds have a longer shelf life because they're a contained seed; however it's more nutritionally beneficial to grind them before eating since it's difficult for the body to crack through the hard outer shell and access the goodness inside.

FLAXSEEDS ARE ALSO RICH IN:

- soluble fibre, which absorbs water and slows down digestion, helping to stabilise blood glucose levels; it also helps to lower cholesterol
- alpha-linolenic acid (ALA), a plant-based omega-3 fatty acid
- protein
- potassium
- some B vitamins including thiamine
- minerals such as copper and manganese.

Though flaxseed oil is a great ingredient, it doesn't pack the perimenopausal benefits of the whole seed. Oil gives us the healthy fats but not the fibrous lignans, so to harness the phytoestrogenic benefits, stick to whole or ground flaxseed. As mentioned above, flaxseeds are best consumed ground as our body is better able to access and absorb their precious nutrients. You can freshly grind the flaxseeds before using them, but I buy ground flaxseed from the supermarket and keep it in the fridge so it stays fresh for longer and the healthy fats don't go rancid.

Note

If you've got diverticular disease (where small pockets form in the colon and become inflamed), you'll have likely been advised to avoid small seeds and grains. Even so, you can still get the health benefits of flaxseeds as long as they're ground.

What the research says

- Plant lignans, found in flaxseeds, can considerably reduce the frequency of hot flushes and vaginal dryness. Even a lower dose of 5 g per day has been shown to decrease the number of hot flushes each week by as much as 44 per cent.
- Eating flaxseeds every day over a three-month period can improve menopausal symptoms and quality of life.
- 40 g of flaxseeds per day for two months has been shown to be as effective as oral oestrogen-progesterone in improving mild menopausal symptoms and lowering glucose and insulin levels.
- A study in 2004 suggested that flaxseed may even be better at increasing oestrogen levels than soy, as it was found to be better able to 'cling on' to oestrogen in the body.

While this research is impressive, it's important to note that a few other studies show no changes in peri symptoms among women who consumed flaxseeds. However, given the way peri symptoms fluctuate in severity and the fact that flaxseeds are packed with many other beneficial nutrients, they can and should be a part of your daily diet regardless.

How much do we need?

In clinic, I usually suggest that clients aim for 1 to 2 tablespoons of ground flaxseeds per day. However, if this is a new addition to your diet, start slowly. As with any high-fibre food, your gut may get upset if you blast straight into the upper doses. I suggest starting with 1 teaspoon per day and building slowly to wherever your tolerance allows. And remember, anytime you add more fibre to your diet, it's really important to up your fluid intake so you don't get constipated.

Personally, I love sprinkling ground flaxseed on my porridge, muesli or yoghurt, and adding some to smoothies. Because my son is allergic to eggs, I also use ground flaxseeds as an egg replacement in meals at home, from pancakes and muffins to meatloaf.

Easy recipe

1 tablespoon ground flaxseed
+ 2 tablespoons water
= 1 egg replacement

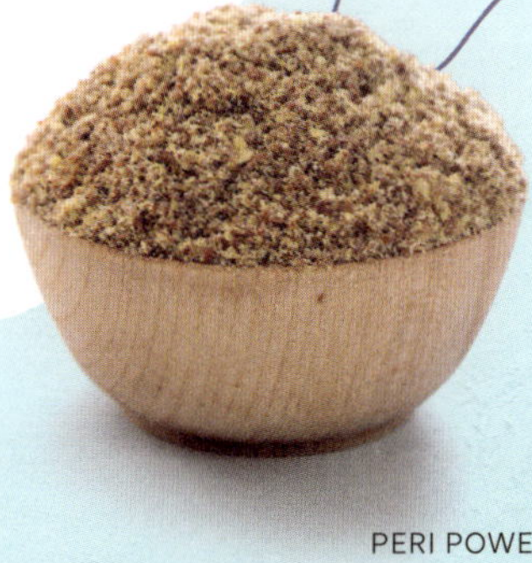

Nuts

A rich source of monounsaturated and polyunsaturated fats, which are unsaturated or 'healthy' fats, tree nuts are also low in carbohydrates and contain moderate amounts of protein. The bioactive components – the parts of the nut that make them so good for our health – include some powerful plant chemicals, antioxidants, vitamins such as vitamin E, minerals such as magnesium and potassium, and fibre.

TREE NUTS INCLUDE:

- almonds
- walnuts
- hazelnuts
- brazil nuts
- pistachios
- cashews
- pine nuts
- macadamias
- pecans.

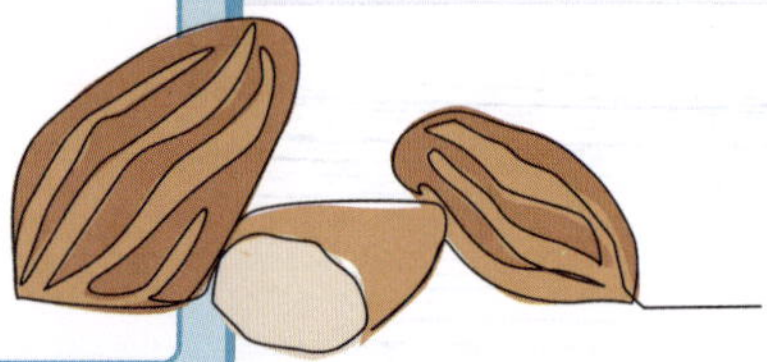

What the research says

Though nuts may not directly affect peri symptoms, they can support our health during this time in a number of other ways.

- Nuts are associated with a 15 per cent reduction in the incidence of cardiovascular disease and a 23 per cent reduction in cardiovascular mortality.
- They're an integral part of the Mediterranean diet (see page 21), an eating pattern known to be beneficial for reducing the risk of major chronic diseases that increase in prevalence during peri.
- They have been shown to have a beneficial impact on carbohydrate metabolism during peri, which can impact the development of metabolic syndrome (see page 70).
- Nuts may play a role in reducing the process of fat accumulation and increase in waist circumference associated with peri.

How much do we need?

It's recommended that we eat 30 g of unsalted mixed nuts per day, but only 2 per cent of Australians hit this target. Many people avoid nuts because they're known to be highly calorific; however, nuts are not associated with higher body weight or waist circumference, and overall they have a neutral, if not slightly positive, impact on our weight. This is likely because they're high in fibre and healthy fats, which makes them satisfying and therefore easier not to overindulge in. Interestingly, we don't absorb between 5 and 26 per cent of the energy from nuts. This is because the fats get trapped in the cell wall of the nut, making it hard for the body to digest and absorb. Consequently, they pass through our gut undigested.

> Nuts are NOT associated with higher body weight or waist circumference.

Berries

Packed full of nutrients, berries contain powerful phytochemicals (plant chemicals) and are a rich source of vitamins, minerals and prebiotics (the fibre that feeds beneficial bacteria in our gut). The phytonutrients that make berries so great for us are the antioxidants anthocyanins and resveratrol. Anthocyanins give blue, purple and black fruits their pigments while resveratrol gives red fruits their pigment. Blueberries, blackberries and raspberries have the highest antioxidant activity of commonly consumed fruits. On average, people who eat more berries seem to live a bit longer than those who don't.

> Berries, particularly blueberries, have been shown to be cardioprotective.

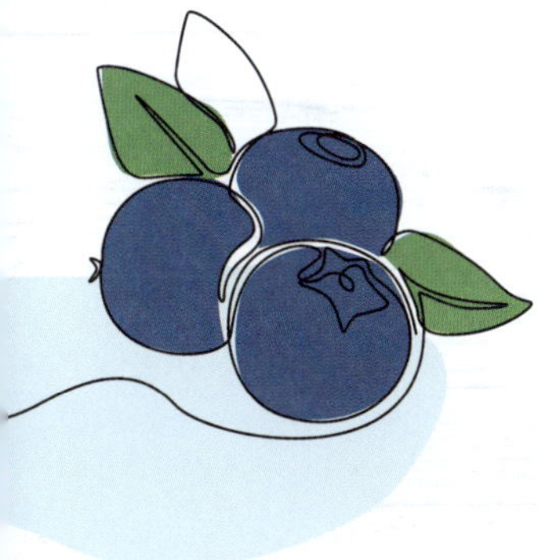

What the research says

- Berries, particularly blueberries, have been shown to be cardioprotective (i.e. they contain nutrients that protect our heart). Blueberries have been shown to reduce the risk of coronary artery disease by 25 per cent, reduce heart attacks by 32 per cent and reduce hypertension by 10 per cent.
- Eating strawberries daily can be helpful for lowering blood pressure, improving the stiffness of the arteries and improving cholesterol profile. This is particularly good for women in mid-late life since we know that menopause and ageing in general are both risk factors for cardiovascular disease.
- The greater the intake of blueberries and strawberries, the slower the rate of cognitive decline may be. Blueberries may also improve executive function, which is the brain's ability to make decisions, stay focused and manage emotions. This may be helpful during peri when brain fog and fluctuations in mood arise.
- A large observational study of women in the peri age group found a positive link between increased consumption of blueberries and a reduced risk of vision impairment.

How much do we need?

So far, there isn't enough data to recommend a specific quantity of berries as part of a peri protocol. However, the studies above involved women eating between a third of a punnet to one whole punnet (125 g) of berries per day. Fresh berries can get expensive, so it's good to know that you can get the same health benefits when you buy them frozen. It's much more cost effective, and they last for months in the freezer. In fact, because berries are picked at their ripest then snap frozen (often on the same day) they retain all their nutrients, unlike fresh berries that can be transported for days to sit on the supermarket shelves and then stay in your fridge for longer.

My favourite way to use frozen berries is in a smoothie because I love how creamy and cold they make it, but they are so versatile. They can be enjoyed as a snack, a healthy dessert, in sweet and savoury salads, on top of cereal, porridge, muesli, overnight oats, pancakes, frozen yoghurt bark – the list is endless!

Extra-virgin olive oil

Olive oil is the freshly squeezed juice of an olive. It's one of the pillars of the Mediterranean diet and 70 per cent of the world's olive oil is produced in that region. Olive oil is associated with a longer life span and many other protective health effects, especially for women in peri.

When buying olive oil, it's important to choose unrefined and unfiltered extra-virgin olive oil that has been cold-pressed. If it doesn't specify 'cold-pressed' on the label, it will be a refined oil, which means it will contain fewer antioxidants and the fat profile will be less than ideal. It can be more expensive than regular olive oil, but a bottle of good-quality, extra-virgin olive oil is worth it. Once opened, it's best used within four to six weeks and stored in a dark pantry or cupboard to preserve those precious antioxidants and prevent the olive oil from degrading.

OLIVE OIL IS HIGH IN:

- **healthy fats:** the monounsaturated fat oleic acid and the polyunsaturated fat linoleic acid
- **polyphenols:** these are a family of phytochemicals (plant chemicals) and include flavonoids, phenolic acids, lignans and stilbenes, which have antioxidant and anti-inflammatory properties. There are two especially potent polyphenols in olives:
  1. oleuropein, which gives olives their bitter taste, is found in the skin, flesh, seed and leaves and has powerful antioxidant and anti-inflammatory properties
  2. hydroxytyrosol, which has several beneficial antioxidant and anti-inflammatory effects on the body, and can also protect the skin and eyes
- **vitamin E:** a fat-soluble vitamin that acts like an antioxidant to remove free radicals, which are chemicals that can damage the body's cells
- **squalene:** an organic compound with potent antioxidant effects.

What the research says

- Extra-virgin olive oil has been shown to increase bone mineral density (in an animal study) by protecting the bone from oxidative stress with its antioxidant and anti-inflammatory effects.
- The polyphenols in extra-virgin olive oil may enhance the growth of bone-forming cells and inhibit the breakdown of bone, which can help to increase calcium levels in the bone.
- Extra-virgin olive oil can protect against cardiovascular disease by lowering 'bad' LDL cholesterol and triglyceride levels and reducing cardiovascular-related inflammatory markers.
- There is limited data on the direct relationship between extra-virgin olive oil and metabolic syndrome in peri. However, there is a lot of information on how it impacts the mechanisms of metabolic syndrome, particularly that extra-virgin olive oil improves insulin sensitivity. A PREDIMED study showed a reversal of metabolic syndrome when having 4 tablespoons of extra-virgin olive oil per day as part of an energy-restricted Mediterranean diet.

> You can absolutely cook with extra-virgin olive oil!

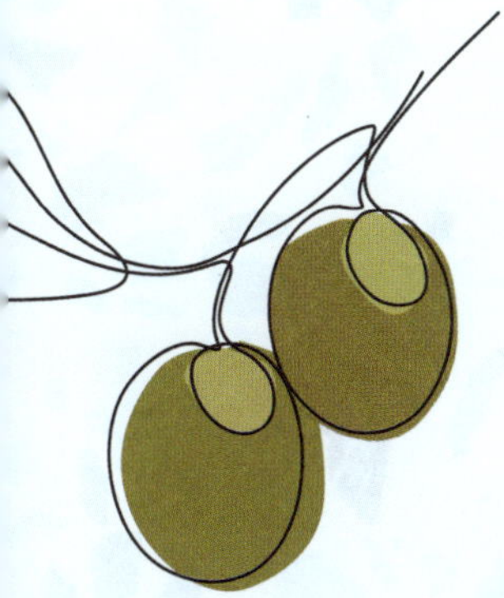

How much do we need?

Consuming as little as half a tablespoon per day of extra-virgin olive oil has been shown to have beneficial effects, especially when it replaces butter, margarine and mayonnaise.

I use extra-virgin olive oil for all my cooking, including pan-frying and roasting, and I also substitute it for butter and coconut oil in all my baking. Loaves, muffins, cookies . . . it's great in all of them. I drizzle it liberally over salads and vegetables, and this is important because not only does that fat make the vegetables taste so much better, the vitamins in those veggies (the fat-soluble A, D, E and K) are better absorbed when consumed with a fat.

I have at least three types of extra-virgin olive oil in my pantry at any one time and I use all of them every day: a robust flavour that I typically use raw, a lighter intensity when I don't want a strong olive oil flavour (such as in baking), and at least one bottle infused with lemon, garlic, chilli or herbs (at the moment, I've got all these on the go!).

* Peri pause

One of the greatest myths about olive oil is that you can't cook with it. You absolutely can! In fact, extra-virgin olive oil is ideal for all types of cooking because the levels of antioxidants and healthy monounsaturated fats in the oil make it more stable during cooking, meaning it's less likely to break down and form harmful compounds.

Omega-3 fatty acids

Omega-3 fatty acids are a type of healthy polyunsaturated fat and they play an important role in cellular function and heart, kidney, eye and skin health. Seafood, particularly oily fish, contains the highest amounts of omega-3. It is also found in plants such as flaxseeds, soy beans, canola oil, chia seeds, hemp seeds and walnuts in the form of alpha-linoleic acid (ALA). Omega-3 fat is essential because our body can't make it, so we have to get it from our diet. If you don't eat oily fish, you can take a fish oil supplement. If you are vegan or choose not to use a fish oil–based supplement, there are vegan options based on algae.

> Omega-3 intake has a beneficial effect on emotional and cognitive behaviours during peri.

What the research says

- A cross-sectional nationwide health and nutrition survey in Korea found that postmenopausal women who had the highest dietary omega-3 fatty acid intake had significantly lower prevalence of depression compared with women with the lowest intake.
- Three high-level studies showed that omega-3 fats may alleviate night sweats for menopausal women.
- Omega-3 fatty acid intake has a beneficial effect on emotional and cognitive behaviours during peri.

How much do we need?

The Heart Foundation recommends we aim to eat two to three 150 g serves of oily fish per week as well as 1 g plant-based omega-3 (ALA) every day.

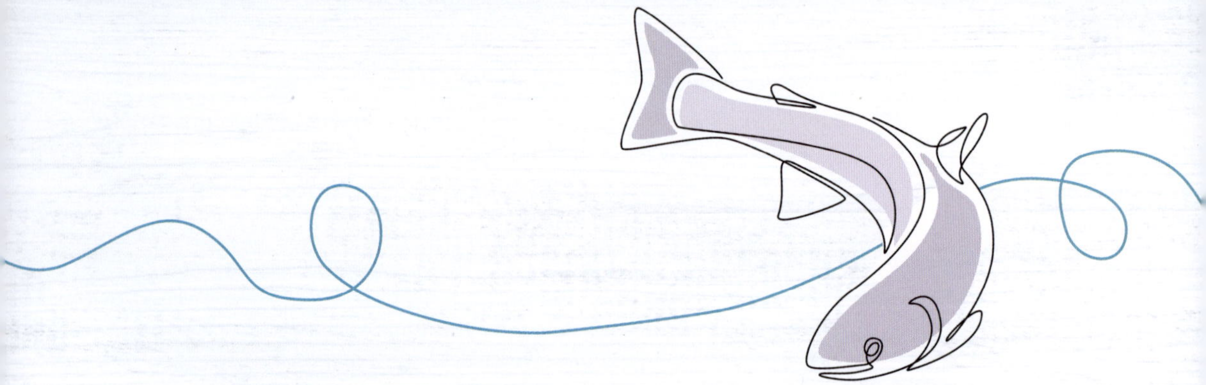

Omega-3 fatty acid counter

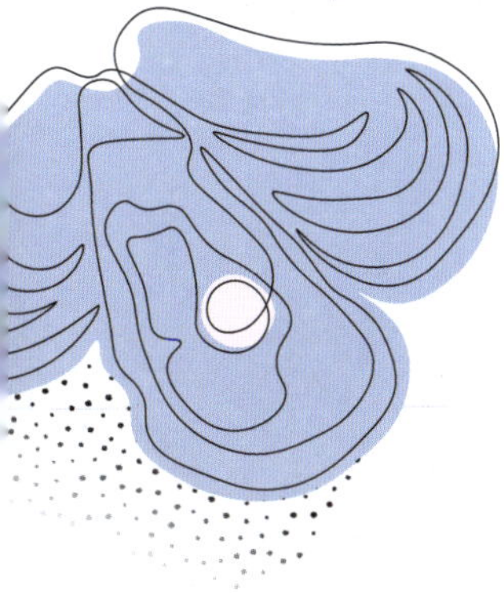

INGREDIENT		EPA (AND DHA) PER 100 G SERVE
Canned salmon	Canned sardines	>1500 mg
Oysters Atlantic salmon Australian salmon Mackerel Sardines Mullet Silver perch Rainbow trout	Bream Mussels Canned tuna Anchovies Pickled herring Squid Calamari	500–1500 mg
Blue-eye trevalla Scallops Prawns Octopus Crab Lobster Moreton Bay bug	Yellow-tail kingfish Australian herring Trevally Tuna Snapper Flounder Mirror dory	300–500 mg
Murray cod Barramundi Smoked cod Flathead	Bass King dory Coral trout Leatherjacket	200–300 mg

INGREDIENT	ALA
Walnuts (30 g)	1,884 mg
Chia seeds (15 g)	2,685 mg
Flaxseeds (1 teaspoon)	922 mg
Canola oil (1 tablespoon)	1,820 mg
Soybean oil (1 tablespoon)	1,434 mg
Flaxseed oil (1 tablespoon)	10,918 mg
Soy and linseed bread (2 slices)	2,480 mg

Low-GI carbohydrates

Low-GI carbs (see page 25) include most whole fruits and starchy vegetables, legumes, nuts and wholegrains, such as rolled oats, wholegrain bread and crackers, rye and barley. They don't cause a spike in blood sugar or insulin (the hormone that shuffles glucose out of our blood and into our cells) in the way refined carbs do. They also tend to be more satisfying because they are digested more slowly, and generally keep us feeling fuller for longer, which is great for weight management and reducing snacking.

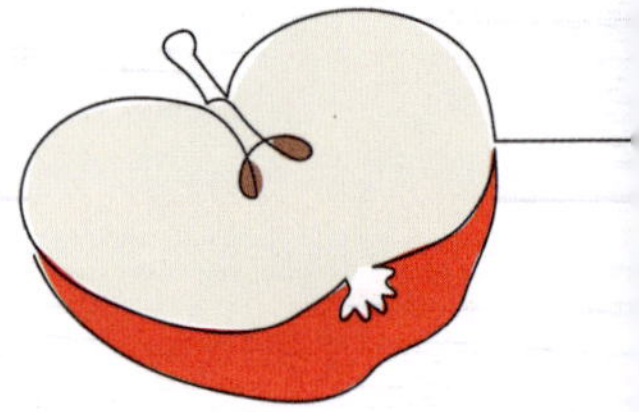

What the research says

- Lower-GI foods have been shown to lower blood sugar levels, which can reduce the severity of hot flushes.
- Researchers who looked at the diet of women through peri found that the risk of developing insomnia was greater in those with a higher-GI diet and a diet higher in added sugars like white and brown sugar, syrups, honey and molasses. They believed the drops in blood sugar and insulin levels that happen after a big spike can trigger waking from sleep.

The easiest way to start switching to lower-GI foods is to make some swaps to your staple foods (see below). Also, make sure to eat fruits whole and unpeeled when their skin is edible. By leaving skins on and not juicing them, the fruit retains more nutrients and that all-important fibre.

> Eat fruits whole and unpeeled.

Swap	For
White bread →	Wholegrain bread
White rice →	Brown or basmati rice
Processed cereals →	High-fibre options (e.g. Corn Flakes for Weet-Bix)
White pasta →	Wholemeal or pulse pasta
Peeled white potato →	Unpeeled potato, purple potato or sweet potato
White crackers →	Wholegrain crackers e.g. Cruskits for Vita-Weats
Rice noodles →	Soba noodles

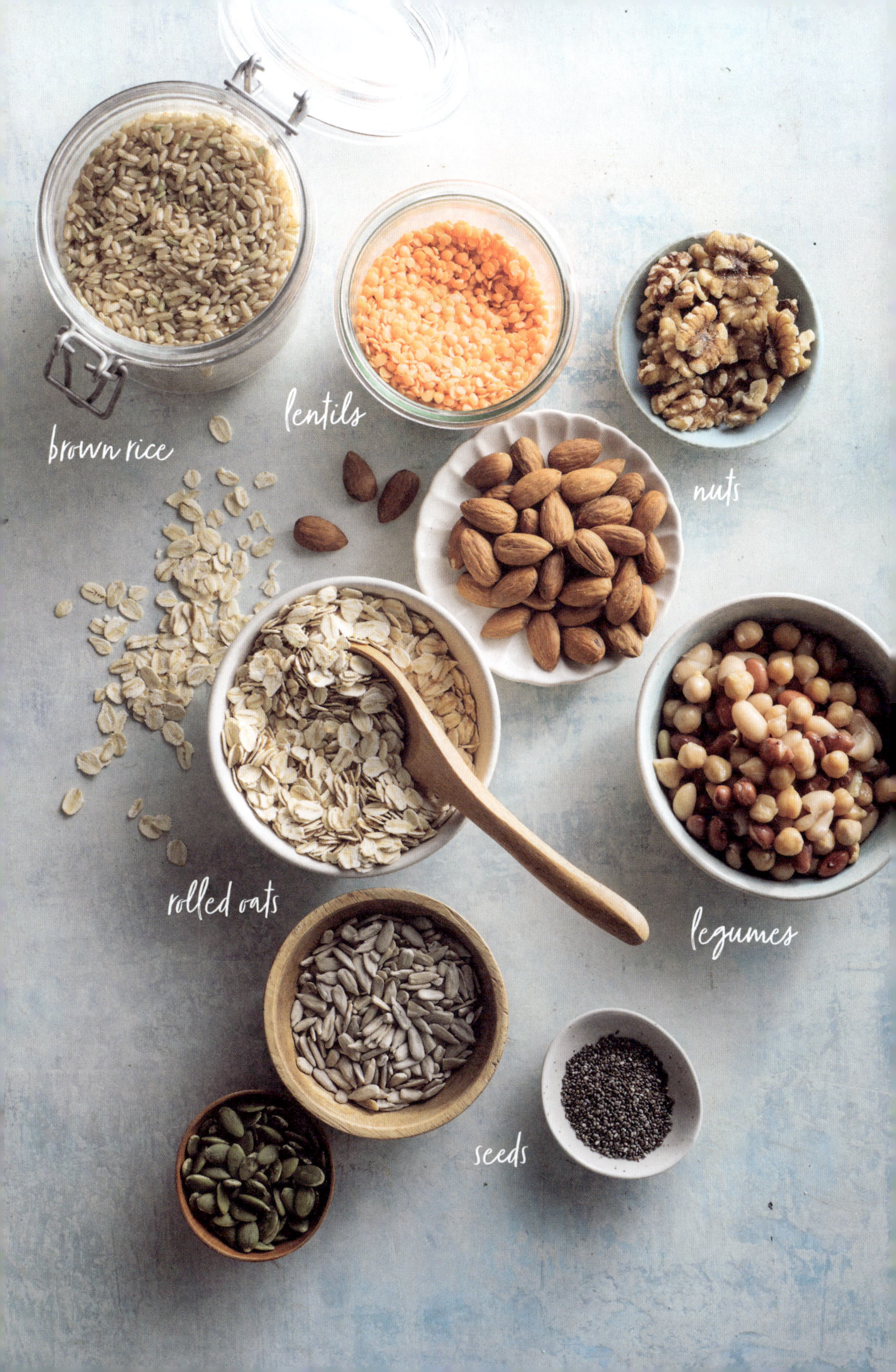
brown rice
lentils
nuts
rolled oats
legumes
seeds

Fibre-rich foods

Fibre is the indigestible part of a plant, and when we consume it, it acts like a big scrubbing brush as it moves through our intestines. It improves the frequency and volume of bowel motions and generally relieves constipation. It's also a prebiotic, which serves as food for the beneficial bacteria in our bowels, which then turn it into by-products that have been shown to be anti-inflammatory. Fibre can also slow the absorption of sugars into our bloodstream, and this helps with energy levels and weight management because we feel fuller for longer.

What the research says

- A random controlled trial of postmenopausal women who ate wholegrains as part of a six-week study showed positive effects on their resting metabolic rate.
- Fibre improves cholesterol levels and reduces the risk of bowel cancer.

How much do we need?

For women, the recommended daily amount of fibre is 25 g per day. By eating more unprocessed plant foods, you will automatically increase your fibre intake. If you find this a challenge, you can start by adding a sprinkle of bran or psyllium husks to your cereal, muesli, yoghurt or smoothie. Adding a small tin of beans to a meal like a salad, soup, stew or curry is a great idea too. Or swap out a packaged snack for a piece of fruit or chopped veggies with dip. Once again, I must stress that if you're increasing your fibre, you should do this SLOWLY over days or weeks. If you add a lot of fibre to your diet immediately, it can cause bloating and an upset tummy.

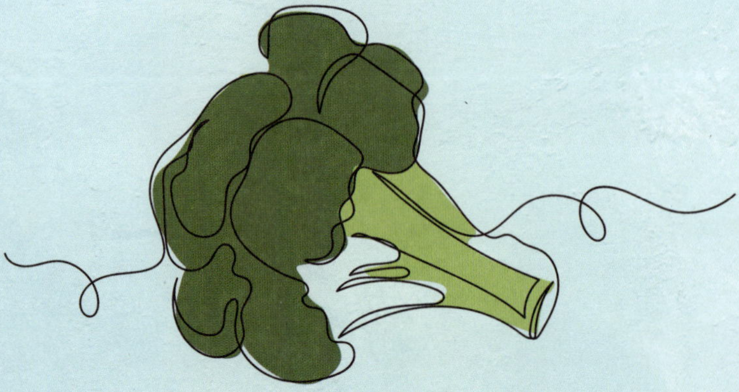

Constipation and the 3 Fs

Ever get a bit constipated before your period, but then notice that you have looser stools once it arrives? This is very common for women because our fluctuating hormones impact bowel function. As a result, women in peri can often experience digestive disruptions. Some might have reflux or indigestion, while others might have bloating and constipation or diarrhoea. If you're bunged up, before you go shopping for an over-the-counter remedy, check that you've ticked off the 3 Fs.

✓ FIBRE

Are you getting the recommended 25 grams of fibre a day for women? If you aren't, food might not be moving through your system efficiently and you may not have enough bulk to create regular, healthy stools – this can lead to constipation. Refer to the fibre counter on page 50 to see if you're meeting the daily requirements. Make sure your fibre intake includes plants that are also good sources of prebiotics to keep your gut bacteria healthy, such as garlic, onion, asparagus, beetroot, fennel, cabbage, legumes, stone fruit, apples, grainy breads, rolled oats, cashew and pistachios.

✓ FLUIDS

Aim for around 2 litres (8 cups) per day because fluids are absorbed by some fibre and help to soften the stool, making it easier to pass. If we're dehydrated, our stools are likely to get hard and in a way, stuck in our bowels. The easiest way to know if you're drinking enough is to monitor the colour of your urine. It should consistently be a light straw colour. If it's darker in colour, then you aren't drinking enough. When tallying your fluid intake, don't just count water. Unsweetened, non-alcoholic drinks (such as herbal teas and sparkling water) also contribute to that overall number, as do soups and broths, fresh veggies, juices and smoothies.

✓ FITNESS

Daily movement is essential for our bowel function as it acts like a massage for the smooth muscle around our intestines, helping to gently move food through our bowels. If you're constipated, a light walk or swim can help to get things moving again, and some gentle stretching and yoga may also be beneficial.

Fibre counter

Remember, the goal for women is 25 grams of fibre a day.

INGREDIENT	FIBRE
Wholemeal pasta (1 cup)	7.9 g
Carrot, unpeeled (1 cup)	6.9 g
Kidney beans (100 g)	6.5 g
Corn (1 medium)	5.9 g
Rolled oats (½ cup)	4.5 g
Wholemeal crackers (2)	4.2 g
Broccoli, unpeeled (1 cup)	3.8 g
Lentils (100 g)	3.7 g
Sweet potato, unpeeled (1 cup)	3.7 g
Almonds (30 g/25 almonds)	3 g
Brown rice (1 cup)	2.7 g
Dried apricots (30 g/5 apricots)	2.5 g
Wholegrain bread (1 slice)	2.4 g
Banana (1 medium)	2.3 g
Apple (1 medium)	2.2 g
Psyllium husk (1 tablespoon)	2.2 g
Popcorn (1 cup)	1.2 g

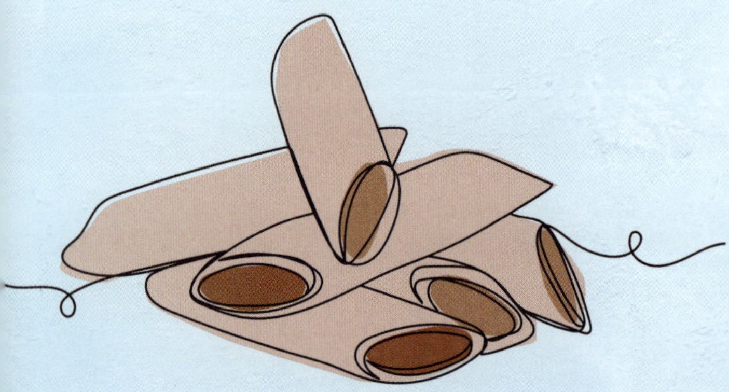

Veg and more veg

> Aim for at least 5 servings of veg a day.

Vegetables have a big role to play in so many areas of the peri diet. Not only are they a major component of the Mediterranean diet and the plant-focused diet we spoke of earlier, they're also rich in antioxidants and fibre, which are particularly important for women in peri. Vegetables such as green leaves are also some of the richest sources of magnesium. Getting adequate magnesium during peri is associated with greater bone mineral density, and it may promote sleep by regulating the body's circadian rhythm. Given their undeniable health benefits, it's kind of shocking that the latest data indicate that nearly 94 per cent of Australians are not getting their recommended intake.

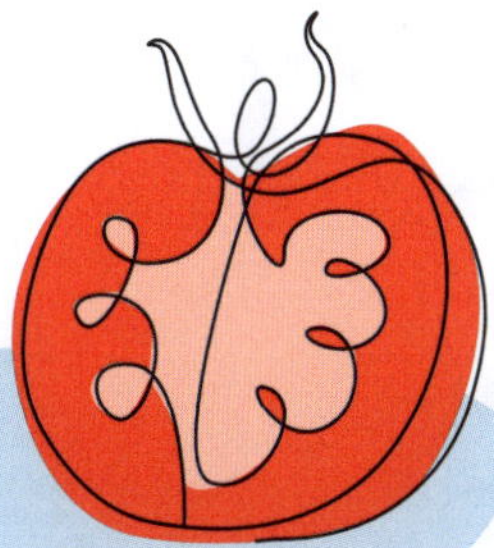

What the research says

- Eating a wide variety of different-coloured veggies every day has been shown to help reduce hot flushes in some women.
- A higher consumption of cruciferous vegetables is associated with an overall reduction in menopause symptoms. Cruciferous veg include broccoli, cauliflower, cabbage, kale, bok choy, rocket, brussels sprouts, collards, watercress and radishes.
- Higher intake of whole plant foods (which includes vegetables) is associated with a reduction in non-specific menopause symptoms.
- One study found that switching to a more veggie-filled diet helped with weight loss for menopausal women.
- The risk of developing insomnia during peri is lower in those who ate more whole vegetables (and fruit).
- A study of postmenopausal women found that those with deficient magnesium were more likely to have moderate levels of depression.
- Another study found that higher magnesium levels were associated with lower inflammatory markers related to heart disease, indicating that magnesium could be protective of heart health.

How much do we need?

Aim for at least 5 servings of veg every day.

A SERVING OF VEG IS:

- ½ cup cooked vegetables
- 1 cup raw green leafy or salad vegetables
- ½ cup corn
- ½ cup cooked legumes (beans, peas or lentils)
- ½ medium potato or sweet potato
- 1 medium tomato.

Fermented foods and probiotics

The gut microbiota is the community of bacteria, fungi and viruses that live mainly in our large bowel. They have many roles including producing certain vitamins, supporting our immune system, helping with digestion and protecting us against harmful pathogens. Dramatic changes or imbalance in this gut microbiota is known as 'dysbiosis', and it's linked to many health conditions, particularly during peri.

Oestrogen has been shown to affect the gut microbiota, which in turn significantly influence oestrogen levels in the body. Oestrogen regulates the gut environment and female reproductive tract by maintaining cell linings, mucus secretion and pH levels, creating the perfect environment for beneficial bacteria such as lactobacilli to thrive. During perimenopause, the drop in oestrogen disturbs many of these processes and this can lead to worsening peri symptoms.

Dysbiosis in the gut can reduce estrobolome – a microbe that regulates the circulating active form of oestrogen by reabsorbing oestrogen in the intestine into the bloodstream. We want the oestrogen in our bloodstream because it helps prevent those peri symptoms. Probiotics may help to enhance estrobolome, which can then modulate those oestrogen levels.

When we eat fermented food such as yoghurt, the beneficial bacterial cultures present in them add diversity to our microbiome and boost our health on many fronts. By consuming probiotics, which are specific, beneficial strains of bacteria that have been added to foods, we increase this diversity and their benefits even further.

> “Beneficial bacterial cultures can boost our health on many fronts.

What the research says

- Beneficial bacterial strains from both yoghurt and supplements in peri and menopause may help to promote absorption of calcium from our gut, supporting bone health.
- Though evidence is limited, researchers believe there may be an association between obesity and the changes to gut microbiota that occur during peri and menopause. If this link is proven, tailoring microbial species that metabolise oestrogens and phytoestrogens may help with weight management.
- There was shown to be a strong association in postmenopausal women and several gut microbial species and markers of insulin resistance, irregular cholesterol levels and inflammation. Studies have also shown a positive effect on probiotic supplementation and cardiovascular risk factors.
- A study found postmenopausal women who ate probiotic yoghurt every day saw improvements in anxiety, stress and quality of life.
- The pH level in the vagina declines in peri, which can increase the risk of vaginal infections. Lactobacilli may help to maintain optimum pH levels and reduce the risk of vaginal infections.

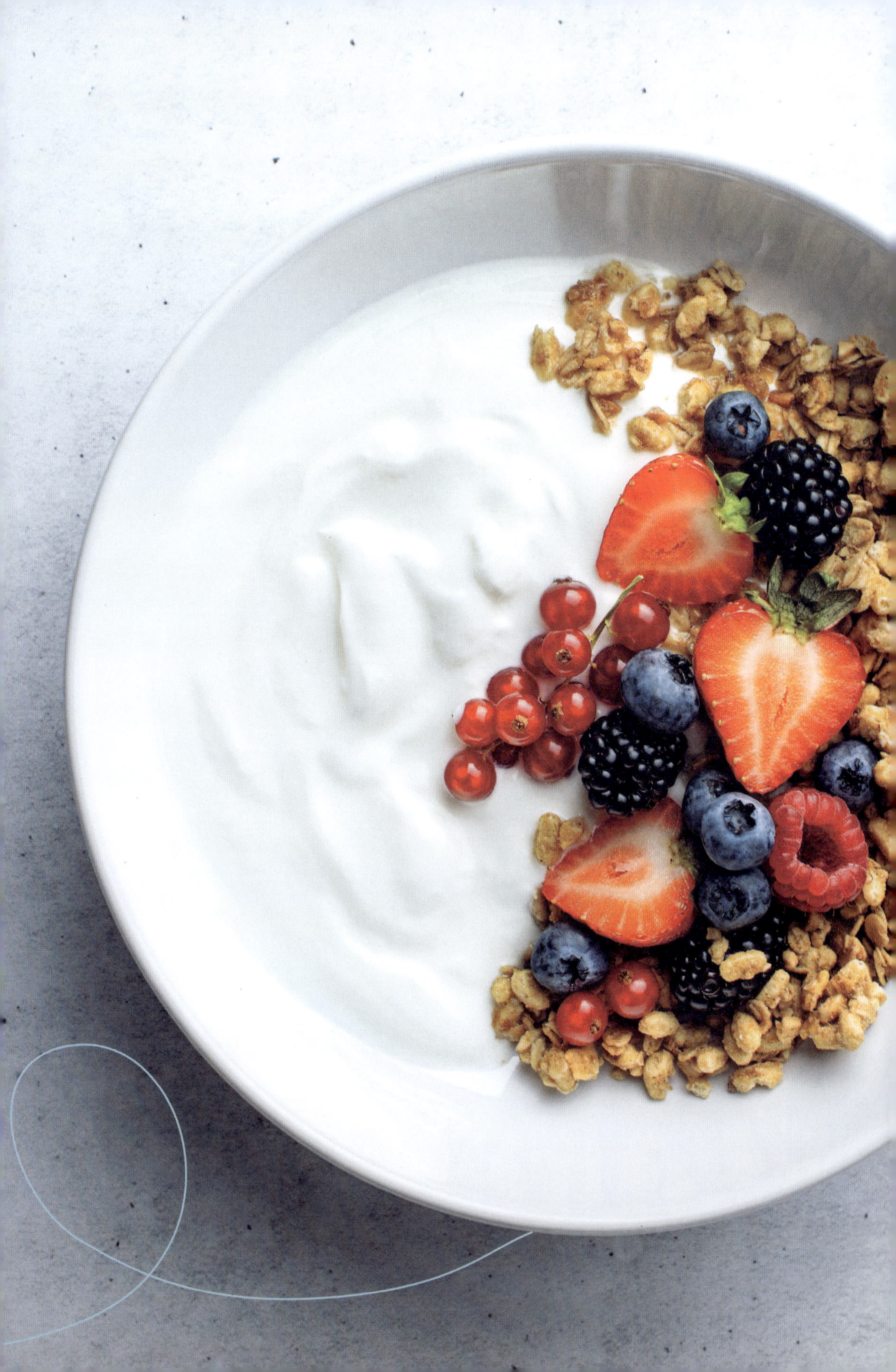

How much do we need?

Aim for a 150 g serve of probiotic yoghurt every day as part of your diet. You can also take a multi-strain probiotic during peri. There are no specific recommendations on which strains are best for perimenopause; however, a good starting point is a probiotic that contains bifidobacterium and lactobacillus. Exactly how much of a difference probiotic supplements make to our overall health and peri symptoms is unknown. But since they are considered to be safe in most cases (check with your doctor first, particularly if you have an immune condition), they can be an additional tool in your peri toolbox if you want to try them.

Probiotic yoghurt:

It may surprise you to learn that not all yoghurts are probiotic yoghurts. All of them do contain bacterial cultures that develop in the fermenting process of yoghurt-making, but which strains are used and how much of them end up in the final product is unknown.

Probiotic yoghurts, on the other hand, have specific strains of healthy bacteria added to them in doses that have been scientifically tested and shown to have specific health benefits. There are only a handful of probiotic yoghurts on the market, and the best way to find them is to look at the label and scan the nutrition panel. There you should find the name of several long and hard-to-pronounce bacterial strains in very high numbers (up in the billions, usually) using the measurement of CFU or 'colony forming units'.

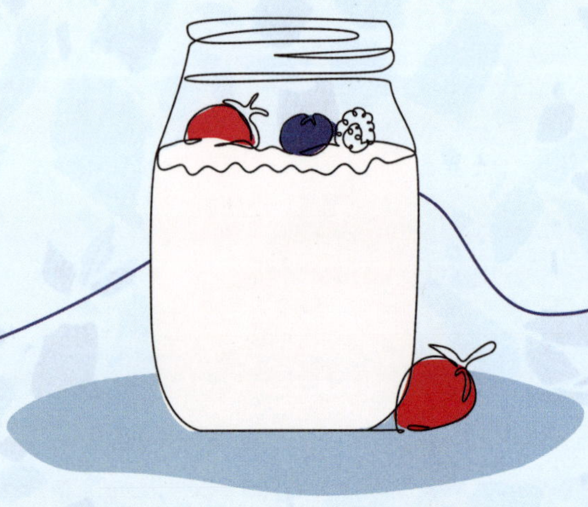

What yoghurt should I choose?

Yoghurt has got to be one of the most confusing foods on the market. Many of my patients find this section of the supermarket overwhelming because there are so many different choices. To simplify things as much as possible, let's break yoghurt down into three main categories.

1

GREEK YOGHURT:

This refers to yoghurt made using a straining process that further removes some of the liquid component of a yoghurt. The result is a thicker, creamier yoghurt that is generally higher in protein because the watery element has been taken out. There are many varieties within this category: flavoured, plain, sweetened and unsweetened, full cream and low-fat or skim.

2

SWEETENED VS UNSWEETENED YOGHURT:

Plain or natural yoghurt contains naturally occurring sugars in the form of lactose or milk sugar, so even if a yoghurt is tart and unsweetened, the nutrition label will still contain the naturally occurring sugars, but no added sugars. Typically, flavoured yoghurts like vanilla and berry contain added sugars on top of those natural sugars to further sweeten the yoghurt. You can also now get flavoured yoghurts that have sweeteners such as stevia added to them to make them taste sweet, without the sugar content.

3

LOW-FAT VS FULL-CREAM YOGHURT:

Full-cream yoghurt is made from full-cream milk and contains around 4–5 per cent fat, or 8–10 grams per 200 gram serve. Low-fat yoghurt contains around 2 per cent fat and 4–5 grams fat per 200 gram serve. And skim or fat-free yoghurt has had almost all the fat removed and contains just 0.1 gram of fat per serve.

Ultimately, which yoghurt you choose will come down to your health goals and your preferences. I generally recommended low-fat and fat-free products for those with a history of high cholesterol or heart conditions, or those needing to trim out excess calories (aka energy) from their diet. On the other hand, if that isn't a concern of yours and you're otherwise healthy and have a good diet, fat is filling so you may prefer the creamy texture of full-fat yoghurt and enjoy the fact that it's more satiating.

Must-have ingredients

Keeping your pantry and fridge stocked with peri power foods (see Chapter 3) along with other key staples means you'll always have quick access to healthy and nourishing meals. You don't need to overhaul your kitchen in one go; you can slowly replace refined carbs with wholegrains, build up your range of canned legumes and spices, and introduce new items over time. Don't forget to stock your freezer, too. Edamame, berries and seafood are wonderful peri staples.

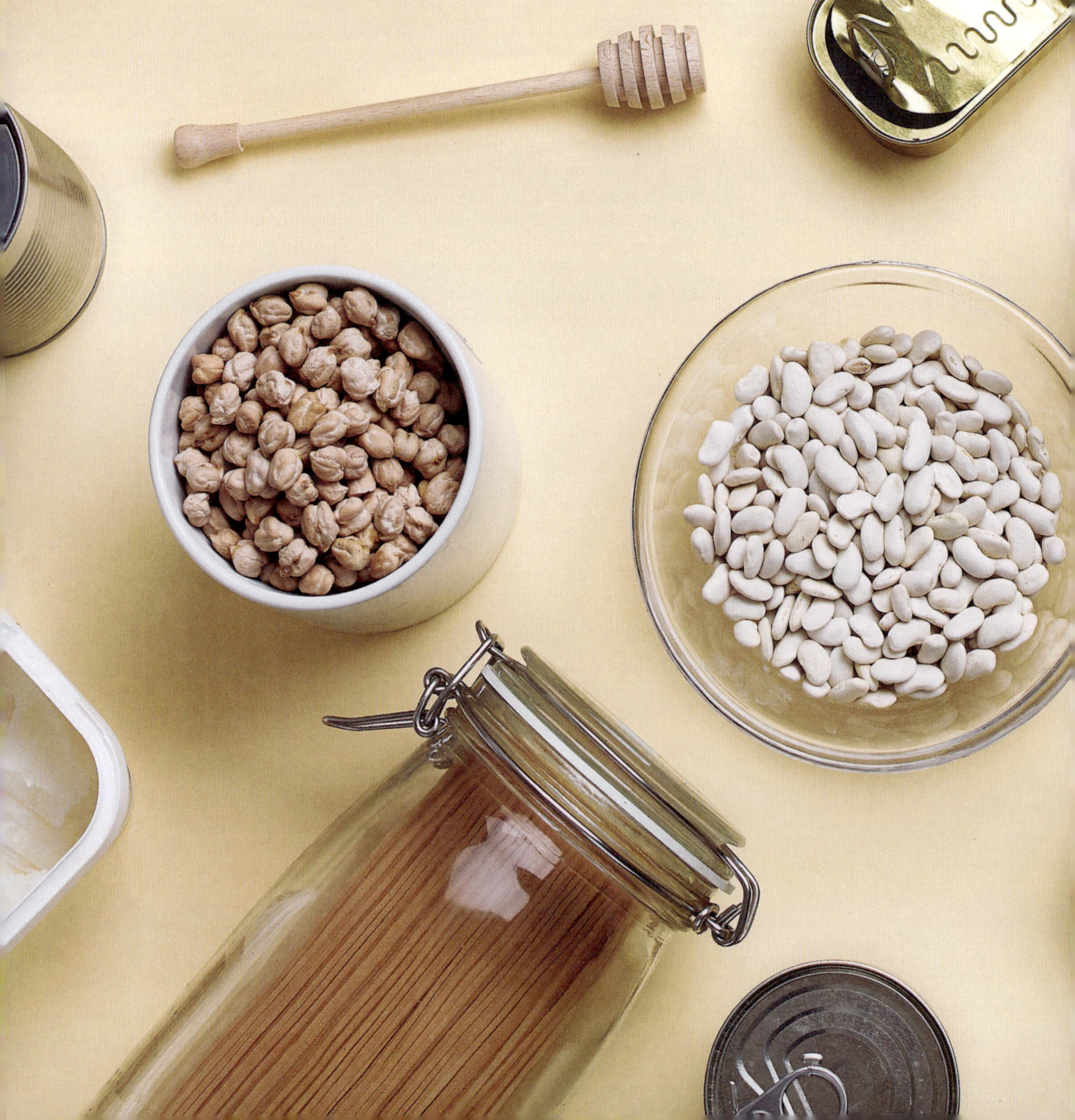

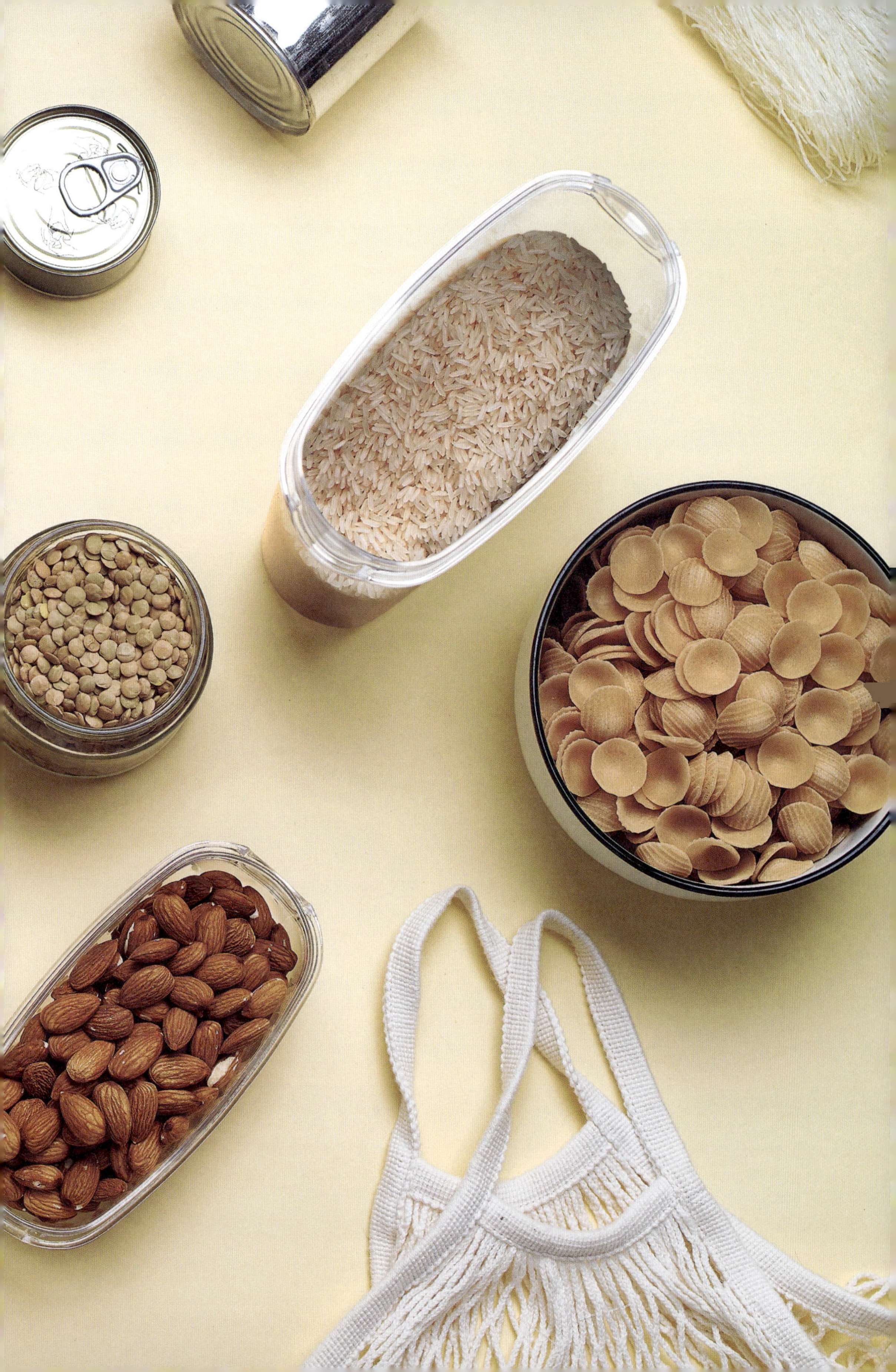

IN THE PANTRY

Oils and sauces

- ◯ Extra-virgin olive oil – you can have a darker coloured oil for raw in salad dressings and lighter colour for cooking
- ◯ Sesame oil
- ◯ Avocado oil
- ◯ Red wine vinegar
- ◯ White wine vinegar
- ◯ Apple cider vinegar
- ◯ Balsamic vinegar
- ◯ Mustard
- ◯ Soy or tamari sauce

Spices and herbs

- ◯ Ground cinnamon
- ◯ Dried thyme, rosemary, oregano, parsley, mint
- ◯ Ground black pepper
- ◯ Turmeric
- ◯ Cloves
- ◯ Garlic powder
- ◯ Onion powder
- ◯ Nutmeg
- ◯ Cumin
- ◯ Cardamom
- ◯ Fennel seeds
- ◯ Paprika – smoked and sweet
- ◯ Sea salt – iodised if you need it
- ◯ Sumac
- ◯ Garam masala
- ◯ Chilli flakes

Baking

- ◯ Maple syrup
- ◯ Honey
- ◯ Coconut sugar
- ◯ Baking powder
- ◯ Baking soda
- ◯ Vanilla extract or concentrate
- ◯ Almond meal or flour
- ◯ Chickpea flour
- ◯ Wholemeal flour
- ◯ Spelt flour

Pulses and lentils

Canned or dried:

- ◯ Chickpeas
- ◯ Red kidney beans
- ◯ Black beans
- ◯ White beans
- ◯ Butter beans
- ◯ Borlotti beans
- ◯ Cannellini beans
- ◯ Four-bean mix
- ◯ Adzuki beans
- ◯ Pinto beans
- ◯ Black-eye beans
- ◯ Lentils
- ◯ Split peas

Grains

- ◯ Brown rice
- ◯ Basmati rice (preferably brown)
- ◯ Quinoa
- ◯ Barley
- ◯ Wholemeal or spelt pasta
- ◯ Rice noodles
- ◯ Rolled oats
- ◯ Wholegrain crackers – such as Ryvitas, Vita-Weats
- ◯ Wholegrain wheat, rye or spelt bread – look for a brown bread that is dense with grains and seeds

Vegetables

- ◯ Canned crushed, diced or whole tomatoes
- ◯ Tomato paste
- ◯ Passata
- ◯ Canned corn kernels
- ◯ Minced garlic
- ◯ Minced ginger

Fruits

- ◯ Unsweetened dried cranberries
- ◯ Dates – medjool
- ◯ Sultanas or currents
- ◯ Dried apricots

Fish and seafood

- ◯ Canned tuna – in olive oil, brine or springwater, flavoured
- ◯ Canned salmon – red or pink, plain or flavoured
- ◯ Canned sardines
- ◯ Canned oysters

Nuts and seeds

- ◯ Almonds – whole, slivered and flaked
- ◯ Walnuts
- ◯ Pecans
- ◯ Brazil nuts
- ◯ Cashews
- ◯ Hazelnuts
- ◯ Pine nuts
- ◯ Pistachios
- ◯ Natural nut spreads
- ◯ Peanut butter
- ◯ Almond spread
- ◯ Cashew spread
- ◯ ABC spread (almond, brazil and cashew)
- ◯ Flaxseeds – whole or ground
- ◯ LSA (ground linseeds, sunflower seeds and almond)
- ◯ Pumpkin seeds (pepitas)
- ◯ Sunflower seeds
- ◯ Hemp seeds
- ◯ Sesame seeds
- ◯ Chia seeds
- ◯ Tahini

IN THE FRIDGE

- ◯ Skim or light cow's milk
- ◯ Calcium-fortified plant milk (soy, almond or oat)
- ◯ Plain probiotic yoghurt
- ◯ Cottage cheese
- ◯ Ricotta cheese
- ◯ Creamed cheese
- ◯ Feta cheese
- ◯ Parmesan or pecorino cheese
- ◯ Cheddar or tasty cheese (preferably reduced-fat)
- ◯ Olive oil spread
- ◯ Eggs – preferably free-range and organic

IN THE FREEZER

- ◯ Blueberries
- ◯ Raspberries
- ◯ Strawberries
- ◯ Mixed berries
- ◯ Frozen mango
- ◯ Frozen banana pieces
- ◯ Edamame
- ◯ Broad beans
- ◯ Peas
- ◯ Corn
- ◯ Salmon fillets
- ◯ Chicken breast
- ◯ Chicken tenderloins
- ◯ Prawns

Kitchen tools

Air fryer

This is such a tidy, efficient way to quickly make a meal without needing to add much or any extra fats. I love to cook salmon fillets and sweet potato wedges in the air fryer, but it has so many uses. Most proteins like chicken schnitzel and tofu work really well, as well as any vegetables you can bake – such as cauliflower, brussels sprouts, broccoli, potato with its skin, onion, cherry tomatoes and capsicum. You can use no oil at all, or just add a little spray of extra-virgin olive oil or a light drizzle for flavour.

Nutribullet

(Or another similar brand.) I loathe lugging out the food processor or Thermomix just to make a quick smoothie. I also love making batter such as with my Weekday pancakes (see page 106) in the Nutribullet. You can drink or pour straight from the blender cup so it's minimal washing up and light and compact for easy storage and use.

Chapter 4

Optimising health in peri and beyond

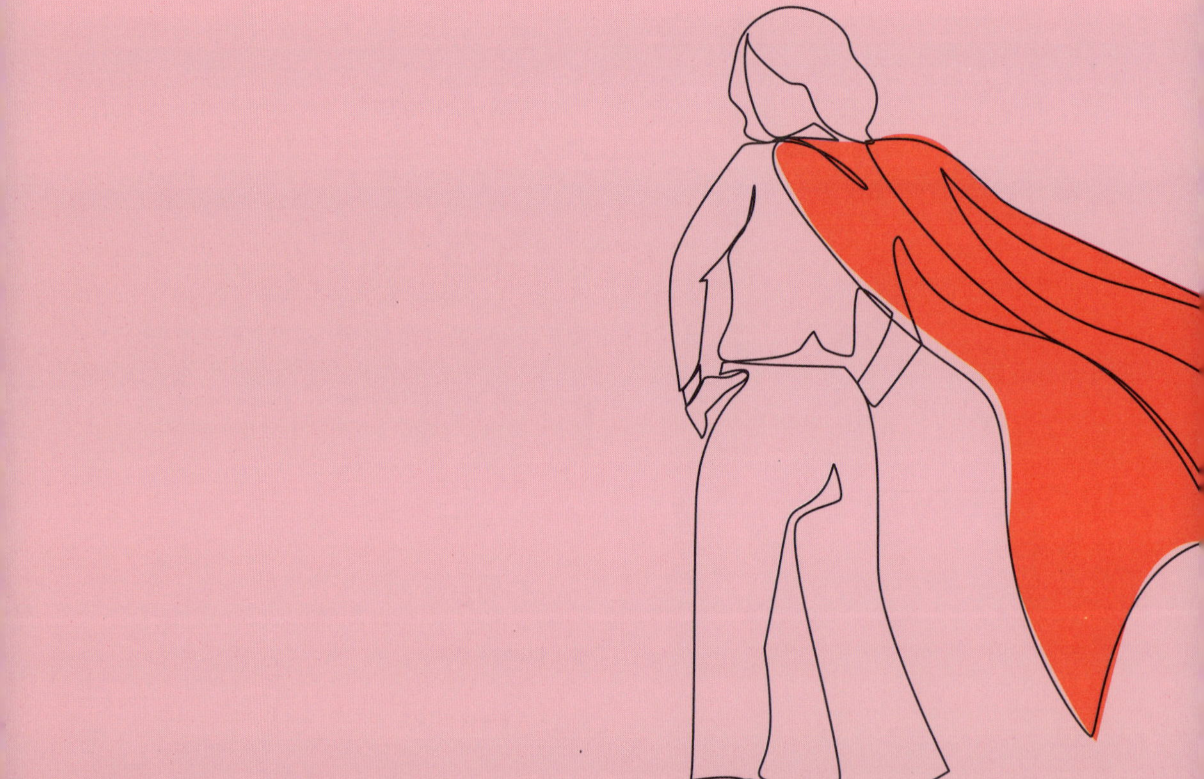

As we explored in Chapter 1, we can experience a range of troublesome symptoms during peri. It is also an optimal time to address other health concerns that can arise now and affect us over the years to come. Being mindful and proactive about these concerns early on can help to prevent issues in the longer term. If you're already into your menopause journey, it's never too late. Just like saving money, the best time to get started is today.

Preserve your bone health

One of the primary concerns during this stage of life is bone health. Women lose around 10 per cent of their bone mass in the first five years of menopause. It's also estimated that one in every two Caucasian women will experience an osteoporotic fracture in their lifetime. Fractures can become a greater risk for peri women, and several factors play into this including genetics, low bone mineral density to begin with, a history of fractures, not using hormone replacement therapy, having three or more chronic illnesses, and smoking.

Osteoporosis is a condition where a loss of bone mass occurs over time, making bones more brittle and susceptible to fracture. As oestrogen levels decline during peri, bone resorption (or bone loss) accelerates, particularly during late peri. The prevalence of osteoporosis in women varies depending on ethnicity. In a US study of 2,000 women, Chinese and Japanese women had the lowest risk, non-Hispanic Caucasians a higher risk and African-American women the highest risk of developing osteoporosis.

Interestingly, having a higher body weight or body mass index (BMI) has been shown to have a protective effect on the bones. Research showed that the rate of bone loss was found to be 35 to 55 per cent higher in women with lower weight compared with women with a higher weight.

There are two types of bone loss that occur as we age: peri bone loss, which is related to the decline in oestrogen, and age-related bone loss, which men also experience. However, the mechanisms of age-related bone loss in men are different than for women throughout their menopause transition. Over our lifetime, our bones undergo a constant remodelling process. As we age, this process shifts from bone formation to more bone loss, leading to a reduced bone mass and increased risk of osteoporosis. If you want to know more about your bone density, ask your doctor about getting a referral for a DEXA scan, which is a type of X-ray that measures bone density.

CALCIUM

Calcium is the nutrient that gives bones their strength and structure, and dairy products are one of the best sources of calcium, so getting enough of it is essential for bone health. Yet a common thing I see at clinic is that women are consuming less and less dairy, usually because they've been told it isn't good for them or that it contains a lot of sugar. But when a woman simply cuts out dairy from her diet without considering where else she's going to get that calcium from, this can become a major issue. I'm seeing women in their thirties being diagnosed with osteopenia (decrease in bone density) as well as osteoporosis.

> Getting enough calcium is essential for bone health.

Another common reason why women cut out dairy is because they experience gut issues and suspect or know that dairy is causing those problems. Dairy is anything made from cow's milk, so yoghurt, cheeses, cream, butter, custard and ice cream are all included. If someone has a dairy allergy, they're allergic to the protein in ALL dairy foods. This is most commonly seen in children, who usually grow out of this allergy.

A lactose intolerance, on the other hand, is an intolerance to lactose (the natural milk sugar) found in cow's milk products. To digest and break down lactose so it gets absorbed into our bloodstream, we need an enzyme called lactase. If we don't have enough of this enzyme in our small bowel, we have a lactase deficiency. Consequently, lactose passes into the large bowel undigested and, usually within a couple of hours, causes a rush of fluid into the bowel triggering an urgent, watery stool that can also cause bloating, gurgling and discomfort on its way down.

Lactose intolerance doesn't have to mean no dairy

While lactose is present in all dairy products, the amount is often negligible, as the chart opposite shows. So, even if you have been diagnosed with lactose intolerance, there is still a full range of dairy products you can enjoy. Milk is the highest in lactose, followed by yoghurt, both of which are readily available in 'lactose-free' varieties in the supermarket. Lactose-free products are regular dairy foods, such as plain cow's milk, that have had the lactase enzyme added to them for easy digestion. Cheese naturally contains very little lactose and can be eaten freely if you have a lactose-intolerance. This means you can continue to eat your dairy foods but also easily meet your calcium needs.

A lactose-intolerance can be formally diagnosed following a gastroscopy procedure; however, informally, the best way to know if you have a lactose intolerance is to drink some milk and see how you feel over the next few hours.

Everyone has a different tolerance level to lactose and this may also change over time depending on the health and environment of your gut and ability to produce lactase. Most people with a lactose intolerance can tolerate the equivalent of half a glass of regular cow's milk at a time. However, I recommend starting with two tablespoons. If you don't seem to have a reaction, build your way up gradually from there to determine your tolerance level.

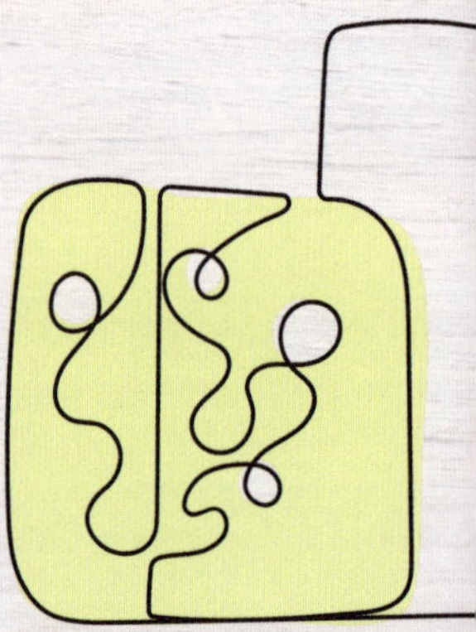

Lactose content of dairy products

INGREDIENT	LACTOSE
Regular milk (1 cup/250 ml)	15.75 g
Yoghurt, natural (200 g)	10 g
Ricotta cheese (120 g)	2.4 g
Ice cream (50 g)	1.65 g
Cream (1 tablespoon)	0.6 g
Cream cheese (22 g)	0.55 g
Camembert (40 g)	0.4 g
Swiss-style cheese (40 g)	0.4 g
Cheddar cheese (40 g)	0.4 g
Parmesan cheese (40 g)	0 g

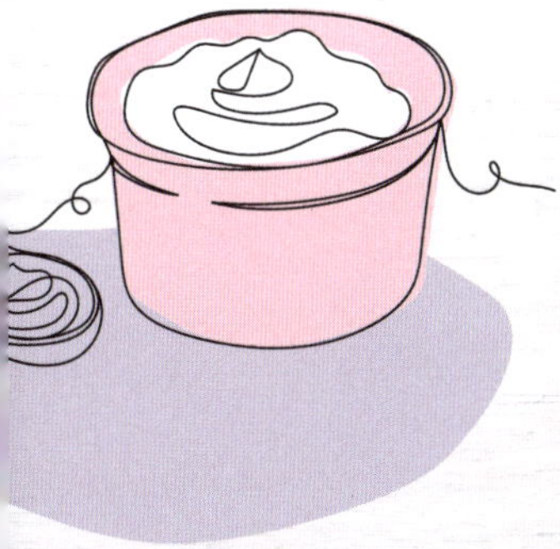

How can I get calcium from dairy without it affecting my cholesterol?

The main nutrient that impacts cholesterol is saturated fat, which is found in animal and dairy products, but there are ways to minimise the saturated fats in dairy. Choose skim or low-fat milk and yoghurt over full-fat varieties. Opt for low-fat cheeses and go for fresh varieties such as ricotta and cottage cheese over harder cheeses. Switching from butter to olive oil and avoiding ice cream, sour cream and cream will also have a huge positive impact on your cholesterol levels.

How much do we need?

Before menopause, women need 1,000 mg of calcium each day – this is the equivalent of three serves of dairy foods. Once we reach menopause, however, we need 1,300 mg per day to balance out the bone losses that occur. This is the equivalent of four servings of dairy per day.

If you can't meet this requirement with diet alone, you may need to take a supplement. Most commercial supplement brands contain up to 600 mg of calcium per dose, which is nearly half the requirement for a menopausal female. It's always best to check with your doctor or dietitian before taking any supplement.

Calcium counter

INGREDIENT	CALCIUM
Skim milk (200 ml)	240 mg
Full-cream milk (200 ml)	236 mg
Plant milk, e.g. soy, oat, almond milk, NOT calcium-fortified (200 ml)	0–26 mg
Plant milk, e.g. soy, oat, almond milk, calcium-fortified (200 ml)	240 mg
Yoghurt, natural (150 g)	207 mg
Yoghurt, flavoured (150 g)	197 mg
Hard cheese e.g. cheddar, parmesan (30 g)	240 mg
Soft cheese e.g. brie, camembert (30 g)	120 mg
Feta, mozzarella cheese (30 g)	135 mg
Cream cheese (30 g)	90 mg
Fresh cheese e.g. ricotta, cottage cheese (200 g)	138 mg
Cream (30 ml)	21 mg
Custard made with milk (120 ml)	111 mg
Vanilla ice cream (100 g)	124 mg
Raw green leafy vegetables e.g. kale, bok choy (50 g)	40 mg
Dried fig (60 g)	96 mg
Canned fish, with the bones e.g. salmon, sardines (60 g)	240 mg
John West Calcium canned tuna (95 g)	800 mg
White beans, cooked (200 g)	132 mg
Chickpeas, cooked/canned (200 g)	99 mg
Almonds (30 g)	75 mg
Tofu set with calcium – check ingredients (120 g)	126 mg

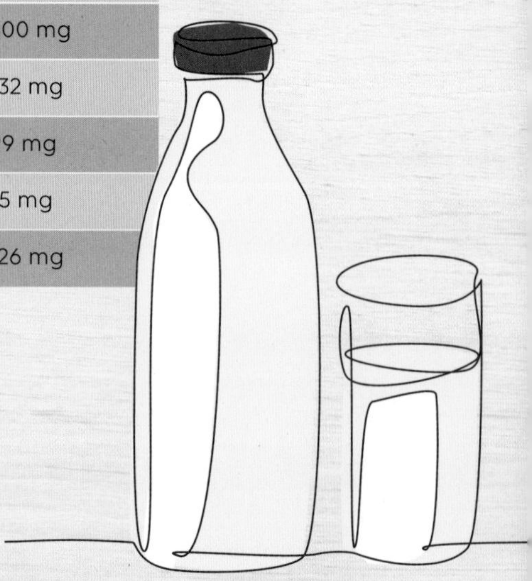

VITAMIN D

Vitamin D is a fat-soluble vitamin. Our main source of it is UVB light from the sun; we store it in the oil on our skin before it gets absorbed into our bloodstream. One of vitamin D's primary functions is to increase calcium absorption from the intestine, as well as supporting the growth and maintenance of our bones.

Given the links between sun exposure and skin cancer, not to mention other damaging effects on the skin, many people are avoiding sun exposure and covering up as much as possible. Unfortunately, this means they miss out on their one major source of vitamin D, and we're seeing greater rates of vitamin D deficiencies with over 30 per cent of adults estimated to have a moderate to severe deficiency.

> One of vitamin D's primary functions is to increase calcium absorption.

How much do we need?

The Cancer Council has great online resources that provide specific recommendations for safe sun exposure in different locations and during different times of the year. However, if you feel this is too unpredictable or want to generally keep out of the sun, you may need to rely on a supplement. Discuss this with your doctor or health care professional.

It's best to begin with a blood test to check your vitamin D levels. If they are low, then you may need to supplement. A standard daily dose would be around 1,000 IU; however if you're severely deficient, you may be recommended an alternative dosing regimen that you can discuss in more detail with your doctor.

What the research says

In addition to the way it supports bone health, supplementing with vitamin D has been shown to have a number of positive effects for women in peri including the following:

- A protective effect against genitourinary symptoms such as vaginal dryness, pain and difficulty with intercourse and urination.
- A protective effect against atrophy (shrinking) of the vaginal wall and subsequent bacterial infections.
- A decrease in 'bad' LDL cholesterol levels and triglyceride levels.
- A lower risk of metabolic syndrome and hyperglycemia (high blood sugar levels).
- Improved glycaemic markers (blood sugar levels), inflammation, bone turnover and body fat measures.

VITAMIN K

Vitamin K is most commonly known for the role it plays in blood clotting, but it's also involved in maintaining bone mineral density and, along with vitamin D, it has been shown to reduce fracture rates. Vitamin K deficiencies are associated with higher risk of bone fractures and lower bone mineral density.

Like vitamin D, vitamin K is fat soluble. It's synthesised by plants, particularly green leafy vegetables, as well as fruits, grains and dairy. Natto, the fermented Japanese food made from soy beans, is especially high in vitamin K. Our body also produces some – it's made in the gut by certain bacteria. Because it's available in so many foods and we also make our own, deficiencies are quite rare.

Due to vitamin K's role in blood clotting, if you're on a blood clotting medication like Warfarin, make sure you discuss this with your doctor before increasing your dietary intake or supplementing.

Vitamin K is involved in maintaining bone mineral density.

THE BEST SOURCES OF VITAMIN K INCLUDE:

- natto (see page 37)
- collard greens
- turnip greens
- spinach
- kale
- broccoli.

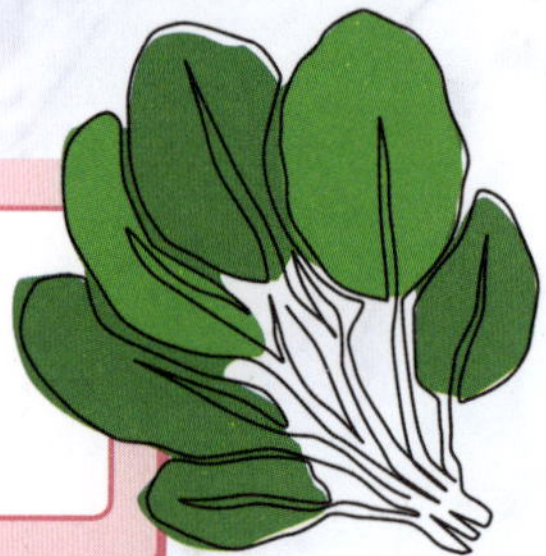

EXERCISE

Exercise is always important, but during peri it becomes even more so for a number of reasons – one of the biggest being bone health. The types of exercise that support bone health during peri are:

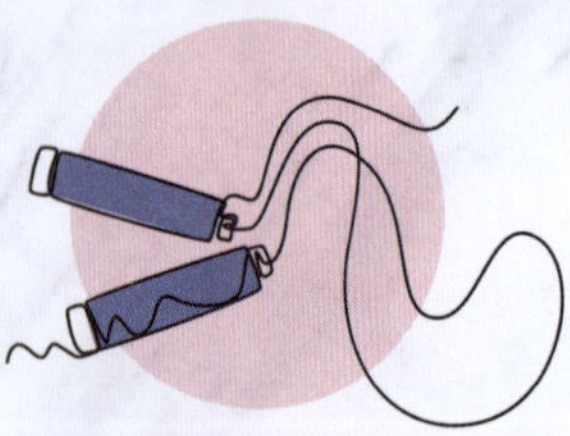

Weight-bearing exercise where your feet hit the ground, such as walking, skipping, running, playing tennis or dancing.

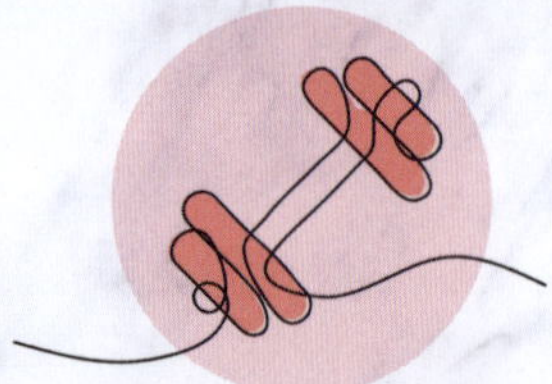

Resistance or strength exercises where you lift free weights, use weight machines, bands, do certain types of yoga or Pilates, or do body-weight exercises like squats.

These exercises put pressure on the bones, which stimulate them to produce more bone tissue. (We'll talk about exercise in greater detail in Chapter 6.) Exercise improves overall fitness, muscle strength and balance, which in turn reduces the likelihood of falls and fractures.

Keep an eye on iron

Two of the major causes of iron deficiency in peri are heavy bleeding and changes in diet. Periods can be erratic during this time and if they are more frequent than usual, we lose more blood and therefore more iron. If we don't correct for this by increasing the iron in our diet or by taking a supplement, our iron levels will continue to drop over time, in some cases leading to iron deficiency anaemia. Many women cut out or reduce the amount of red meat in their diet for a variety of reasons including health, environment and cost. The intentions are good, but since red meat is one of the densest sources of bioavailable (easily absorbed by our body) iron sources, reducing our consumption can lead to deficiency over time if not corrected for with other sources.

SYMPTOMS OF IRON DEFICIENCY INCLUDE:

- fatigue
- weakness
- pale skin
- headache
- feeling light-headed
- feeling dizzy
- shortness of breath
- cold hands and feet
- brittle nails
- cravings to eat unusual items like ice.

If you suspect you may have an iron deficiency, ask your doctor for a blood test to check your levels. If you're unable to build back your iron levels with diet alone, oral supplements are available. In cases where iron is very low, an iron infusion can restore levels very quickly.

How much do we need?

Iron requirements during peri can be confusing because periods can change so much. We might go for months without having one, and then have stretches of time where it comes every couple of weeks. Additionally, our periods can vary from light to heavy, and when blood loss is high, iron requirements are higher, too. For this reason, during peri it's essential to keep a close eye on iron levels by having them checked regularly with your doctor. You may need to respond to changes in your menstrual cycle by increasing your dietary intake and possibly supplementing when your periods are heavy or regular, and backing off on your iron intake when they're not.

Iron requirements vary a lot between premenopause and postmenopause. Generally speaking, women with regular periods need 18 mg of iron per day, and women in menopause only need 8 mg per day. The general dietary recommendation for women with regular periods is three or four 120 g extra-lean red meat meals per week (around 550 g in total).

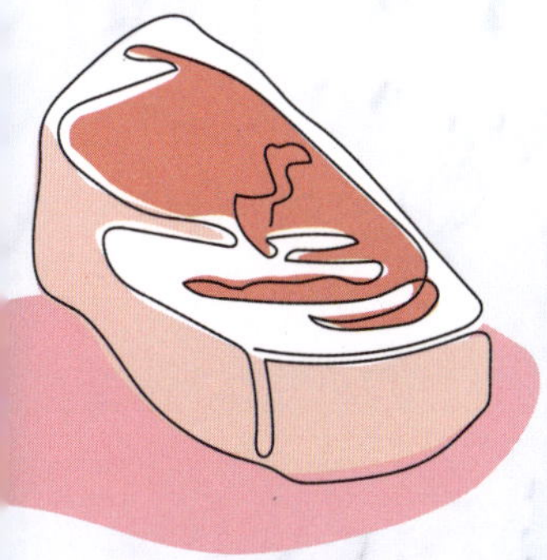

Iron counter

ANIMAL SOURCES	IRON
Chicken liver (100 g)	11 mg
Beef (100 g)	3.5 mg
Kangaroo (100 g)	3.2 mg
Lamb (100 g)	2.5 mg
Salmon (100 g)	1.28 mg
Canned tuna (100 g)	1.07 mg
Lamb brains (100 g)	1.0 mg
Pork (100 g)	0.8 mg
Chicken (100 g)	0.4 mg
Snapper (100 g)	0.3 mg

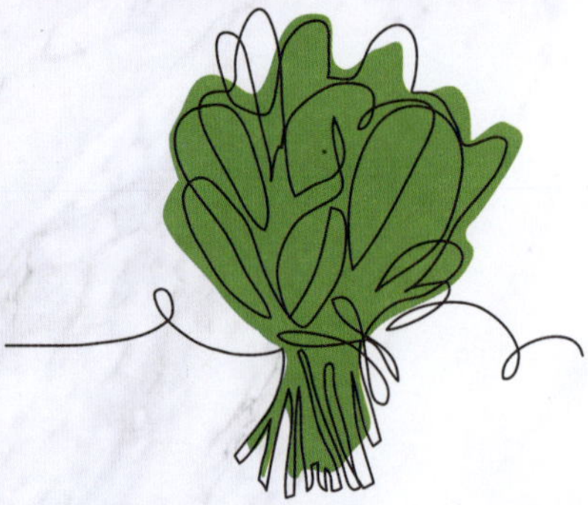

PLANT SOURCES	IRON
Weet-Bix (30 g)	4.2 mg
All Bran (30 g)	3.2 mg
Kidney beans (1 cup)	3.1 mg
Green lentils (1 cup)	3 mg
Tofu (100 g)	2.9 mg
Chickpeas (1 cup)	2.7 mg
Cooked wholemeal pasta (1 cup)	2.3 mg
Cashew nuts (30 g/20 nuts)	1.5 mg
Raw spinach (1 cup)	1.2 mg
Rolled oats (30 g)	1.1 mg
Almonds (30 g)	1.1 mg
Dried apricot (30 g/5 dried apricots)	0.93 mg
Broccoli (1 cup)	0.86 mg
Cooked brown rice (1 cup)	0.7 mg
Wholegrain bread (1 slice)	0.4 mg

Top tip: **Eat foods that contain vitamin C with iron-rich foods to boost absorption:**

- lemon or lime juice
- orange
- broccoli
- capsicum
- tomato and canned tomato and concentrates
- pineapple
- blueberries
- strawberries
- kiwi.

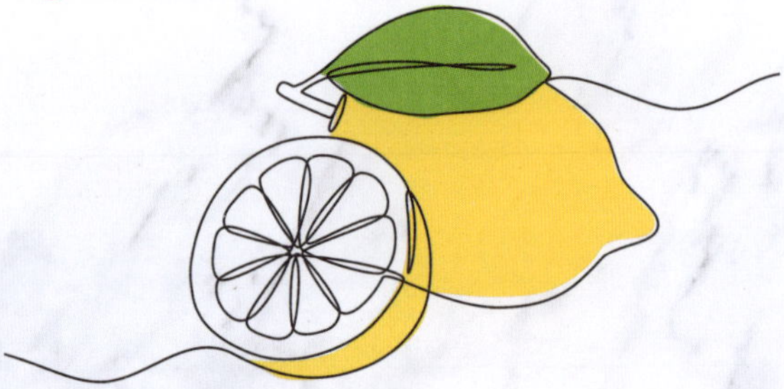

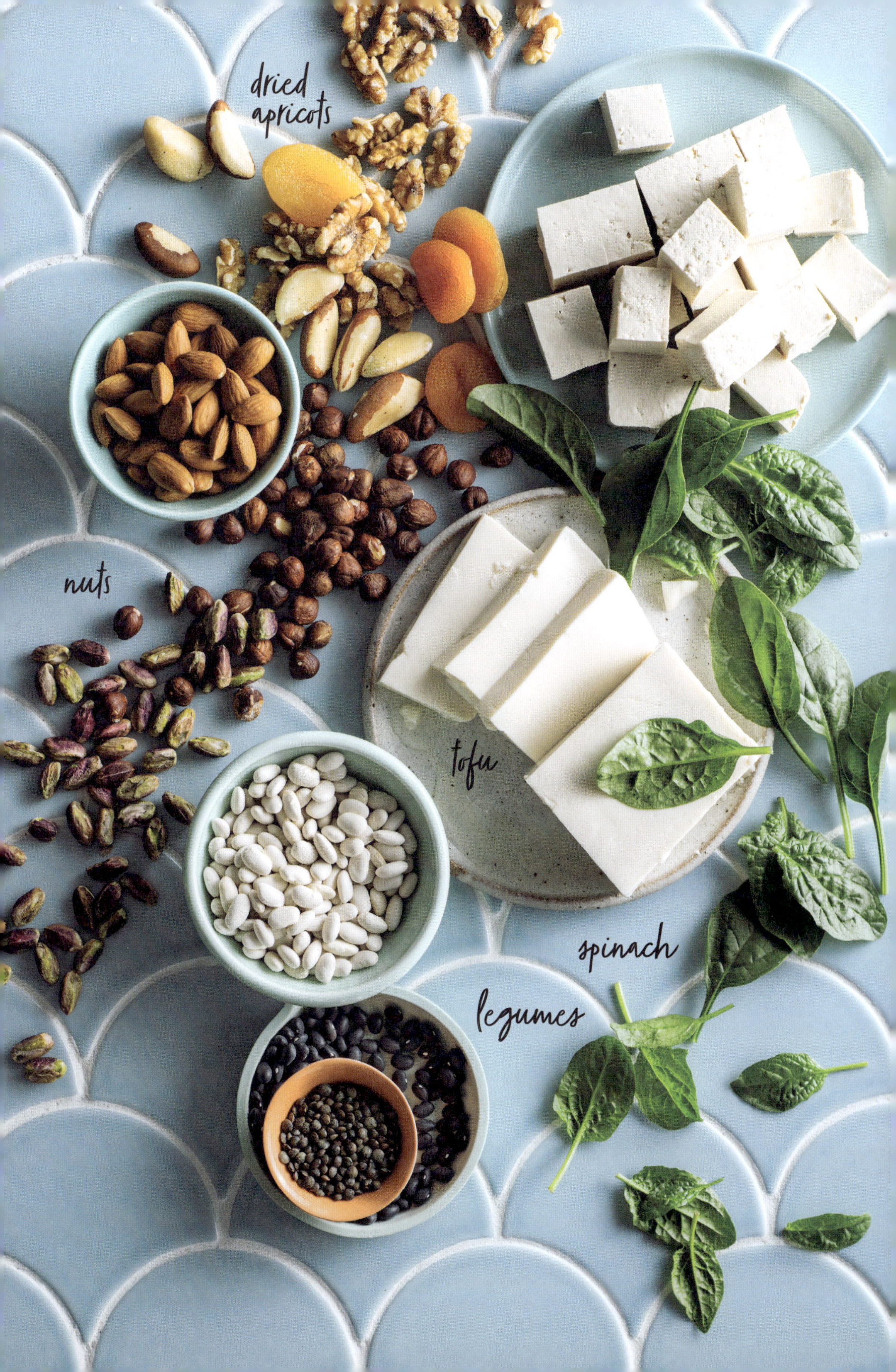
dried apricots
nuts
tofu
spinach
legumes

Other health concerns

BLOOD SUGAR MANAGEMENT

During peri, women can experience severe fluctuations in blood sugar levels after a meal because oestrogen and progesterone affect the way the cells in our muscles and tissue respond to insulin. This means that sugar (or glucose) remains in the bloodstream for longer, and this can mean poor blood sugar control and an increased risk of pre-diabetes and diabetes.

HEART HEALTH

Age is an independent risk factor of cardiovascular disease (CVD). The incidence of CVD in adults aged between 40 and 59 is around 40 per cent, and this increases to 75 per cent for those between the ages of 60 and 79. It's probably no great shock to hear that women are at greater risk of cardiovascular disease than men due to the decline in our oestrogen levels starting in peri and the subsequent risks that come with that, including obesity and diabetes.

Ageing can cause changes in the heart and blood vessels, which means our heart can't beat as fast when we're active, and that makes exercise more challenging. Research also suggests that fat metabolism changes during peri, meaning that our blood fat levels (cholesterol) increase as we get older.

BRAIN HEALTH

Ageing affects our brain in a number of ways. Certain parts of the brain shrink, particularly those involved in learning and complex mental activities. The neurons that are responsible for communication between different parts of the brain may also become less effective. Additionally, the blood flow to the brain may decrease, while inflammation increases, which can affect mental function.

METABOLIC HEALTH

Metabolic syndrome occurs when a person has a cluster of conditions known to be risk factors for type 2 diabetes and CVD. This cluster includes irregular blood sugar and cholesterol levels, increased blood pressure and excess abdominal weight. Excess abdominal weight is a trigger for insulin resistance, and insulin resistance is believed to be the link underpinning the clustering of these risk factors. In the next chapter, we'll discuss how declining oestrogen in peri leads to unwanted abdominal weight gain, which can trigger the conditions that lead to metabolic syndrome.

What to avoid in peri

It's essential that we still enjoy a range of foods and drinks during peri. We don't want to feel restricted and then overdo it; we also don't want to feel as though we're missing out on life's pleasures, or that we're unable to fully enjoy social and special events. But everyone is different when it comes to how well they can tolerate certain foods and drinks at this time. During peri, it becomes more important to be careful about consuming alcohol, caffeine and spicy foods because all three have been linked to hot flushes, and alcohol and caffeine are also known to disrupt sleep.

Other items to not necessarily avoid entirely but to tread carefully with include high added-sugar sweets and desserts, ultra-processed and packaged foods, and fried takeaway foods. These foods contribute a lot of extra calories to the diet with little nutritional value, making weight management difficult. They can also disrupt the gut microbiome and contain unhealthy fats that are not good for our cardiovascular system.

WHAT ABOUT CAFFEINE?

The great news for those of us who love a morning coffee is that caffeine is generally not harmful. In fact, most of the products it's found in are really good for us – freshly ground coffee, teas and dark chocolate. However, how that caffeine affects us and how efficiently we're able to clear it from our system is very individual. You might be able to have a latte before bed and fall sound asleep, while I might drink one weak coffee with breakfast and still be jittery at dusk. This comes down to many factors, and the most dominant one is probably genetics. Caffeine has an average 'half-life' of five hours. This means that half of the caffeine is cleared from our system in five hours, but the rest of it can remain in our system for up to 12 hours in some people. So, if you have a coffee with lunch, that means caffeine may still be in your body until midnight.

Many people are aware that coffee is high in caffeine and by the time most of us reach peri, I think most of us have our caffeine management more or less under control. However, it can build up without realising it. A common scenario I see at clinic is a mum who has a cup of tea when the kids go to bed, along with a couple of rows of dark chocolate. Unfortunately, this combination equates to the same amount of caffeine in a café-style latte and is almost certain to disrupt sleep.

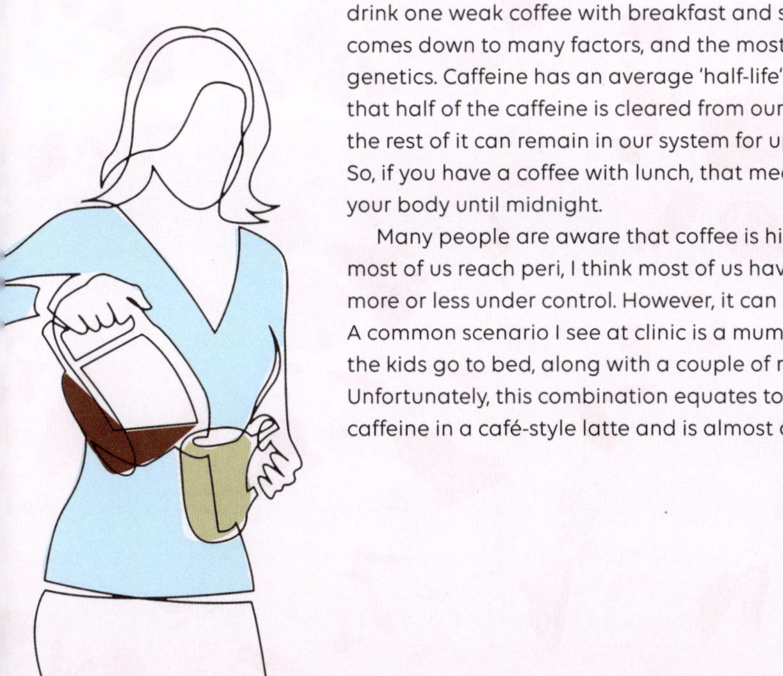

What the research says

- In one study, caffeine was associated with increased vasomotor symptoms (hot flushes and night sweats) in menopausal women.
- Peri women who consume caffeine have fewer problems with mood, memory and concentration, likely because it is known to enhance arousal, mood and attention.

How much do we need?

We don't 'need' any caffeine at all, so whether or not we consume it comes down to choice and personal taste rather than necessity. The US Food and Drug Administration (FDA) recommends no more than 400 mg of caffeine per day. This is an upper limit for all adults, so for peri women who may generally not be able to metabolise caffeine as efficiently, I'd aim to consume less than this recommendation.

Caffeine counter

INGREDIENT	CAFFEINE (MG)
Double espresso or large café coffee	290
Espresso or café coffee (1 shot)	145
Energy drink (250 ml can)	80
Instant coffee (1 teaspoon)	80
Black tea (250 ml cup)	50
Cola (375 ml can)	36
Milk chocolate (50 g bar)	10

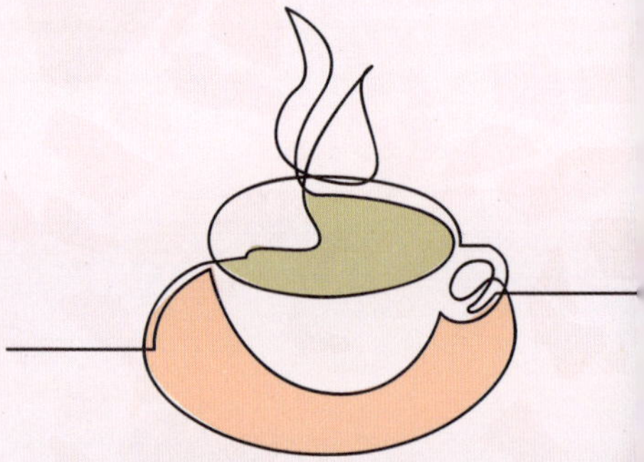

SHOULD I CHOOSE LOW-FAT OR FULL-FAT?

Fats can either be beneficial or harmful for our body. 'Healthy' fats are the unsaturated fats like those found in fish and most plants. Harmful fats are the saturated fats found in many animal foods (meat, dairy, eggs) as well as tropical oils, such as coconut and palm, and processed foods like margarine and deep-fried, takeaway foods. We can handle having some harmful fats in our diet, but we should aim to have mostly beneficial fats. This is one of the reasons that following a plant-focused way of eating can be a great foundation during peri; as animal foods get subbed for ingredients like soy milk, tofu and pulses, our intake of harmful fats decreases.

Fat is the most energy-dense of the macronutrients. Where protein and carbohydrates contain 4 calories per gram, fats contain more than double that at 9 calories per gram. If our goal is to lose weight, it makes sense, then, that restricting our energy (i.e. calorie) intake by following a low-fat diet might be a good way to do this. Even so, it's important not to lower fat intake too much because these fats are essential for hormone production and for slowing digestion, helping us to feel fuller for longer. Beneficial fats like those omega-3 fatty acids we discussed on page 44 are essential nutrients, and especially beneficial during peri.

What the research says

- A low-fat, vegetarian diet has been shown to lower total, low-density lipoprotein (LDL or 'bad') and high-density lipoprotein (HDL or 'good') cholesterol levels in premenopausal women. The women in this study ranged in age from 22 to 48 years old, so although they weren't all women in peri, it's safe to assume a decent portion of the participants were.
- Another trial following women on low-fat diets showed greater loss in body fat at the one-year mark, and again at the three-year mark compared with a control group.

How much do we need?

In general, less than 20–25 per cent of your total energy should come from fats – so if you're eating 1,500 calories a day, that means fat should account for no more than 300–375 of those calories. Ideally, that portion will be from beneficial fats from fish, seafood, nuts, seeds and healthy oils. If you're sticking with animal products, you can reduce your intake of harmful fats by choosing lean and extra-lean cuts of meats as well as skinless poultry, skim or low-fat dairy. Try to avoid those processed fats in fried takeaway foods and baked goods as much as possible by making those occasional.

Look out for hidden fats!

If an ingredient list includes 'vegetable oil' but doesn't specify what that oil is, you can almost guarantee that it's palm oil. Health foods often contain coconut oil, but despite the tsunami in popularity it has enjoyed in recent years, it's best to avoid it, particularly during peri.

Chapter 5

Weight *management* during peri

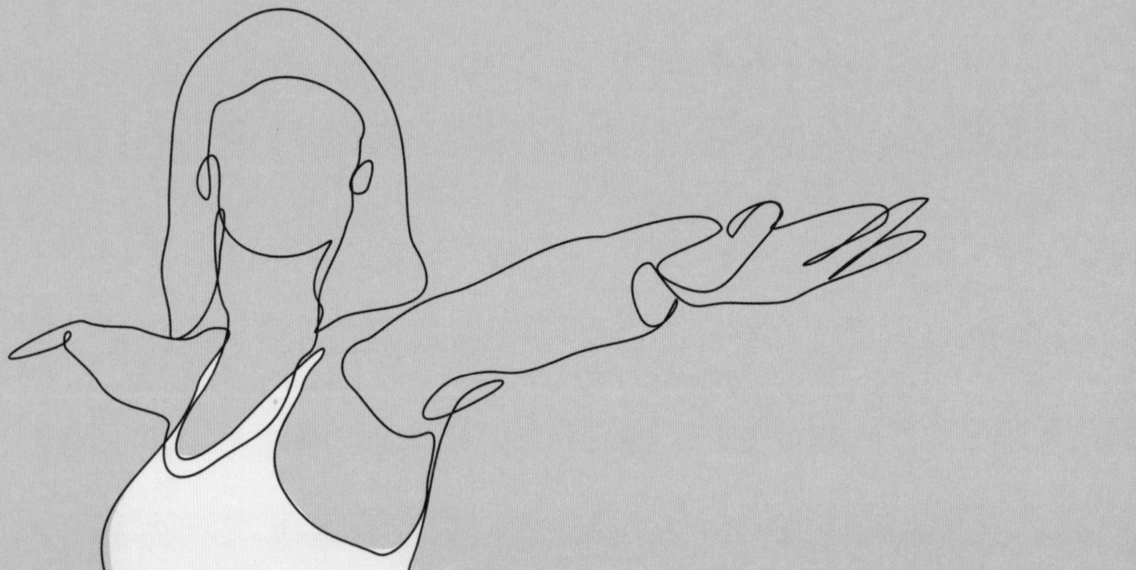

Weight gain is a well-documented part of peri, along with an increase in waist size and changes in body shape. It can be one of the most distressing symptoms of peri for many women.

What makes this weight gain so distressing is that, in most cases, it occurs without any changes to diet or exercise. Interestingly, research shows that the greatest increase in body fat and decrease in lean muscle occurs in perimenopause, not menopause.

As a dietitian who specialises in weight management, this reflects what I see in clinic. Patients aren't doing anything differently – their diet and exercise patterns are the same as they have been for years – yet they are still gaining weight. From my observations, the amount of weight women put on during this time falls between 3 and 10 kg. It can either creep on slowly over years or pile on so quickly that it can be really unsettling.

To add to the worsening metabolic picture, as fat mass increases, muscle and bone mass decline, which causes a very unfavourable change in body composition. This is the mechanism behind the increased risk of many major health issues during peri and beyond.

Along with the physical changes of weight gain during peri come psychological changes. It would be wonderful if we all felt comfortable and happy with our body, but the reality is that most women don't – even before peri. These feelings can be exacerbated by any unwanted changes in body shape, especially if they seem to be out of our control.

Feeling self-conscious about body shape and weight can have negative knock-on effects in several areas of life. Some complaints I hear most commonly from my peri patients are that they used to have a waist but it seems to have disappeared, or they can no longer wear some of their favourite clothes. Because of this, some women don't want to go out or be as social as they were before. Many of my patients feel frustrated and resentful, saying they simply don't deserve to be the shape they are when they are still eating well and exercising regularly.

> The great news is that weight loss during peri leads to improvements in many peri symptoms.

Body changes can also put a strain on a relationship if a woman feels less comfortable being intimate with her partner. She might also feel self-conscious about getting out to exercise. Unfortunately, so many women become less active because of how they feel about themselves, when becoming more active is exactly what helps!

Almost 39 per cent of women enter peri already overweight or obese and then go on to gain on average half a kilogram per year during this time. This weight gain, along with a change in fat distribution that leads to it becoming concentrated around the tummy, increases the severity of menopausal symptoms.

The great news, however, is that weight loss during peri leads to improvements in many peri symptoms, such as hot flushes, mood disorders and sleep disturbances. Though weight loss during peri can be incredibly challenging, it's definitely not impossible.

Once upon a time, weight gain was considered an inevitable part of the ageing process. For many women, certainly in the generation above me, it was thought to be something they'd 'have to' succumb to. Now, however, we know so much more about the peri journey and several theories about why we gain weight have emerged. Some of them are being formally tested right now, and this is exciting because if we can learn exactly why peri women gain weight, we may be able to correct for these biochemical changes and either help to slow down or stop peri weight gain. So, I hear you asking, what are the bodily mechanisms behind these theories?

1 The protein leverage effect

In peri, intermittent low oestrogen levels lead to accelerated protein (lean muscle) breakdown in the body. This triggers an increased appetite as the body tries to access more protein. The theory is that if we don't add more protein to our diet to meet our increased needs, our body will drive up our hunger hormones, so we eat more in an effort to access more protein. This means we end up eating more total energy or calories, and when we consume more energy than our body needs, it leads to weight gain.

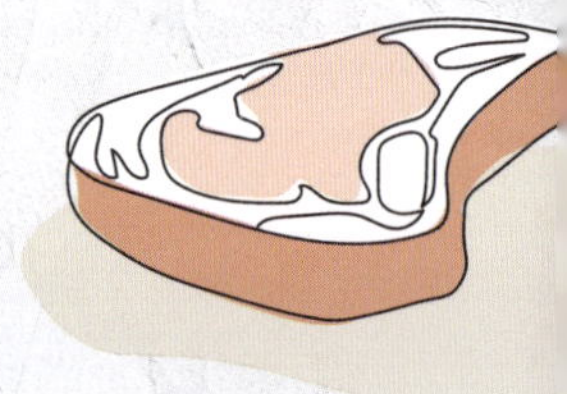

However, if we actively include more protein in our diet, the total amount of energy or calories we eat overall ends up being less, so weight management becomes easier. Supporting this theory is the interesting research showing that this enhanced protein breakdown that happens in peri is completely reversible with oestrogen hormone replacement therapy (HRT).

2 Reduced energy needs

Skeletal muscle is the biggest organ in the body, making up around 45 to 55 per cent of our body mass. It's a major determinant of our basal metabolic rate, i.e. the energy our body uses at rest. Skeletal muscle needs and uses a lot of fuel. As we lose lean muscle tissue during peri, our basal metabolic rate (BMR) reduces. This means that the amount of energy we were once able to burn while resting is reduced. If we keep eating the same amount of food, the energy intake that used to keep our weight stable will now cause weight gain.

3 Change to appetite

Lowered oestrogen and increased androgen levels (male hormones) create a hormone imbalance that disrupts our hunger and satiety signals. This is because oestrogen stops hunger signals, preventing us from overeating. Oestrogen decline is believed to cause more intense hunger signals, which increases food intake and can lead to weight gain.

4 Mood disturbances and life circumstances

Peri and menopausal women commonly report having a negative emotional state. This isn't a direct physiological cause of weight gain; women in their forties often have a lot going on! Peri may be causing mood disturbances, irritability, rage, frustrations and fluctuations in mood. Peri women commonly feel distressed by their body changing and are TIRED from disrupted and disturbed sleep.

Many women use food as a tool to manage these emotional changes, which leads to episodes of emotional eating, driving up their total energy intake and leading to weight gain. Women in peri often have relatively young families; they may also be working, running a household, managing a relationship, looking after ageing parents, balancing financial concerns and many other burdens. This can create a lot of stress, which leads many women to drink alcohol as a way of winding down after a long and difficult day and use food as a source of comfort or distraction. These two things alone can add a lot of extra energy or calories to the diet, leading to weight gain.

5 Reduced activity

As women age, there is a progressive reduction in their physical activity levels. This may be due to sedentary jobs and busy lives that leave them with limited time to exercise. It may also be because of the decline in muscle strength, which limits their ability to not only do daily activities but also exercise to any great capacity. Additionally, the cost of living is high, and so many women experience financial difficulty that makes spending on gyms, personal trainers, exercise studios and classes a luxury that can't be maintained.

RISKS ASSOCIATED WITH PERI WEIGHT GAIN

In addition to liver disease and sleep apnoea, which are both associated with higher weight, several other conditions are linked to weight gain.

Cardiovascular disease

Higher fat mass, particularly abdominal fat, increases cardiovascular risk factors, such as hypertension (high blood pressure), high cholesterol and insulin resistance.

Inflammation

Studies have shown an association between the loss of oestrogen and an increase in the size of fat cells. This fat accumulation tends to focus on the abdominal area and acts as metabolically active tissue, which produces inflammatory cells. This type of inflammation is linked with many chronic diseases, including type 2 diabetes.

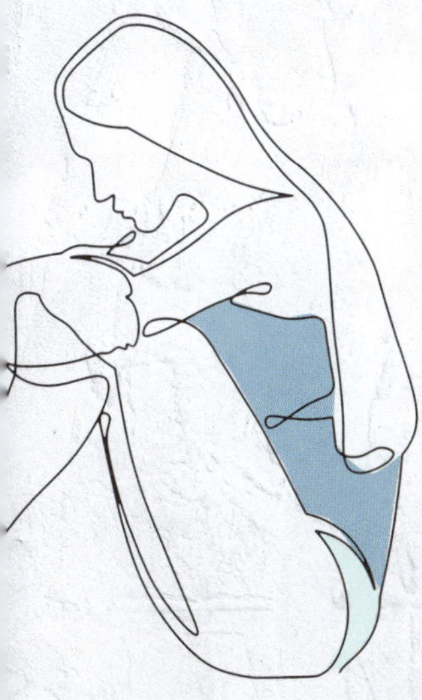

Joint pain and degeneration

Joint pain, particularly in weight-bearing joints like the knees, hips and feet, can become a problem for women in peri, along with back pain, which is often exacerbated by abdominal weight gain and a heavier bust.

Cancer

Higher weight or BMI is associated with breast, endometrium and uterine cancers because of the long-term continuous exposure to oestrogen, which is produced by adipose or fat tissue.

Common strategies for weight management in peri

Exactly how weight management looks will be a little different for each of us; it requires us to take a personal approach to find what works for our lifestyle and body. That said, now that we know more about why weight gain is such an issue in peri, there's a broad prescriptive foundation we can lean on, then adjust to suit us.

You may be going into peri at a weight you feel comfortable with. If so, 'managing' your weight will be about maintaining that current weight. If you've gained a little extra weight already, your goal might be to slow any future weight gain down. If you've been overweight for some time, your focus might be on preventing future weight gain and even trying to lose some weight.

Ultimately, the primary goal should be to stop (or slow) muscle loss, but to achieve weight loss, you'll need to create an energy deficit, and there are two ways to go about achieving this:

1. **Calculate your energy (calorie) needs, then work out what will create an energy deficit for weight loss while still meeting your nutritional requirements, and then track your food intake to stay within those numbers.**

2. **Make adjustments to your current diet or base your food intake on a particular dietary strategy (such as the ones discussed in Chapter 2).**

Whichever way feels the most achievable and sustainable for you is likely to be the best option. To achieve any desired weight loss and maintain that loss forever, you have to choose something you'll be able to stick to pretty easily for a long time. Consistency is the key. Finding a regime that works for you and being consistent with it for as long as it is successful will be the key to your success.

> Finding a regime that works for you and being consistent with it will be the key to your success.

When a patient wants to lose weight, I start by doing a deep dive into their eating habits and routines. My goal is to uncover whatever is causing their weight gain in the first place. Often, the culprits are lack of physical activity, too much snacking, big portions and eating late at night. In addition to finding out the causes, I'll also try to identify any major barriers to their weight loss, e.g. lack of time, lack of confidence in the kitchen, resistance to starting 'yet another diet'.

From there, we can work together to determine which approach will be the most sustainable and achievable based on their current habits and lifestyle. Introducing an energy deficit can either be done by reducing calories in small amounts daily, or intermittently, in larger amounts.

Traditional calorie-controlled diet

This approach involves slightly restricting intake by roughly 500 calories on a daily basis. For example, if your daily energy requirement to keep your weight stable is 2,000 calories, you'd reduce your intake to 1,500 calories a day to lose weight. This approach can be a great option if you like routine and eat in a similar way every day, although it can feel like you're restricting yourself. To avoid feeling that you're having to count every calorie, my top tip is to cut those 500 calories by making minor tweaks such as the following:

- Swap from sugary drinks like soda, cordial and fruit juices to water, unsweetened teas and no-added-sugar drinks.
- Adjust portion sizes so you're eating larger volumes of lower-energy foods such as salad and veggies, fruits and lean proteins, and smaller volumes of more energy-dense foods such as pasta, rice and energy or calorie-dense foods like oils.
- Trim snacks from your routine and make sure you're only eating when you're hungry. So many of our extra calories come from mindless munching.

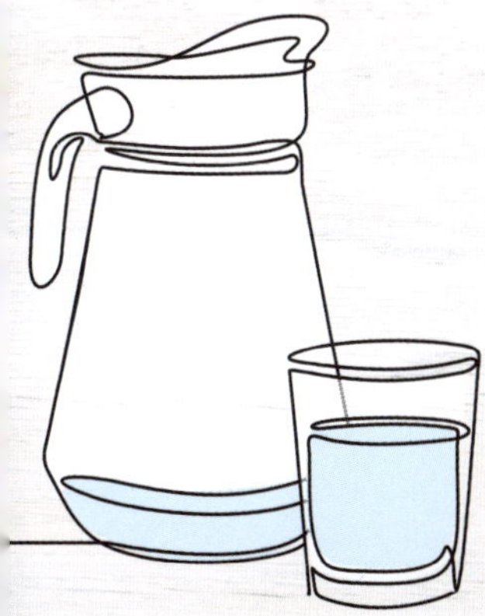

Calorie-counting isn't for everyone. It tends to suit people who are quite scientific and objective about what they eat, not to mention diligent about recording everything they put into their mouth. There are a number of good apps, such as My Fitness Pal, to help you track calories. Please note, though, that they come with a high rate of error, both from discrepancies in calculating energy content of foods but also in individual food recall and logging accuracies. Despite this, it can be a great short-term tool to get a guide of the energy value of common foods and their quantities and keep within an energy target.

Keeping a food diary

This is a less formal way to track your calorie intake. Instead of counting the calories, you simply log what you're eating. Even doing this for just a few days can be incredibly enlightening and eye-opening, especially if you're not entirely sure what you eat most days. When I ask my patients what they ate today or yesterday, most can't recall what they had for lunch, or how many mouthfuls of their kids' leftovers they ate, not to mention the choccy their co-worker gave them or the mouthfuls of dinner they ate while prepping and cooking. This isn't surprising since so much of what we consume happens mindlessly or is so involuntary and routine that it's difficult to remember. Keeping a food diary keeps you accountable to every mouthful, and this can highlight where you're doing great work nutritionally, and where there may be gaps or areas of excess eating that need work.

Intermittent fasting

Intermittent fasting has been shown time and again to be a safe and effective weight-loss tool, although as with any strategies for weight loss, it's not for everyone. There are a number of styles of intermittent fasting, but the two most popular fasting regimes for perimenopausal women – not to mention the two most comprehensively studied – are 16:8 and 5:2. These are the styles of intermittent fasting that I consider safest for women in peri and beyond.

16:8 intermittent fasting

This method of intermittent fasting is a daily routine where you extend your overnight fast by fasting for 16 hours each day and narrowing your eating window to 8 hours. So for example, if you normally finish eating and drinking by 7 pm, count back by 8 hours and you would break your fast at 11 am. For most people, simply achieving a 12-hour overnight fast is a great starting point. Have a think about what time you usually have your meals and whether holding off on breakfast, or having dinner earlier would work for your lifestyle. This strategy is brilliant for women who are naturally not that hungry as soon as they wake up or later in the evening and can comfortably fast over that period. It's particularly useful for women who generally have a very long eating day, for example a 7 am breakfast and 8 pm dinner, and therefore have more time to eat over the course of a day. I also love it for women who tend to nibble late at night as the time restrictions draw boundaries around eating times, and this simple change can trim lots of excess energy (calories) without adding complicated rules and restrictions.

5:2 intermittent fasting

This method of fasting is slightly different in that you eat 'normally' five days of the week and eat around a quarter of your daily energy needs (around 500 calories for a female) on two non-consecutive low-calorie fasting days, e.g. Monday and Thursday. This type of fasting can be great for busy women who aren't particularly hungry on days they're rushing around, and for women who are happy to put in two hard days a week in order to enjoy the freedom to eat as they normally do the rest of the week. I recommend this regime to a lot of my peri and menopausal patients when their excess weight is stubborn and hard to shift. I find that it gives them a great metabolic boost that can really help to kick-start their weight loss.

> 5:2 can really help to kick-start weight loss.

High-protein, lower-carbohydrate way of eating

This method is very relevant to women in peri because we have higher protein needs. Additionally, we're likely to need less fuel from carbohydrates as we're generally less active than we were in previous decades. Protein is filling and satisfying, so we're likely to feel fuller for longer after a high-protein meal and need less to eat between meals. This alone can reduce overall energy intake, which is essential for weight loss. Revisit page 32 to calculate how much protein you need each day and where you can get it from in your diet. As for carbohydrates, there are a few approaches you can take to reduce your intake:

- Make carbs a lower percentage (roughly 30–40 per cent) of your total energy intake. This is useful if you're tracking your energy or calorie intake and there are many apps that can break this down for you.
- Reduce carbs at each meal. This can be done in a few different ways:

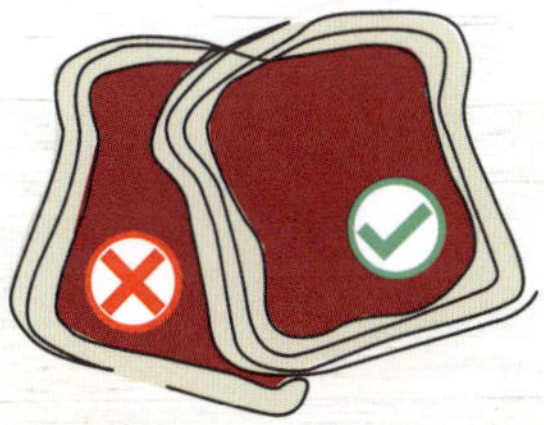

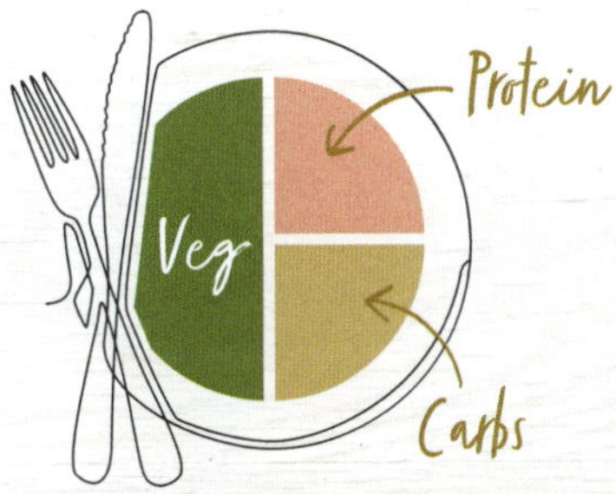

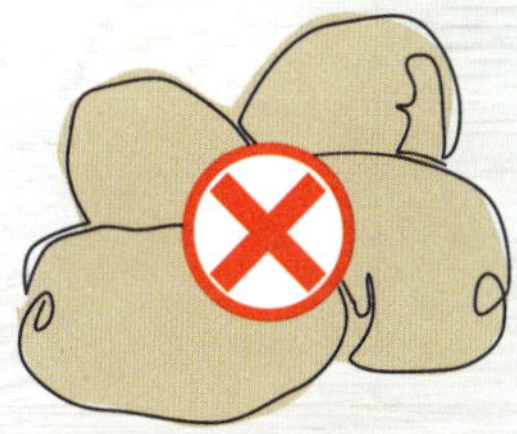

HALVE YOUR CARBS

If you usually eat two pieces of toast with your morning eggs, reduce this to one. If you usually eat 2 cups cooked rice with dinner, reduce this to 1 cup.

FOLLOW THE PLATE MODEL

I use this a lot as a visual aid to avoid weighing and measuring foods, particularly for lunch and dinner. For peri women, the 'half, quarter, quarter' model is ideal. This is HALF the plate non-starchy veggies and salad, a QUARTER of the plate lean protein, and a QUARTER cooked carbohydrates (which usually works out to be around ½–1 cup cooked grains or starchy vegetables, or 1 medium potato).

SKIP NIGHT FUEL

We need carbohydrate fuel during the day – we don't necessarily need it at night. A popular strategy to reduce total carbs and prevent an evening blood sugar and insulin spike is to enjoy carbs throughout the day, then skip the main carb portion with your dinner, such as the potato or the rice, and focus just on protein and veggies. So, for example, you may just have chicken and salad or fish and non-starchy vegetables.

The tidy-up

This is the approach I most commonly take with patients, especially when they already have a healthy foundation diet. In these cases, their weight struggles are usually related to extra foods and drinks that have crept into their routine over time. Rather than overhaul everything, we simply identify where those high-energy foods and drinks have snuck in. Perhaps you've fallen into the habit of having dessert every night or sharing a bottle of wine with your partner after work. Or maybe you mindlessly nibble on the kids' leftover meals and snacks after finishing your own.

Our aim is to keep the foundational foods from the five key food groups – lean proteins, fruit, veggies, dairy and grains – because that's where our body gets the nutrients it needs. Those discretionary or extra foods our body doesn't need get 'tidied' up and reduced or removed. Remember a little treat every now and then is absolutely fine, and even encouraged, so that you don't feel too restricted. It's the daily treats we consume mindlessly out of habit that need trimming. This type of 'tidy up' is easy and can save you hundreds (maybe even thousands) of excess calories each day.

> The 'tidy-up' is easy and can save you hundreds (maybe even thousands) of excess calories every day.

Plant-focused eating

This approach means you're likely to consume less energy purely because plant foods are high in fibre and quite filling, so we tend to eat less of them. Upping your intake of plants is a great strategy to begin with if the quality of your diet is currently poor (i.e. lots of processed foods) and you aren't consuming many plant foods such as fresh vegetables, fruits, wholegrains, nuts, seeds and legumes.

DEALING WITH A WEIGHT PLATEAU:

This happens because our body adapts to changes in our activity and energy intake, so weight loss will slow or come to a stop.

The best strategy around a weight plateau is to MIX IT UP! Change up your diet patterns and your meal choices, and mix up your exercise so you've got some good variety.

You don't have to stick religiously to any one of these eating strategies. It may be that combining one or two of them works better for you. For example, you might decide to try 5:2 intermittent fasting and use a calorie-counting app on your two fasting days to track those 500 calories. Alternatively, you might decide to 'tidy up' your diet by keeping a food diary so you can get clarity about where unnecessary calories are coming from.

But ladies, whichever method you settle on, I implore you to approach your weight management with love and kindness towards yourself. Not only do you deeply deserve to treat yourself with compassion, but research has shown that women with a higher self-esteem, health perception and lower stress and hunger lose more weight over a six-month period when following a calorie-restricted diet.

WEIGHT-LOSS MEDICATIONS

It would be remiss of me not to mention weight-loss medications given how incredibly popular they've become and how regularly they are prescribed by medical professionals. There are many weight-loss medicines but the three most common ones that I see at this current time being prescribed are Ozempic, Saxenda and Duromine (there are more set to blast onto the market soon).

Given how challenging losing and maintaining a stable weight can be for perimenopausal and menopausal women, and how out of control, helpless and desperate it can make them feel, it's not surprising to learn that menopausal women are one of the biggest demographics using these medicines, particularly Ozempic. Since weight gain during peri increases the risk of pre-diabetes, type 2 diabetes and cardiovascular disease, not to mention the frequency of hot flushes and night sweats, the task of weight management can become a little more urgent for women in this group. In addition to the benefits these medications offer, they also come with a long list of side-effects. The most common ones are gastrointestinal, such as nausea and diarrhoea, but they can also impact mood and sleep. There is the risk of much more serious side-effects like thyroid cancers too. Since these drugs have only been available for a relatively short period of time, we've yet to learn what the effects of longer-term use may be.

Ozempic

Ozempic is taken as a weekly self-administered injection, starting with the lowest dose and building up over time, as needed. Its active ingredient, semaglutide, works by mimicking the natural hormone GLP-1 that is released into the gut in response to eating, inducing a feeling of fullness that causes you to eat less and lose weight. Originally, Ozempic was developed for the treatment of uncontrolled type 2 diabetes because it supports the production of insulin. However, it has surged in popularity because of its weight-loss effects. Research has shown an average weight loss of 15 per cent of body weight over two years in overweight and obese women.

Saxenda

Like Ozempic, Saxenda is also injected – but daily rather than weekly – and is also a GLP-1 receptor agonist. It works in the brain to decrease appetite, and thereby reduce food intake, leading to weight loss. Research subjects taking Saxenda over the course of a year lost 5–10 per cent of their body weight.

Duromine

Duromine is a once-a-day tablet that's popular because it's more cost-effective and generally more readily available than the injectable drugs. The active ingredient is phentermine, which is in a class of medications called anorectics. It works on the brain to decrease appetite, and research has shown a greater than 5 per cent body weight loss over four months of taking Duromine.

As a dietitian, my greatest concern with these drugs is weight regain, because as soon as you stop taking these medications, the appetite-suppressing effects stop and weight regain becomes virtually inevitable. One study showed that one year after stopping Ozempic, participants had regained two-thirds of the weight they had lost and my observation in clinic is that most people regain all of the weight they lose – and gain a little extra – within around two years after stopping the medication. This means many people end up heavier than when they started.

Weight-loss medications are a support tool and a complementary therapy to diet, exercise and lifestyle practices. The doctors I work with routinely refer patients prescribed weight-loss medications to me because there's an art to losing weight in an efficient way while taking them. If you do choose to take weight-loss medications, I urge you to see the time that you're on them as an opportunity to set some great healthy habits in stone that you can maintain for life. This way, when you come off the medication, you'll be in the best position to maintain any weight loss you've achieved and enjoy the long-term health benefits that brings.

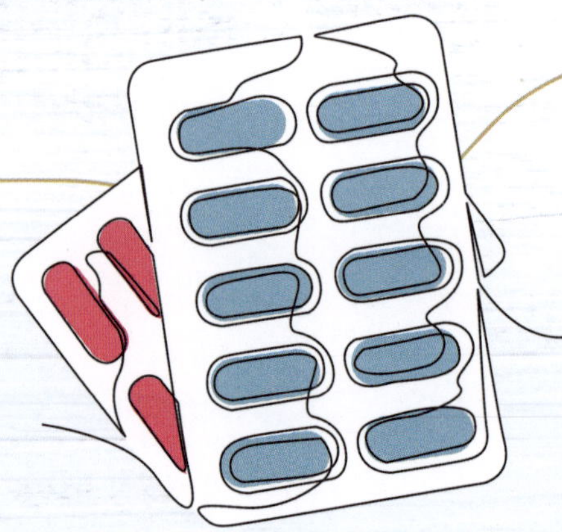

Calculating energy needs for weight loss

If weight loss is a goal of yours, then mapping out how to get there by calculating how many calories you should be aiming at is often the first step on that journey.

Step 1	Step 2	Step 3
Determine your ideal weight	Calculate daily energy (calories) needs	Calculate the energy (calorie) deficit you need for weight loss

Step 1

DETERMINE YOUR IDEAL WEIGHT

Naturally, this step is only relevant if weight loss is a goal of yours. There are two main ways I determine someone's ideal weight:

1. Use your set point body weight
When using this method, I make an informed decision based on a few factors, but even then, the target weight we set may change if the patient discovers they feel comfortable at a weight that's a little higher than the one they had in mind. Alternatively, we might revise this number down slightly if they sail through to this target easily and are keen to continue on their weight-loss journey. A 'set point' is believed to be a weight our body can maintain happily without too much effort. It also tends to be the weight we can get down to fairly easily when following a mild-energy restricted diet. Past that, however, losing more weight can take major effort and be hard to maintain long term. To come up with this number, I usually ask my patient for a sensible and realistic weight they felt comfortable with, or for the weight they tend to return to consistently after weight loss or weight regain attempts. For example, think back to times you may have attempted weight loss. Perhaps you went from 75 kg to 65 kg, but after some time, your weight slowly crept back to 72 kg and you were able to stay there quite comfortably for a long time. This is most likely to be your comfortable set point body weight and perhaps 65 kg is an unrealistic long-term weight goal.

2. Use your body mass index (BMI)
BMI is a clinical calculation used to determine a person's ideal weight for their height. However, since it's used for all adults and both genders, and doesn't take factors such as body composition into consideration, I see it as a very loose guide and mostly use it to get a ballpark 'ideal' weight.

You can calculate your BMI quickly using an online calculator like this one: https://www.gethealthynsw.com.au/healthier-you/tools-and-calculators/bmi-calculator/

What does your BMI indicate?

BMI (ADULTS)	CLASSIFICATION
Less than 18.5	Underweight
18.5 to 24.9	Healthy weight
25 to 29.9	Overweight but not obese
30 to 34.9	Obese class I
35 to 39.9	Obese class II
40 or more	Obese class III

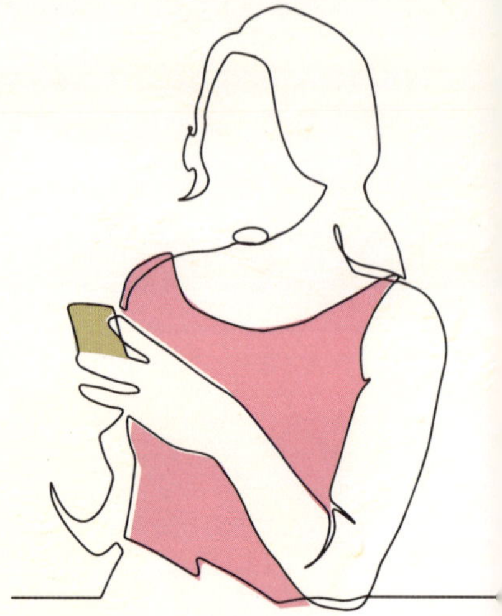

Step 2 CALCULATE YOUR DAILY ENERGY (CALORIC) NEEDS

The formula for calculating your daily energy needs, also known as estimated energy requirements (EER), is quite complex, so rather than do it on paper, I'm going to direct you to an online calculator where you can simply plug in your details and get that number.

Firstly, the equation will figure out your basal metabolic rate (BMR), which is the amount of energy your body needs at rest to keep your organs functioning. This includes your gender, age, weight and height.

Next, it will ask for your activity level based on your job. If you are desk-bound all day, you can choose the first option 'very sedentary.' If, however, you are desk-bound but also exercise vigorously for 30–60 minutes four or five days a week, you'll want to choose the activity the next level up. The number this calculator gives you is the amount of energy you need to maintain your weight. Remember, though, these are crude calculations, and should be used as a guide only.

Calculator:

https://www.eatforhealth.gov.au/nutrition-calculators/daily-energy-requirements-calculator#results

Once you have this number, you can use that to work out the reduced amount of calories you need for weight loss.

Seek advice

If you have medical considerations that may affect your energy use, such as chronic kidney disease or an eating disorder, please seek the advice of your doctor and accredited practising dietitian first.

Step 3 CALCULATE THE ENERGY (CALORIE) DEFICIT YOU NEED FOR WEIGHT LOSS

Again, this can be done in a few ways:

1. Base it on your ideal weight

If you want to lose weight, plug your ideal weight into the EER calculator above. By doing this you'll find out what the total energy intake for that smaller body is.

I urge you not to make this 'ideal' number too low. Many of my perimenopausal patients strive to be the same weight they were at their wedding 20 years ago, or the weight they once got down to when they went on a crash diet in the past, even though they were unable to maintain it.

I will mention, though, that this method of calculation will give you the lowest energy deficit number. You may find, especially if you only have a small amount of weight to lose (e.g. less than 5 kg), that the deficit this calculation gives you is not significant enough to achieve a considerable weight loss.

2. Reduce your EER by 20 per cent

This method will provide a moderate energy deficit. Once you know what your daily energy requirements or needs are for your current weight, calculate what 20 per cent of that is, and then reduce that from your daily total. For example, if your EER is 1,800 calories per day, 20 per cent of that is 360 calories. Deduct that from your total for the day and your calorie target for weight loss would be 1,440 calories per day.

3. Shave off 500 calories

This is a simple and fairly standard tactic that gets used a lot for weight loss. It's most likely to give you the greatest energy deficit. It can be quite a stretch for some people, though, and if your EER is already reasonably low you may find cutting 500 calories out every day too much. I recommend not going below 1,200 calories per day as a weight-loss target.

Patient example

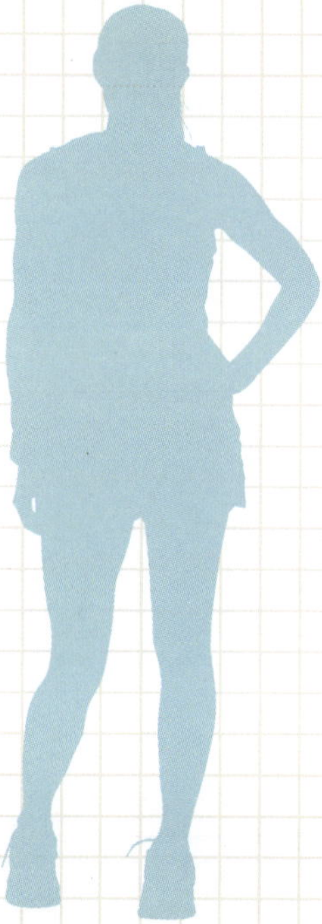

Name: Jenny

Age: 48

Height: 1.62 cm

Current weight: 74 kg

Ideal weight: 65 kg

This was Jenny's happy weight throughout most of her adult life that she was able to maintain quite easily before COVID lockdowns when she gained nearly 10 kg. She is now in peri and finding it incredibly difficult to lose weight.

When I calculated Jenny's BMI based on this 'ideal' weight to see if it was a realistic clinical target, it sat within the normal BMI range for someone of Jenny's height and age. Therefore, it was an ideal weight loss goal.

CURRENT BMI

= 28

BMI AT JENNY'S IDEAL WEIGHT

= 65 (1.62 x 1.62)

= 24.8

We plugged Jenny's information into the EER calculator. She's a teacher and is moderately active in her job, and also goes for the occasional walk and Pilates class when she has time. I put her activity level at 1.4 'sedentary work and no strenuous leisure activity'. To maintain her current weight, Jenny needed:

2,028 calories (or multiply by 4.18 for kilojoules = 8,476 kJ)

For weight loss, I reduced this by 20 per cent:
1,622 calories (6,781.6 kJ)

> Remember, weight loss is always more successful and sustainable when it is not too extreme or too hard.

Our food choices are governed by so many factors including the weather, our habits and our finances. But during peri, it's common for women to feel very fatigued and moody due to the peri hormone fluctuations, and food and alcohol may begin to be a comfort or reward after a hard day. For this reason, it's important to keep in mind that females are generally more vulnerable to dramatic dietary change and energy intake. When a female becomes too lean, or follows a diet that's too limited, they might stop having their period (known as amenorrhea). For this reason, and particularly due to the (often severe) fluctuations in hormones during peri, it's really important that we approach weight management in a gentle and sustainable way.

It's important to be kind to ourselves as this can be a really difficult time for many women. If weight loss is too extreme, eventually we will get diet fatigue and our hunger hormones will crank up, making us hungrier and leading us to regain any weight we've lost. Remember, weight loss is always more successful and sustainable when it is not too extreme or too hard.

HOW FAST SHOULD I EXPECT TO LOSE WEIGHT?

If you consider that our body is programmed to store fat as a way of protecting ourselves from times of limited access to food, it's easier to understand why weight loss is so difficult: you're effectively working against your body's natural processes. And during peri, trying to override those processes becomes considerably harder.

For many women, maintaining their current weight and preventing future weight gain is a win in itself. Others, though, will feel uncomfortable when carrying more weight than they're used to and unable to wear their favourite clothes, and be keen to lose weight quickly. As a general rule however, around 0.5–1 kg a week is considered to be a healthy and safe rate of weight loss, though many women will see that range and think, *But I want to lose weight faster*. I get it! But when you consider that 1 kilo of body fat is equivalent to 7,700 calories (32,200 kJ), that's a huge energy deficit that's needed to lose a kilogram of fat every week.

Cutting your diet by around 500 calories is a much more realistic daily deficit. If you do this consistently, over a week this equates to 3,500 calories, which would equal a weight loss of just under 0.5 kg. If you're able to exercise efficiently on top of this, that deficit will increase and drive a slightly greater weight loss.

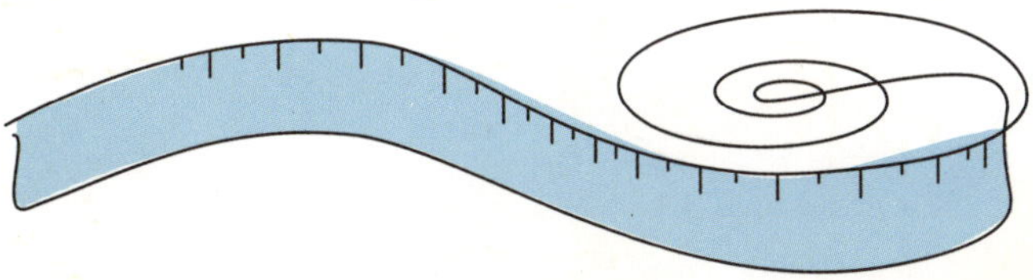

Chapter 6

Exercising to support your journey

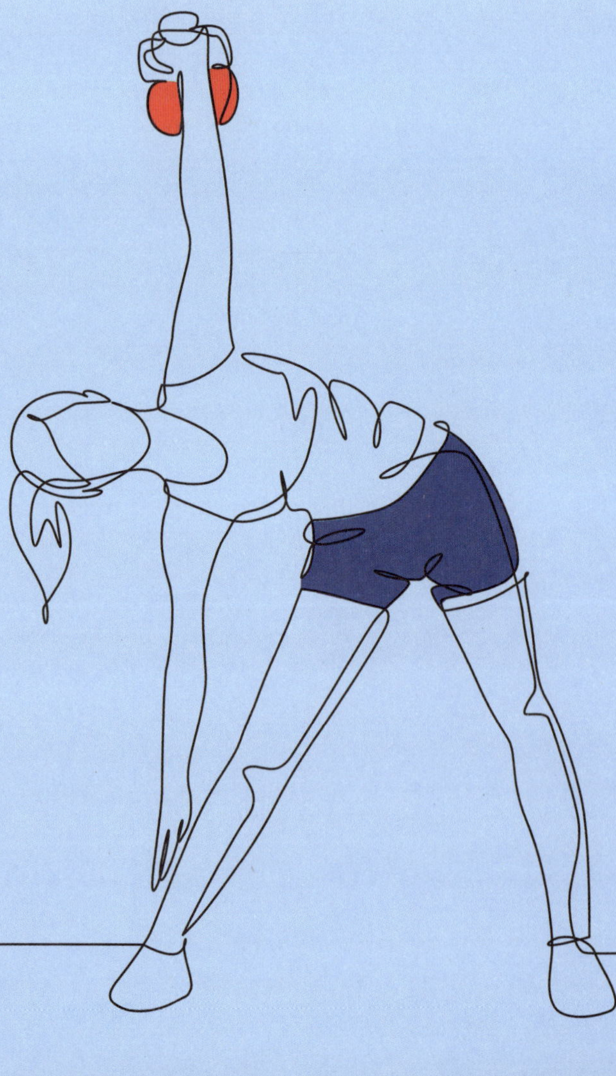

Exercise plays an essential role in managing the symptoms of peri and the natural body changes that occur during this time. Exercising regularly is beneficial during every phase of life, but in peri it can be even more important.

For starters, exercise is a natural mood booster, plus it slows down the decline in bone density that begins in peri. Aerobic exercise (aka 'cardio') raises the heart rate and improves cardiovascular health and fitness. It's also been shown to improve anxiety and depression in perimenopausal women as well as sleep quality. And the more frequent the exercise (more than 3 times per week), the greater this effect. Resistance training, such as lifting weights, stimulates the muscle to help preserve that precious lean tissue that naturally declines during peri. Strength training also helps to increase muscle performance.

What exercise looks like for you depends on what you enjoy. I truly believe that the exercise you choose to do should be something you love doing because it's far easier to be consistent and stick with something you enjoy.

One of the biggest benefits of exercising during the peri years is that it can help to manage the symptoms and changes that happen through peri. If we experience significant decline in muscle and bone during peri, for example, we'll be left to contend with those biochemical changes for the remainder of our lives. In fact, this has been confirmed in research that the benefits of these peri-specific exercise interventions must be maintained diligently in order to achieve and maintain their benefits.

This is why I think a great way to approach exercise in peri is to create a foundation of movement and activity based on exercise you love to do. The same way you build your diet on the foundations of an eating pattern that naturally appeals to you, your exercise regime should be built around something that feels natural and enjoyable. That might be yoga, walking, Pilates, dancing or weight-training, or skiing, swimming, cross fit and more. Whatever that thing is for you, engage in that activity most often – it will be easier to maintain because it's enjoyable.

When selecting your activities, however, bear in mind that the exercise you NEED now must meet certain criteria to mitigate the changes happening during peri. So, in addition to whatever enjoyable foundation exercise you've chosen, consider how to add or integrate some peri-specific exercise, too.

This might mean you need to either switch some sessions around or add some peri-specific exercise sessions to your repertoire and increase your sessions per week. Have a think about what might be missing from your exercise. Are you doing plenty of low-intensity cardio like walking, but little to no strength exercise? Or are you doing Pilates a few times a week but no cardiovascular movement?

How often should you be exercising?

- **Aerobic exercise (aka cardio):** brisk walking, jogging, aerobics, cycling, swimming, etc. at least 3 days per week.
- **Resistance training (aka strength training):** weightlifting with dumbbells or body weight exercises like squats at least twice a week.

How long should your workouts be?

- **Aerobic:** either 30–60 minutes or 8–10,000 steps.
- **Strength:** 30–40 minutes per session.

Initially, we need to exercise consistently for at least 8 weeks to establish a habit and see and feel the benefits. In all the research I've studied, the overarching message is that the more often we exercise, the better the outcome in managing the symptoms of peri, particularly when it comes to mood, sleep, bone density and weight. It also shows that the beneficial effects of exercise on peri symptoms will wear off eventually if the exercise isn't consistently maintained.

SLEEP AND EXERCISE

Not only is exercise important metabolically, it's also been shown to help with other pesky and disruptive symptoms of peri, including insomnia. Exercise can be a simple and cost-effective way to manage sleep disturbances during peri, while also potentially avoiding pharmaceutical therapies.

The key seems to lie in the consistency and intensity of the exercise. In the research, it seems lighter-intensity exercise doesn't improve sleep quality as significantly as higher-intensity exercise does. However, this is likely to be quite personal as well and you may find that lighter-intensity exercise for you does in fact help to improve your sleep.

Exercise targets for improved sleep

- Higher-intensity training at least three times a week.
- Sessions should last between 30–60 minutes.

Try this consistently for at least three months.

MOOD AND EXERCISE

Frustration, rage and irritability, as well as depression and anxiety, are common symptoms of peri. Exercise, particularly high-intensity aerobic exercise, has been shown to be very effective in reducing depression and anxiety scores and, as with sleep disturbances, is considered a cost-effective and natural remedy or treatment for peri-related mood disorders. To reap these mood-boosting benefits, exercise vigorously more than three times per week, and find a way to make this a habit so you can continue to get the benefits long term.

OSTEOPOROSIS AND EXERCISE

Exercise has been shown to play an important role in both preventing and treating osteoporosis in peri and menopause. Once again, the type of exercise is quite specific and prescriptive. Weight-bearing exercise like walking, running, aerobics and skipping as well as strength exercise has been shown to have a significant impact on bone mineral density, and reducing the risk of osteoporosis and osteopenia.

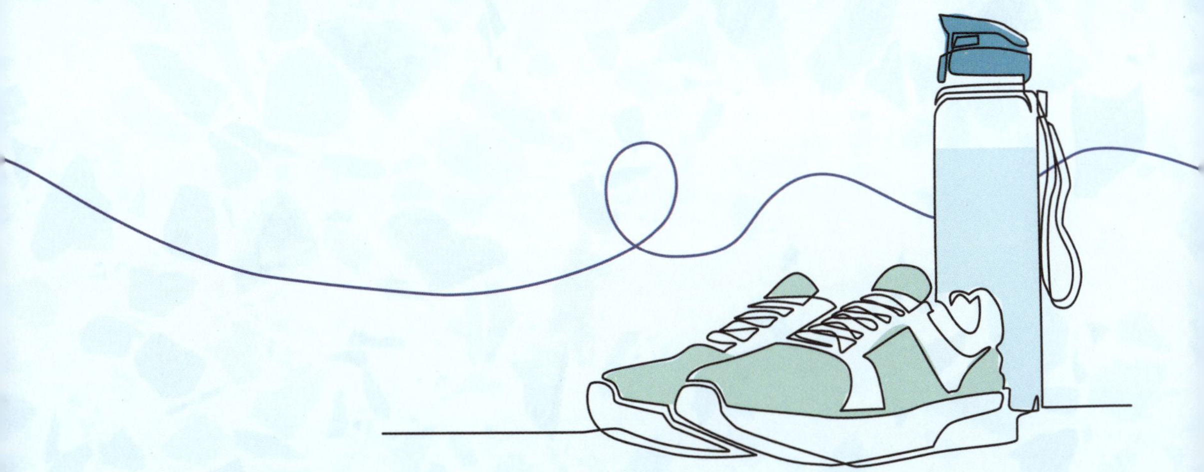

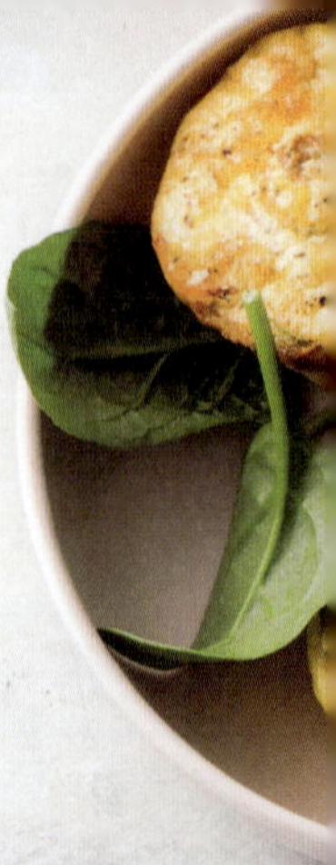

Conclusion

Awareness of perimenopause is growing and more research is finally under way. The more we learn, the more tools and insight we gain. The research and suggestions in this book might seem daunting when viewed all at once, especially as peri often coincides with one of the busiest and most stressful times in a woman's life. But it is a long process. Give yourself grace and be kind. You don't have to sort out all the areas of life we've talked about in one go. Start with something easy that feels manageable (e.g. tweaking your diet, trying intermittent fasting, upping your protein, doing some strength-training) and then gradually add to that when you feel up for it.

Try to embrace this transition as part of your natural evolution as a woman, rather than something to be dreaded. It's not easy, but there's so much life to be enjoyed during these years and on the other side of them, especially if you take good care of yourself.

Don't ignore your body and how you feel. Don't try to power through life the same way you did in your twenties and thirties. Adjust to make the most of your life as it is now and keep an eye on how you want to move through the world in the decades to come. Visualise the type of older woman you wish to become and work backwards from there. What lifestyle tweaks could you make over the next year or two to ensure that vision becomes reality?

Now you're all up to date with the latest research and recommended patterns of eating for peri, it's time to put it all into practice in the kitchen. In the following section, you'll find loads of easy, delicious recipes featuring a range of power peri foods (hello, tofu!), with the goal of supporting your health and well-being in peri and beyond.

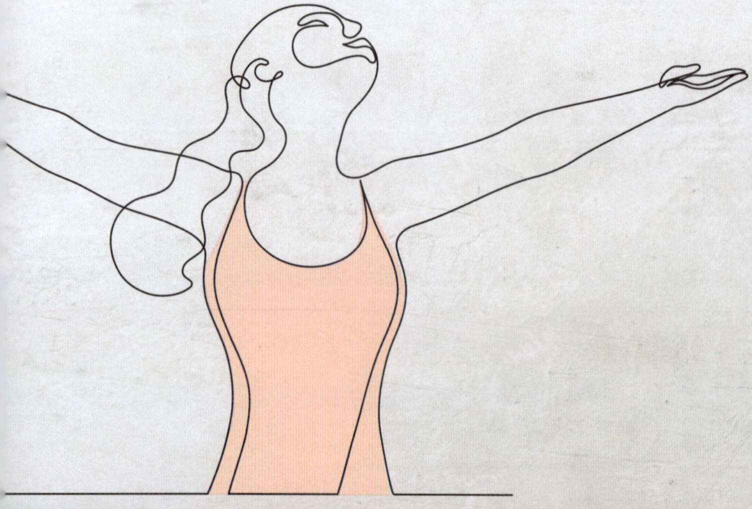

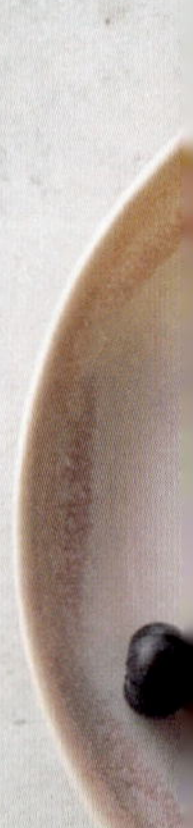

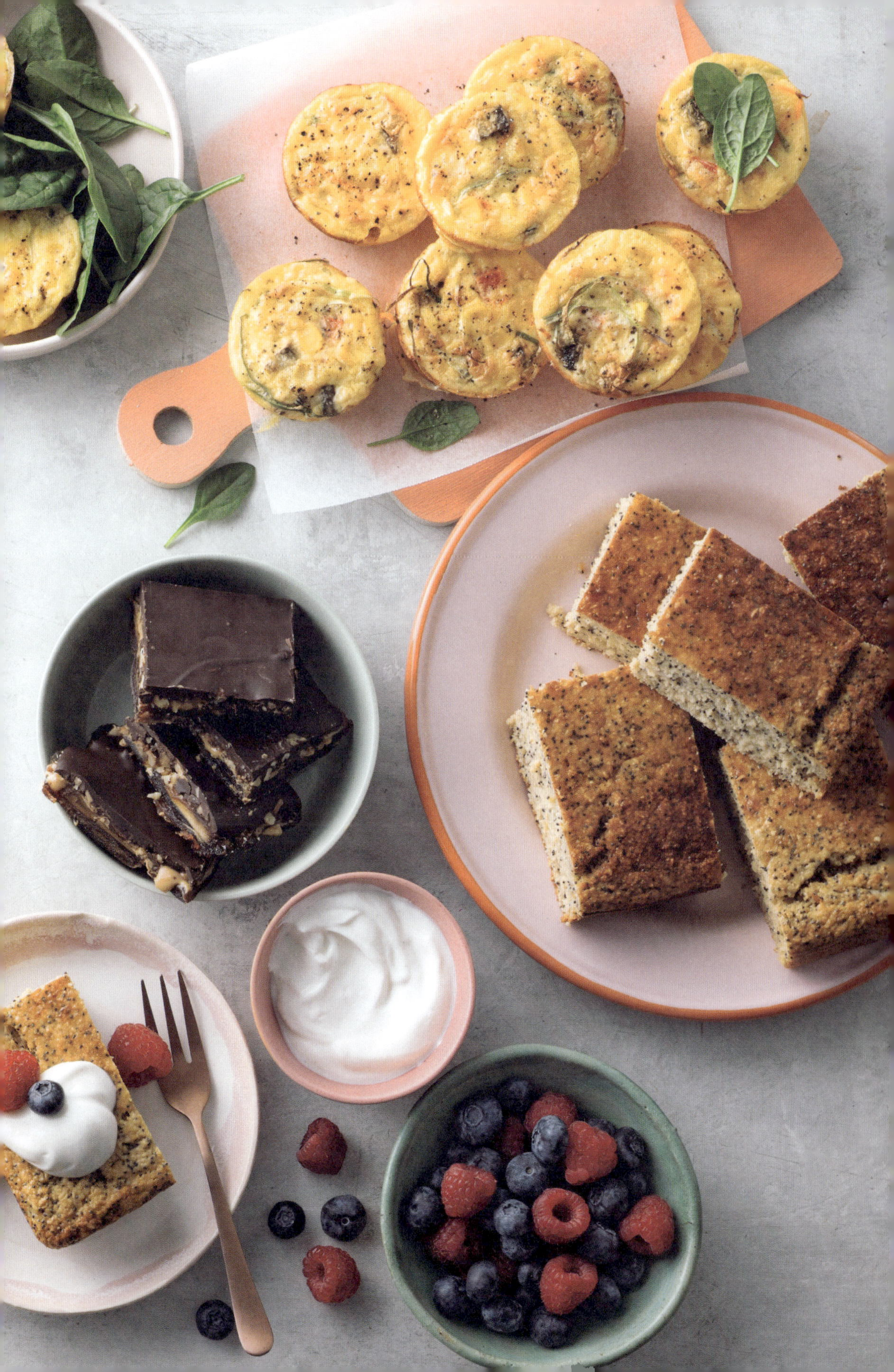

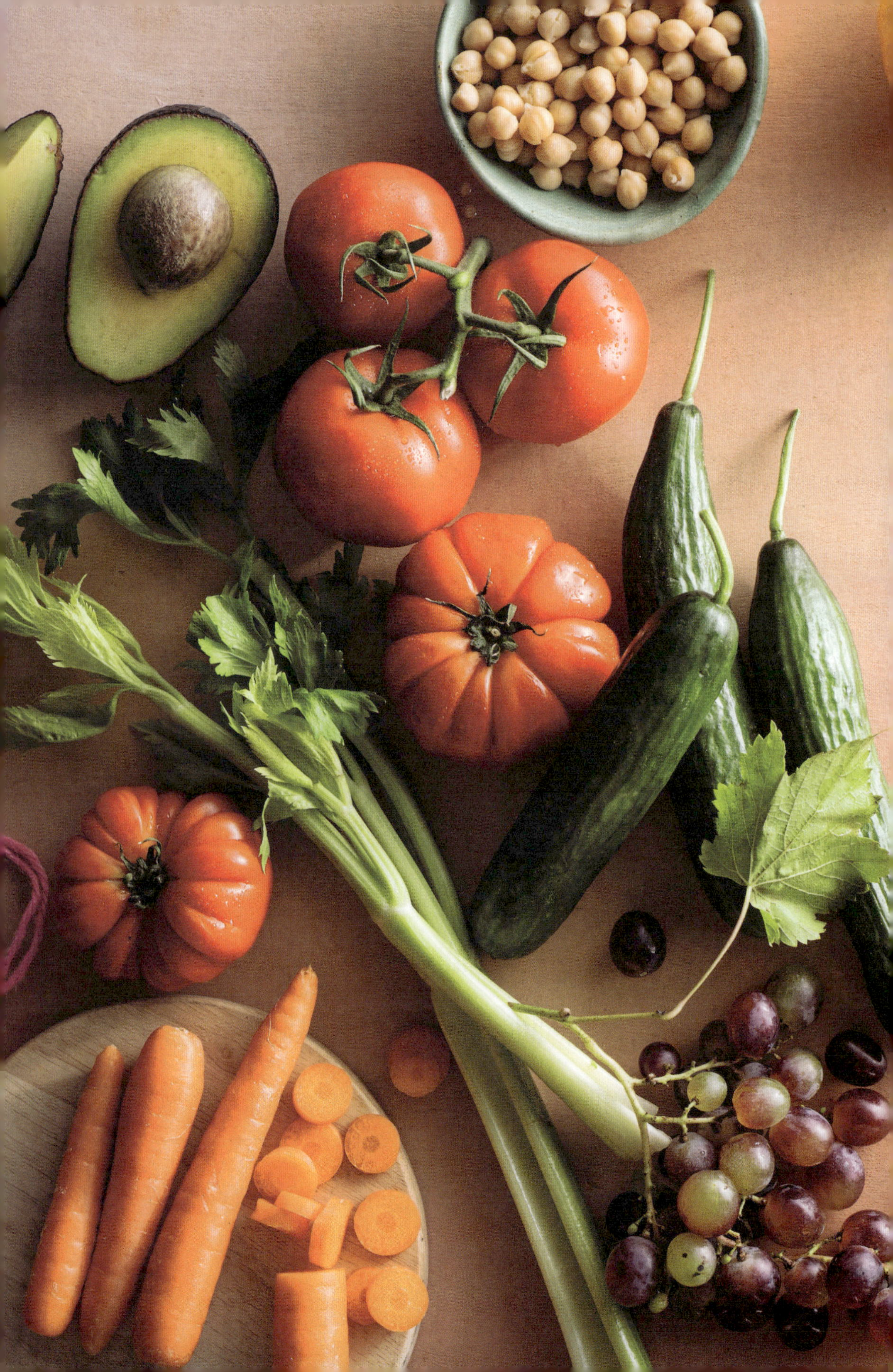

RECIPES

01

BREAKFAST

Getting enough protein at breakfast is so important. Eggs are an amazing source of this peri power nutrient. Try to incorporate dairy and soy milk, cottage cheese or yoghurt, too. Each recipe in this chapter contains at least 20 grams of protein to make sure you're breaking your fast in the best way possible and setting yourself up for the rest of the day.

Serves 1

PERI-BERRY SMOOTHIE

I love a smoothie meal – you can throw all kinds of goodness into the blender, plus it's preferable to juicing as it retains all that excellent fibre (see pages 48–9). You'll notice that this smoothie contains most of the major peri foods: soy milk, berries, fermented dairy yoghurt, spinach and flaxseeds. A true peri-power mix!

- 250 ml (1 cup) soy milk (see Notes)
- ½ frozen banana
- 75 g (½ cup) frozen mixed berries, plus a couple extra to garnish (optional)
- ½ teaspoon ground cinnamon
- 125 g (½ cup) plain probiotic yoghurt (see Notes)
- small handful of baby spinach leaves
- 1 teaspoon ground flaxseeds

Place all the ingredients in a blender and process until smooth. Garnish with extra berries, if you like.

NOTES

Soy milk: Choose a brand of soy milk that specifies 'whole soybeans' in the ingredients list so you can reap the benefits of the whole food.

Probiotic yoghurt: Though all yoghurts contain natural cultures thanks to the fermentation process they undergo, not all contain gut-boosting probiotics. Probiotics are strains of bacteria scientifically proven to have health benefits in certain doses. These are added to the yoghurt to provide specific strains and doses of probiotics.

When shopping for a probiotic-rich yoghurt, look at the nutrition information panel. A good probiotic yoghurt will have around three different probiotics specified at the bottom of the panel, and will also detail their CFU, which is the dose of colony forming units used in the recipe. Anything above 1 billion CFU indicates a probiotic-rich yoghurt.

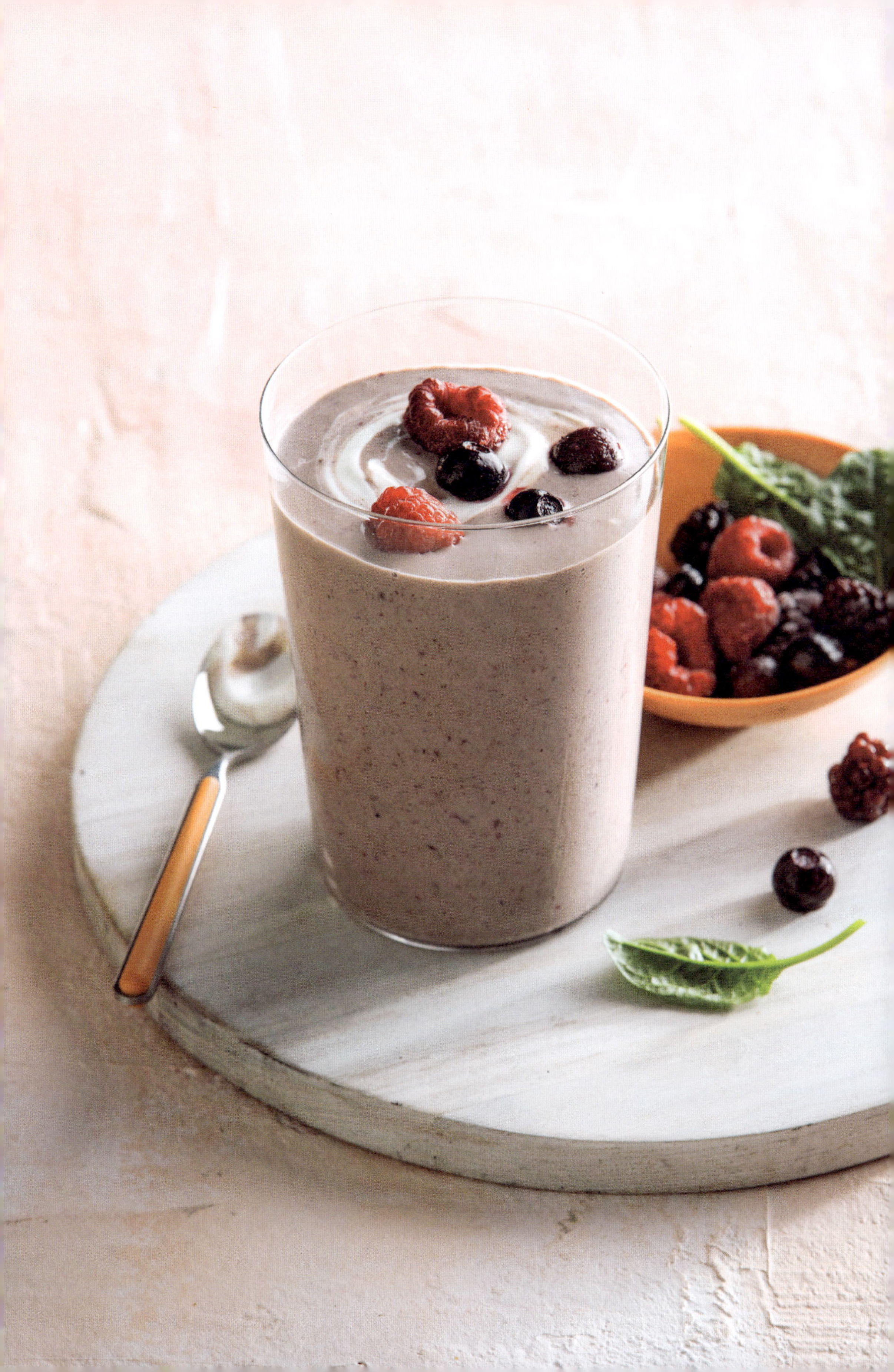

Serves 2

PERI-FRIENDLY MUESLI, FRUIT AND YOGHURT

I've taken thousands of diet histories in my time and one of the most popular breakfast options by far is muesli with fruit and yoghurt, especially in the warmer months. While this can be a wonderfully healthy way to start the day if done right, it can also become a carbohydrate-dense and calorie-laden meal with not a lot of protein if the proportions aren't considered. That's why I'm sharing this super simple recipe here – to show you how to tweak the quantities in a perfectly peri-friendly way.

- 1 tablespoon almonds
- 4 walnuts
- 4 Brazil nuts
- 1 tablespoon pumpkin seeds
- 500 g (2 cups) plain Greek-style or probiotic yoghurt (see Note on page 100)
- 1 teaspoon vanilla extract
- 2 teaspoons maple syrup
- 150 g (1 cup) mixed berries

To serve (optional)

- extra seasonal fruit, such as peach, nectarine, fig, kiwi, etc

Place the nuts and pumpkin seeds in a small frying pan and toast over medium heat until they start to colour and become fragrant. Transfer to a chopping board and, once cool enough to handle, roughly chop with a large knife.

Mix the yoghurt, vanilla and maple syrup in a bowl, then divide between serving bowls.

Top each bowl with mixed berries and extra seasonal fruit, if you like, then sprinkle over the toasted chopped nuts and seeds.

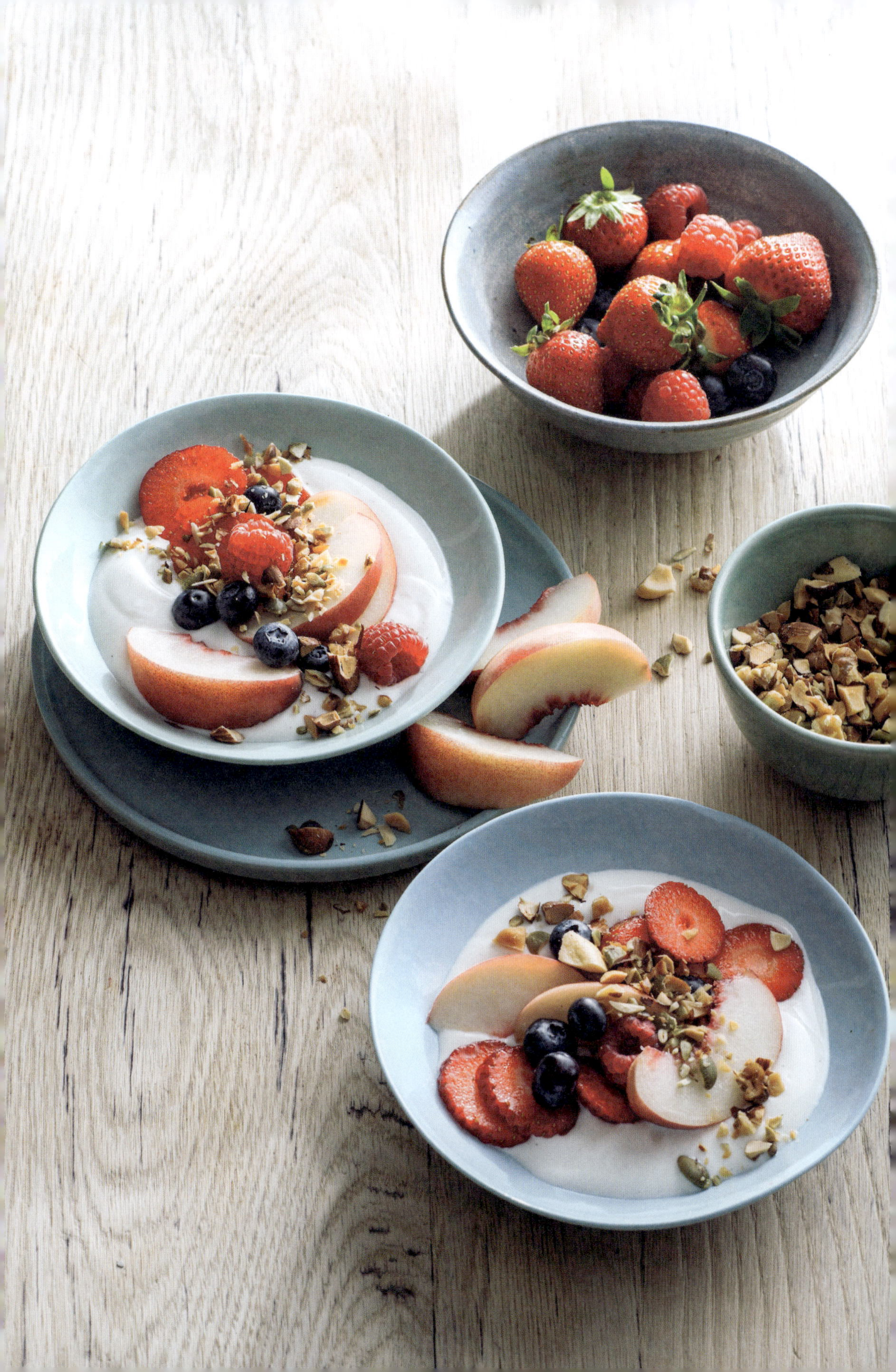

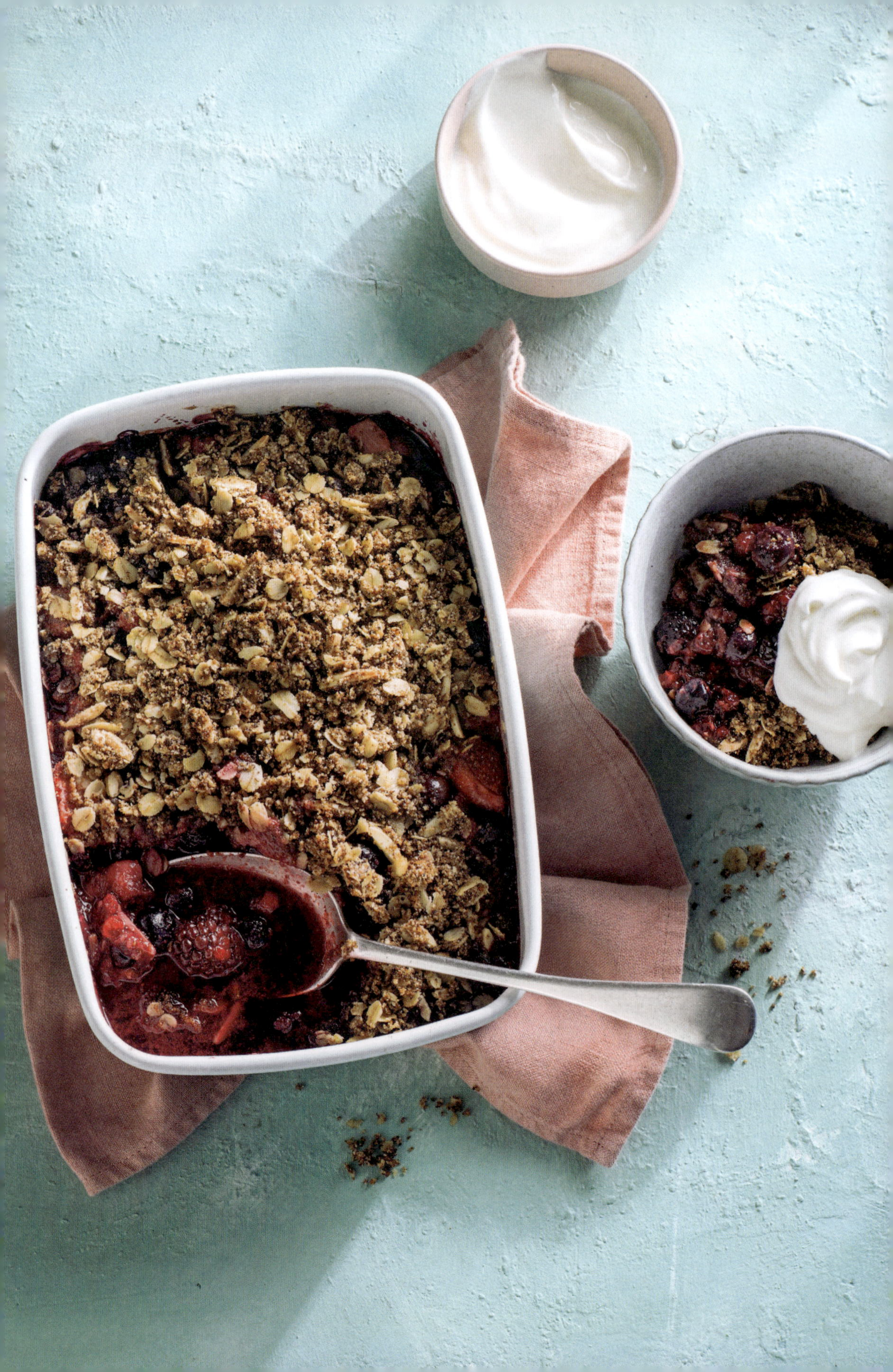

Serves 6

BERRY BREAKFAST CRUMBLE

Who says you can't have dessert for breakfast? I adore this warm and crunchy baked crumble, complete with oozy berries and a deliciously nutty topping. A few clever subs – replacing the usual butter, flour and refined sugar with olive oil, almond meal and a little coconut sugar – and you've got a nourishing start to a chilly day.

1 kg frozen mixed berries
2 tablespoons cornflour
80 ml (⅓ cup) maple syrup
1 teaspoon vanilla extract
plain Greek-style yoghurt, to serve

Crumble topping
75 g (¾ cup) rolled oats
55 g (½ cup) almond meal
30 g (⅓ cup) ground flaxseed
40 g (⅓ cup) slivered almonds
75 g (⅓ cup) coconut sugar
½ teaspoon baking powder
1 teaspoon ground cinnamon
80 ml (⅓ cup) extra-virgin olive oil
pinch of sea salt

Preheat the oven to 180°C.

Place the berries, cornflour, maple syrup and vanilla in a bowl and combine well. Spread over the base of a small baking dish.

For the crumble topping, place all the ingredients in a large bowl and rub the mixture together with your fingers until combined.

Sprinkle the crumble topping evenly over the berry mixture in the baking dish. Bake for 30–40 minutes, or until the top is golden and the berry mixture is syrupy and bubbling.

Serve topped with a dollop of yoghurt.

Serves 1

WEEKDAY PANCAKES

Just a few ingredient tweaks and these quick blender pancakes are not only super easy to make on a busy weekday morning, they're also good for you. With a healthy dose of fibre, protein and slow-release carbohydrates, they deliver all the taste of the breakfast favourite without the energy crash afterwards.

1 tablespoon extra-virgin olive oil

Pancakes

50 g (½ cup) rolled oats
60 g (¼ cup) cottage cheese
1 egg
½ small banana
½ teaspoon ground cinnamon
½ teaspoon baking powder

Toppings

maple syrup
mixed berries
plain yoghurt

Process the oats in a blender until a fine powder forms. Add the remaining pancake ingredients and process again until well combined.

Preheat the olive oil in a frying pan over medium–high heat and swirl it around the pan to evenly coat. Pour in half the batter to make one large pancake. Cook for a few minutes until bubbles start to appear on the surface, then flip over and cook for another minute or two before transferring to a plate.

Repeat with the rest of the batter, then serve with your choice of toppings.

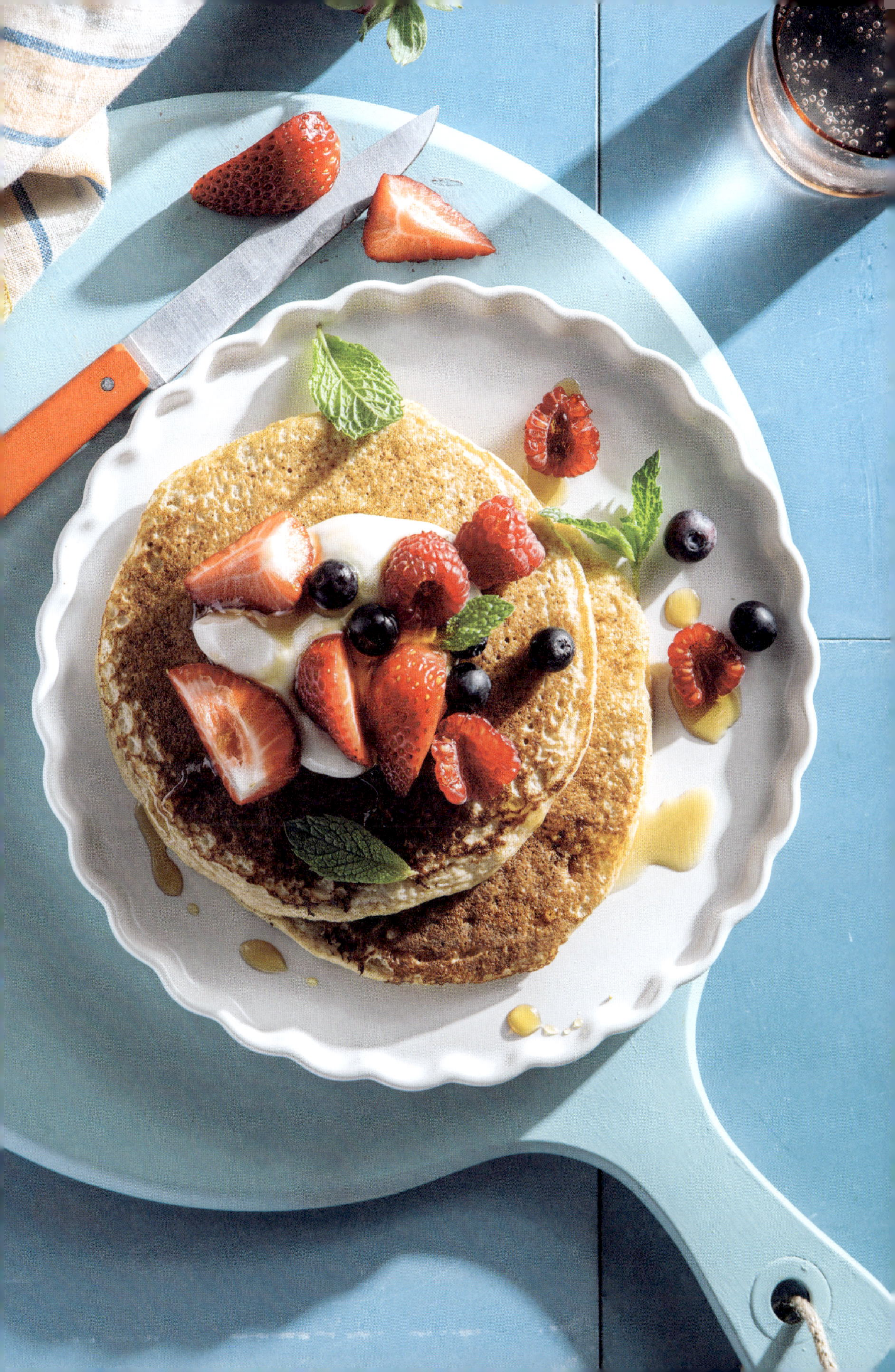

Serves 1

SPINACH FETA OMELETTE WRAP

I've been making these quesadilla-inspired breakfast wraps on repeat lately. They're just so easy, you can't get it wrong! Spinach and feta is a classic combination but feel free to play around with the fillings – try cherry tomatoes, onion, capsicum, zucchini, even smoked salmon.

- 2 eggs
- 1 tablespoon milk of your choice
- sea salt and freshly ground black pepper
- 2 teaspoons extra-virgin olive oil
- 1 high-fibre or wholegrain wrap
- 25 g (½ cup) baby spinach leaves
- 1 tablespoon crumbled feta
- lemon wedge, to serve
- chilli sauce or low-sugar barbecue sauce, to serve (optional)

Whisk the eggs and milk in a small bowl with a pinch of salt and pepper.

Heat the olive oil in a frying pan over medium–high heat. Pour in the egg mixture and tilt the pan so the mixture is evenly distributed.

Place the wrap gently on the egg so that it sticks, then cook for 30 seconds. Flip the whole lot over like a pancake, so the wrap is on the bottom.

Scatter the spinach leaves and feta over half the omelette. After 1–2 minutes, or when the wrap is golden underneath, use a spatula to fold it in half so the wrap is on the outside. Serve with a lemon wedge and your favourite chilli or barbecue sauce, if you like.

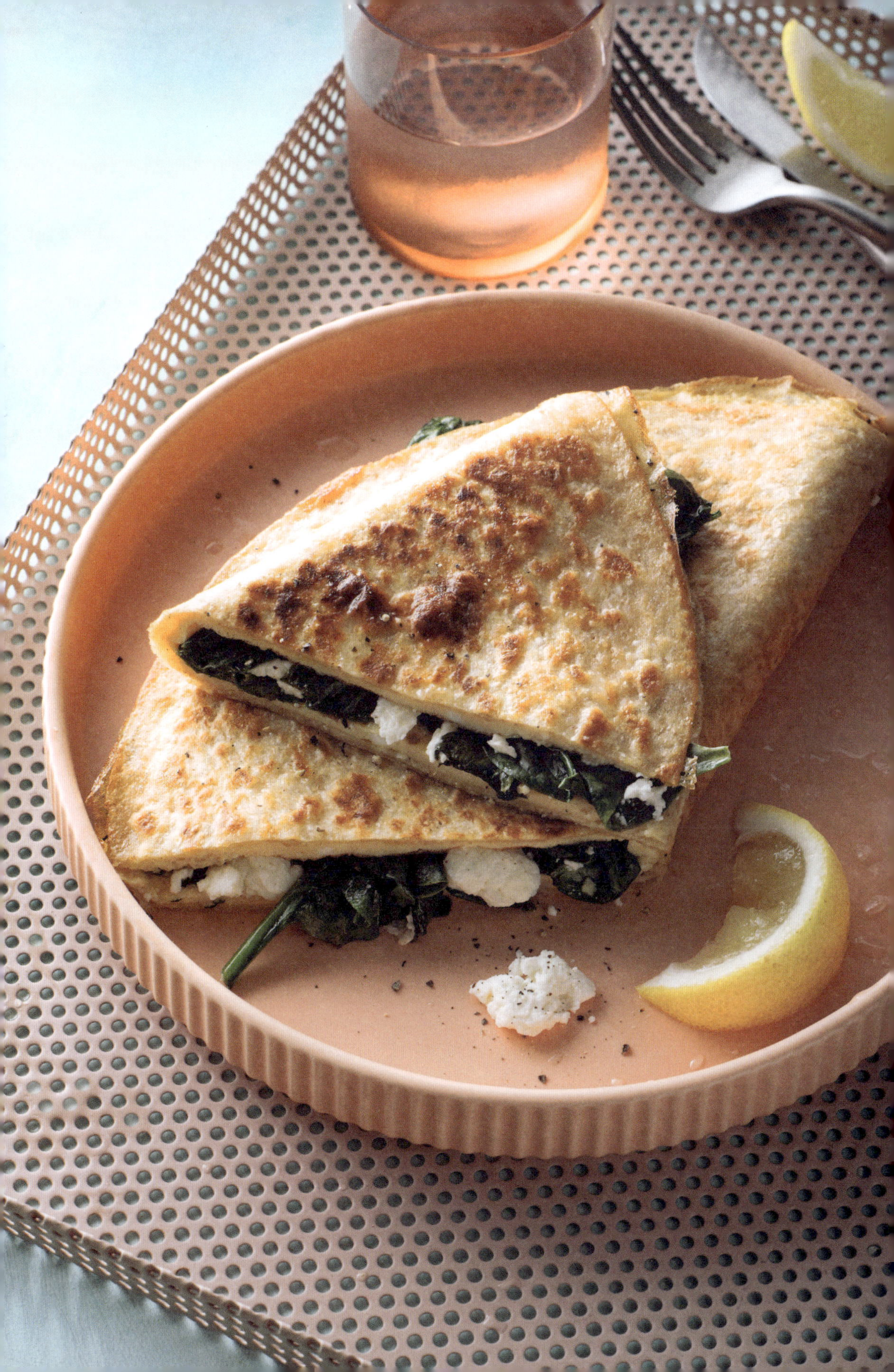

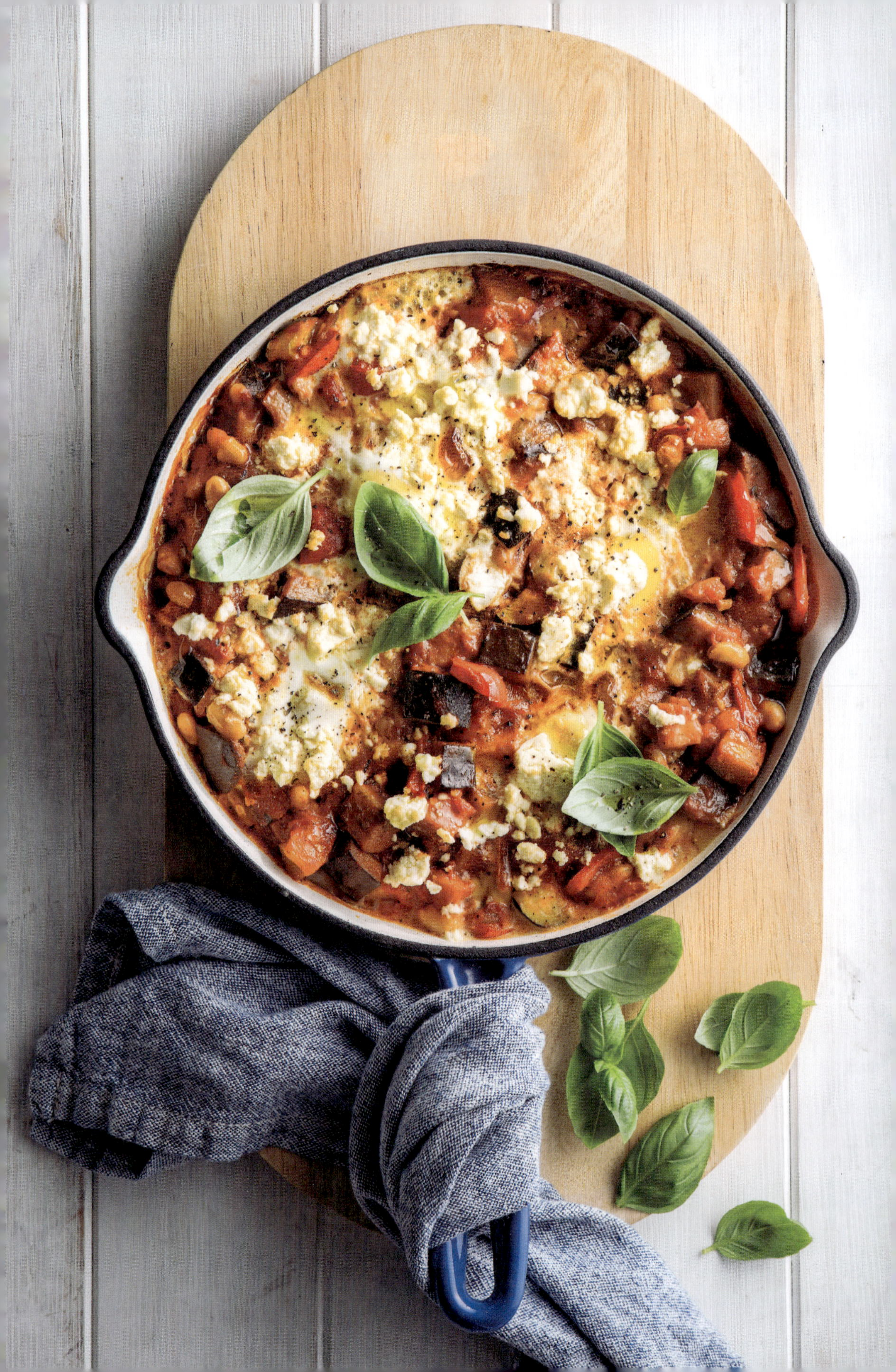

Serves 2

RATATOUILLE SHAKSHUKA

If you're after a hearty breakfast that's going to keep you going for hours, look no further. This recipe transforms any leftover bean ratatouille from the dinner on page 151 into the shakshuka of your dreams!

⅓ batch of Bean ratatouille (see page 151)
4 eggs
50 g feta
sea salt and freshly ground black pepper

To serve (optional)
basil leaves
2 x 40 g slices of grainy toast or wholemeal pita
dried chilli flakes or hot sauce of your choice

Reheat the leftover bean ratatouille in a small ovenproof frying pan over low–medium heat. Use a spoon to evenly spread the ratatouille over the base of the pan, then make four small indents with the back of the spoon.

Carefully crack an egg into each indent, reduce the heat to low and place a lid on the pan for 1–2 minutes.

Preheat the grill to medium.

Remove the lid from the pan. Sprinkle the shakshuka with the feta. Place the pan under the grill for 3–5 minutes, or until the eggs are just cooked and the feta starts to turn golden. Season with salt and pepper.

Divide between two plates and scatter with basil leaves, if you like. Serve with toast or pita and top with chilli flakes or hot sauce.

Serves 1

CURRIED TOFU VEGGIE SCRAMBLE

Who says you have to stick with eggs if you want a high-protein savoury breakfast? Tofu scrambles up so well and packs a real protein punch, too. This particular recipe also has a built-in quality carb in the form of potato with its fibre-rich skin on. This will keep your energy resources charged and your stomach satisfied for hours.

- 1 tablespoon extra-virgin olive oil
- 1 potato, diced into 1 cm pieces
- 1 spring onion, finely sliced
- 200 g firm tofu
- ½ teaspoon minced garlic
- ¼ teaspoon ground turmeric
- ¼ teaspoon curry powder
- 90 g (1 cup) mushrooms (button or cremini work well), brushed clean and quartered
- sea salt and freshly ground black pepper
- handful of baby spinach leaves (optional)

Heat the olive oil in a frying pan over medium–high heat, then add the diced potato and cook, stirring regularly, for 5–7 minutes, or until the potato starts to turn golden.

Add the spring onion to the pan, then roughly crumble the tofu over the top. Use a fork to break up any larger pieces, if necessary. Add the garlic, turmeric and curry powder and toss to coat the veg and tofu in the spices.

Add the mushrooms to the pan, season with salt and pepper and continue to cook until the mushrooms have softened and any liquid they've released has evaporated.

Add the spinach leaves, if using, then turn off the heat and stir until the spinach has wilted. Serve immediately.

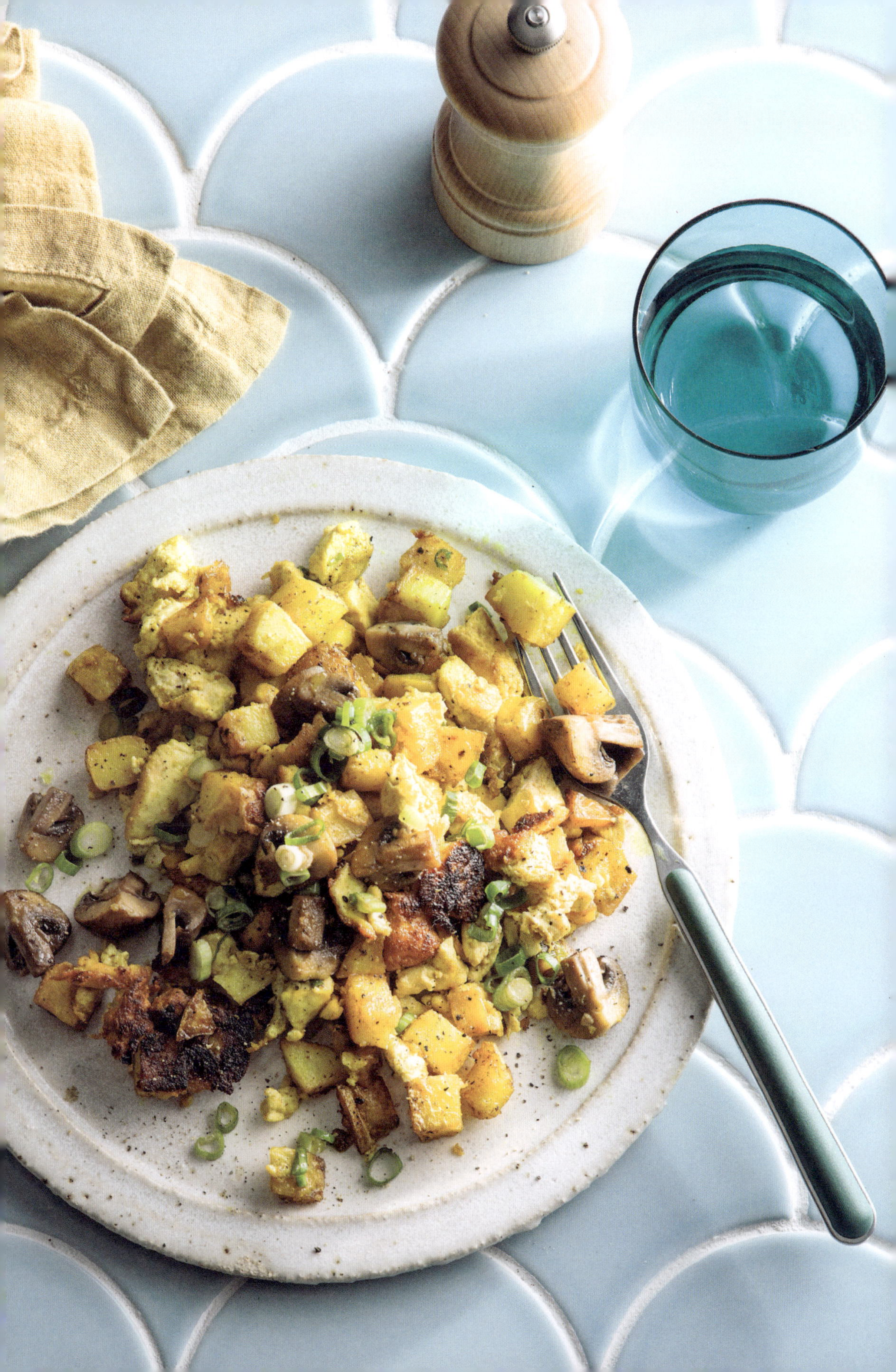

WHIPPED RICOTTA FOR EVERY MOOD

The best thing about having whipped ricotta in the fridge is that it can be tweaked to satisfy any season and craving – warm or cold, sweet or savoury. It can also bend to whatever ingredients you happen to have on hand. Apparently, this ricotta keeps for a long time in the freezer, too. I haven't tried freezing it yet, but if you do, let me know how it goes.

To turn the ricotta into a brilliant satisfying snack (or mini meal), spread it on a dense, dark, seeded rye bread and load up with the toppings on the opposite page. Not only is rye bread rich in nutrients, it also has a low-GI rating (see page 25) and it's packed with gut-loving prebiotics. You should be able to find a nice rye bread (or even sourdough rye) from the supermarket or bakery. If you're slicing a whole loaf, aim for around 40 g per slice as a portion. And if rye isn't for you, then a regular wholegrain, spelt or grainy gluten-free bread will also be wonderful.

Whipped ricotta

Makes enough for 8 slices

500 g (2 cups) low-fat ricotta (see Tip)
1 tablespoon extra-virgin olive oil

Put the ricotta and olive oil into a food processor or blender. Process for 1–2 minutes, or until smooth and creamy. Scrape down the sides every 10–15 seconds and blend until the ricotta is a light, fluffy and even consistency. Store in an airtight container in the fridge for up to 4 days.

To serve, spread 2 heaped tablespoons ricotta on a slice of toast and top with any of the opposite ideas.

TIP FOR A DAIRY-FREE VERSION

Swap the ricotta recipe here for two batches of the tofu-based 'ricotta' on page 158. When making, omit the onion and garlic powders and the salt to create a more neutral-flavoured base for your toppings.

Serves 1

Savoury toppings

Smoked trout

Spread **whipped ricotta** on toast. Flake over 50 g **smoked trout or salmon** and top with sliced **cucumber**, a squeeze of **lemon juice**, a few **caper**s and some **dill**.

Sautéed pesto tomatoes

Dice up 1 large **tomato**. Heat 1 teaspoon **olive oil** in a frying pan. Add the tomato and 1 teaspoon good-quality **pesto** and sauté for 1–2 minutes, or until warm and the tomato is starting to soften. Spoon over your **ricotta toast**.

Mashed edamame and avocado

Thaw 90 g (½ cup) podded **edamame** and add to a bowl with ¼ **avocado**, 1 finely sliced small **shallot**, the juice of ½ **lime** and a good pinch of **sea salt** and freshly **ground black pepper**. Mash together roughly with the back of a fork, then pile on top of your **ricotta toast**.

Beetroot hummus and cucumber

Spoon dollops of **beetroot hummus** onto your **ricotta toast** and top with thin slices of **cucumber**.

Sweet toppings

Banana and cinnamon

Arrange thin slices of **banana** over your **ricotta toast**. Sprinkle with a pinch of **ground cinnamon**.

Mixed berry sauce

Cook 150 g (1 cup) **frozen mixed berries** in a small saucepan over medium heat with 1 teaspoon **chia seeds** and 1 teaspoon **maple syrup**. Simmer, stirring occasionally, until the sauce thickens. Allow to cool and thicken into a warm jam, then spread a spoonful or two over the **ricotta toast**.

Apple slices and crushed walnuts

Arrange thin slices of ½ **apple** over the **ricotta toast**. Sprinkle a small handful of crushed **walnuts** and 1 teaspoon **honey** on top, if you like.

Pan-fried peaches

Slice up 1 ripe **peach** (a **nectarine or apricot** will also work). Heat 1 teaspoon **olive oil** in a small frying pan over medium heat and add the peach slices. You can add a few **thyme or mint leaves** too. Once soft and starting to caramelise a little, pile on top of the **ricotta toast**.

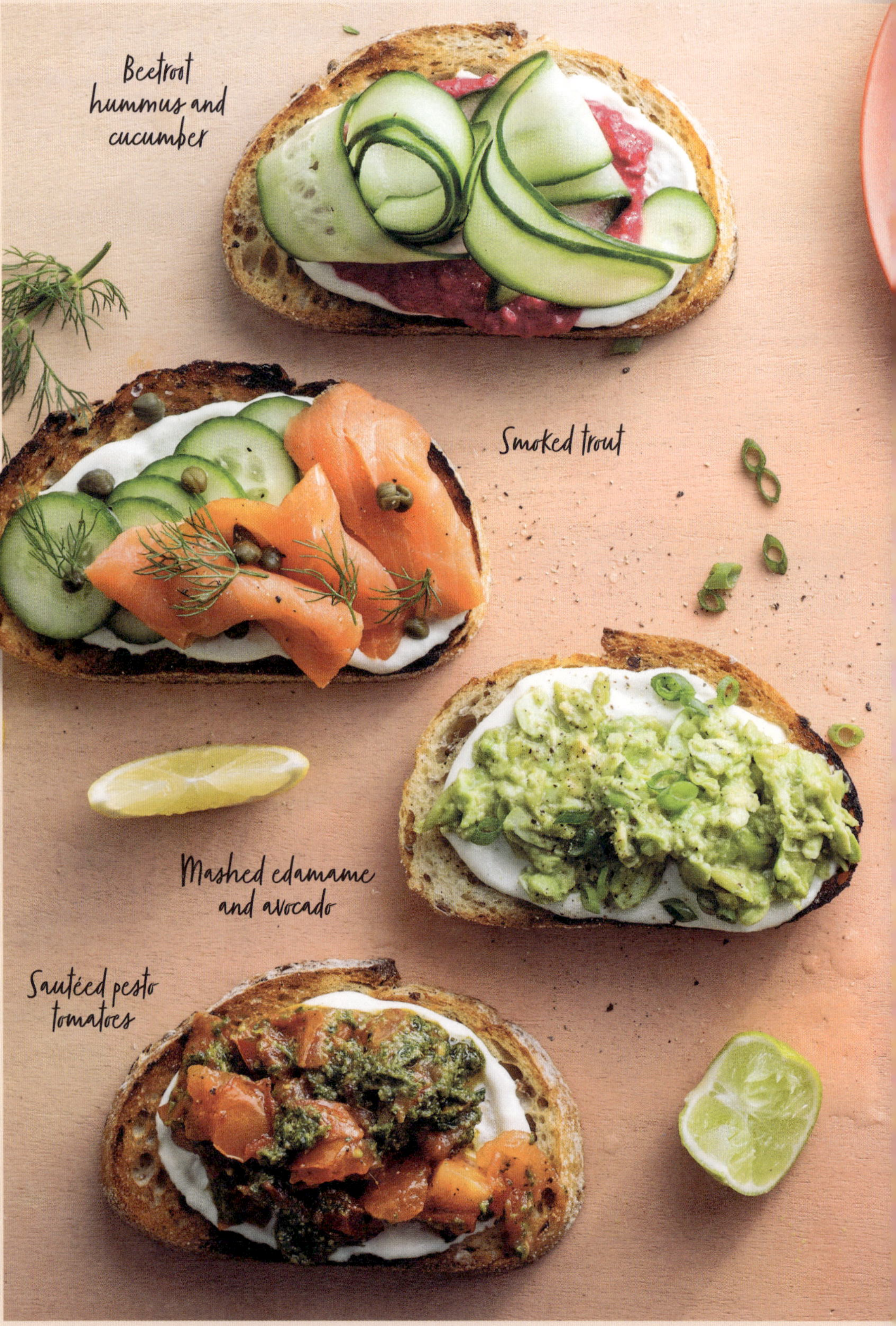
Beetroot hummus and cucumber
Smoked trout
Mashed edamame and avocado
Sautéed pesto tomatoes

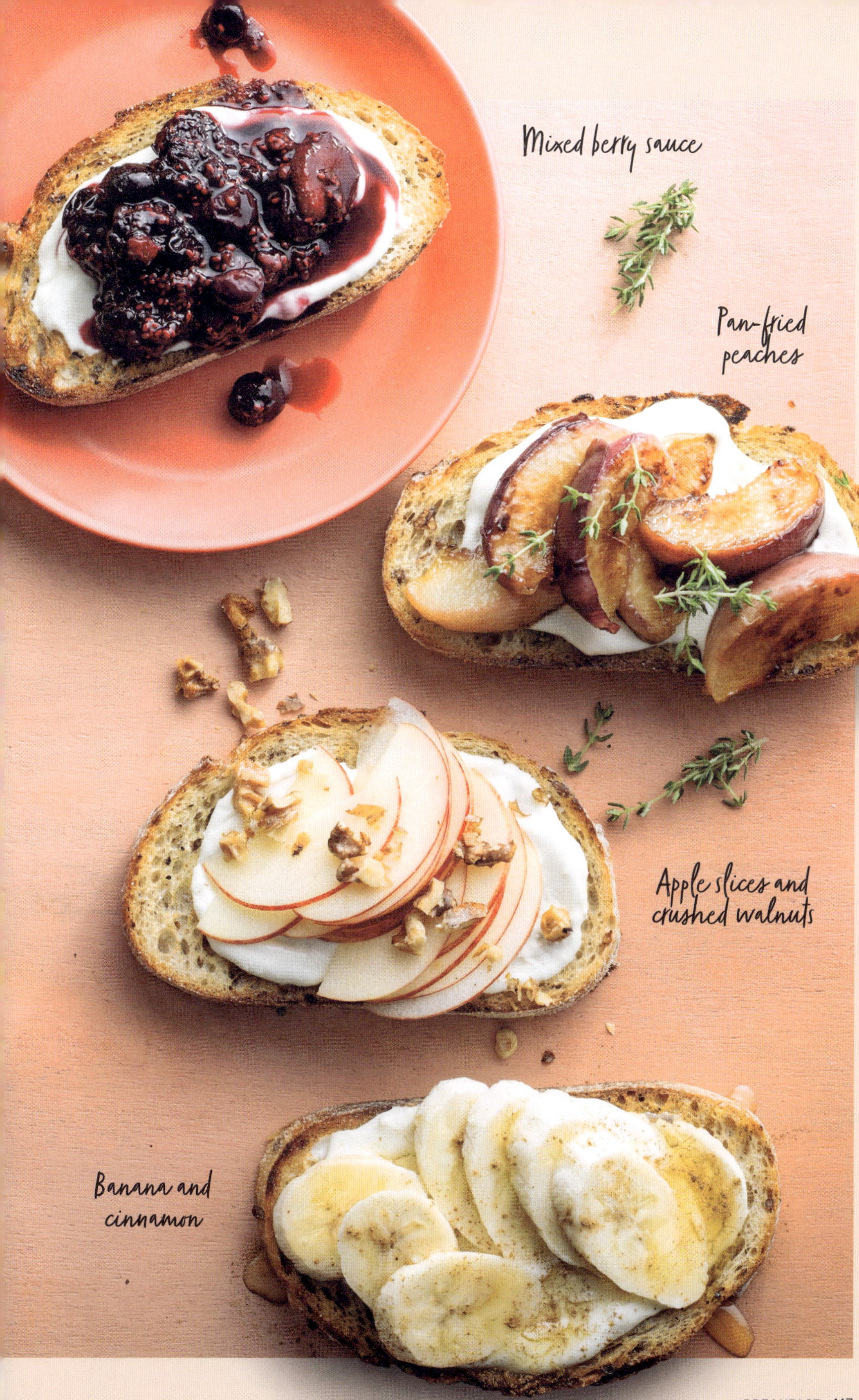
Mixed berry sauce
Pan-fried peaches
Apple slices and crushed walnuts
Banana and cinnamon

Serves 2

HEALTHIER FRENCH TOAST

With the simplest swaps, you can make a typically indulgent meal into a nutritious peri-friendly breakfast. Here, the traditional brioche or French bread is swapped for wholegrain, and the custard is lightened up with milk rather than cream. The flavour is still rich and delicious, but the underlying calorie count and nutritional profile come up smelling like roses too!

2 teaspoons extra-virgin olive oil
4 x 40 g slices of wholegrain, spelt or rye bread

French toast mixture

2 eggs
125 ml (½ cup) milk of your choice
1 tablespoon maple syrup
1 teaspoon vanilla extract
¼ teaspoon ground cinnamon

Toppings (optional)

seasonal fruit
plain Greek-style yoghurt
maple syrup

Whisk all the ingredients for the French toast mixture together in a wide, shallow bowl until well combined.

Heat the olive oil in a large frying pan over medium heat.

Lay a slice of bread in the egg mixture and leave to sit for 10 seconds or so to absorb plenty of liquid, then turn over and wait for another 10 seconds.

Transfer the eggy bread to the frying pan and cook for 1–2 minutes on each side, or until golden. Repeat the process with the remaining slices.

Serve 2 slices of French toast per person with your choice of toppings.

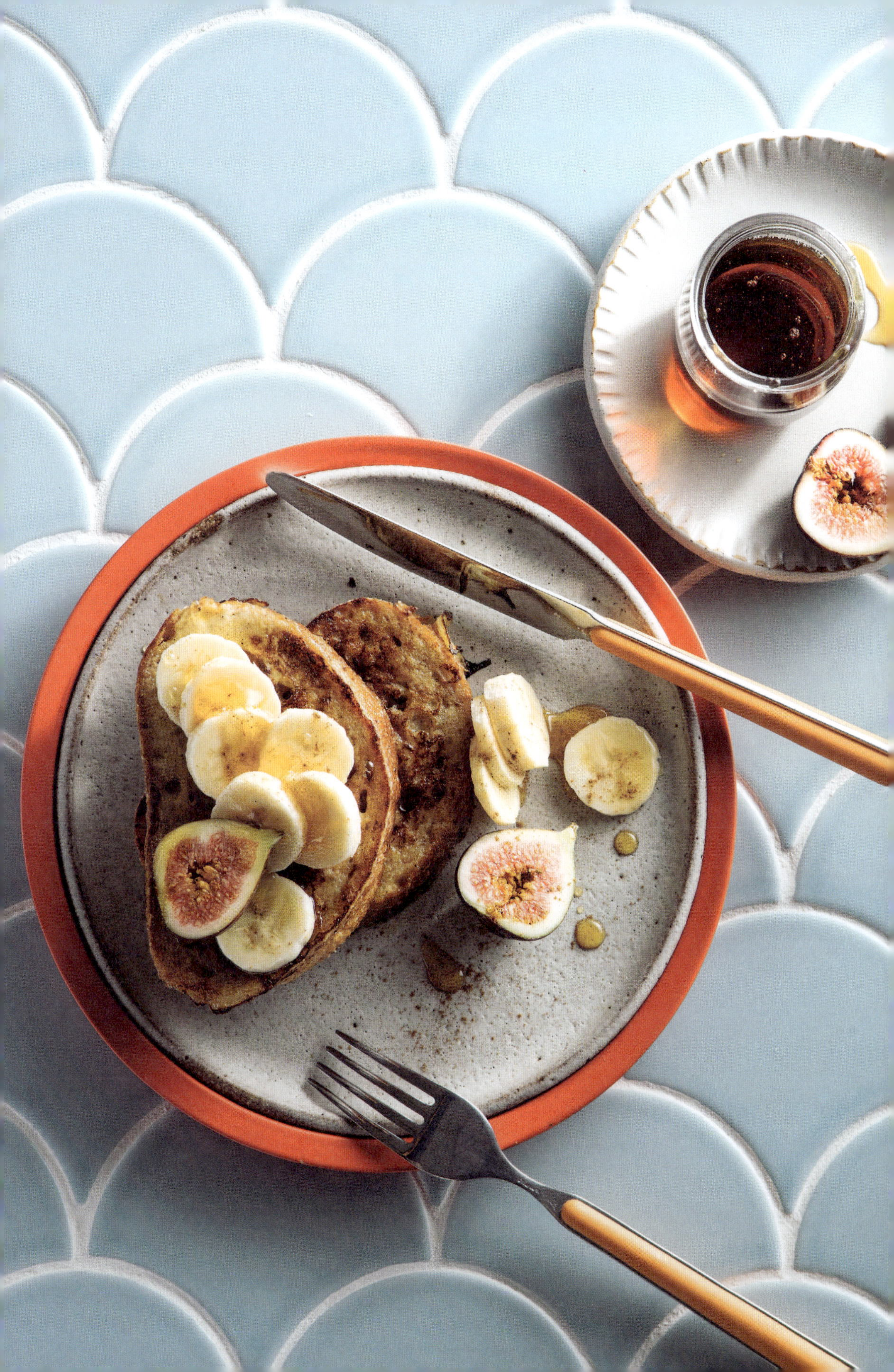

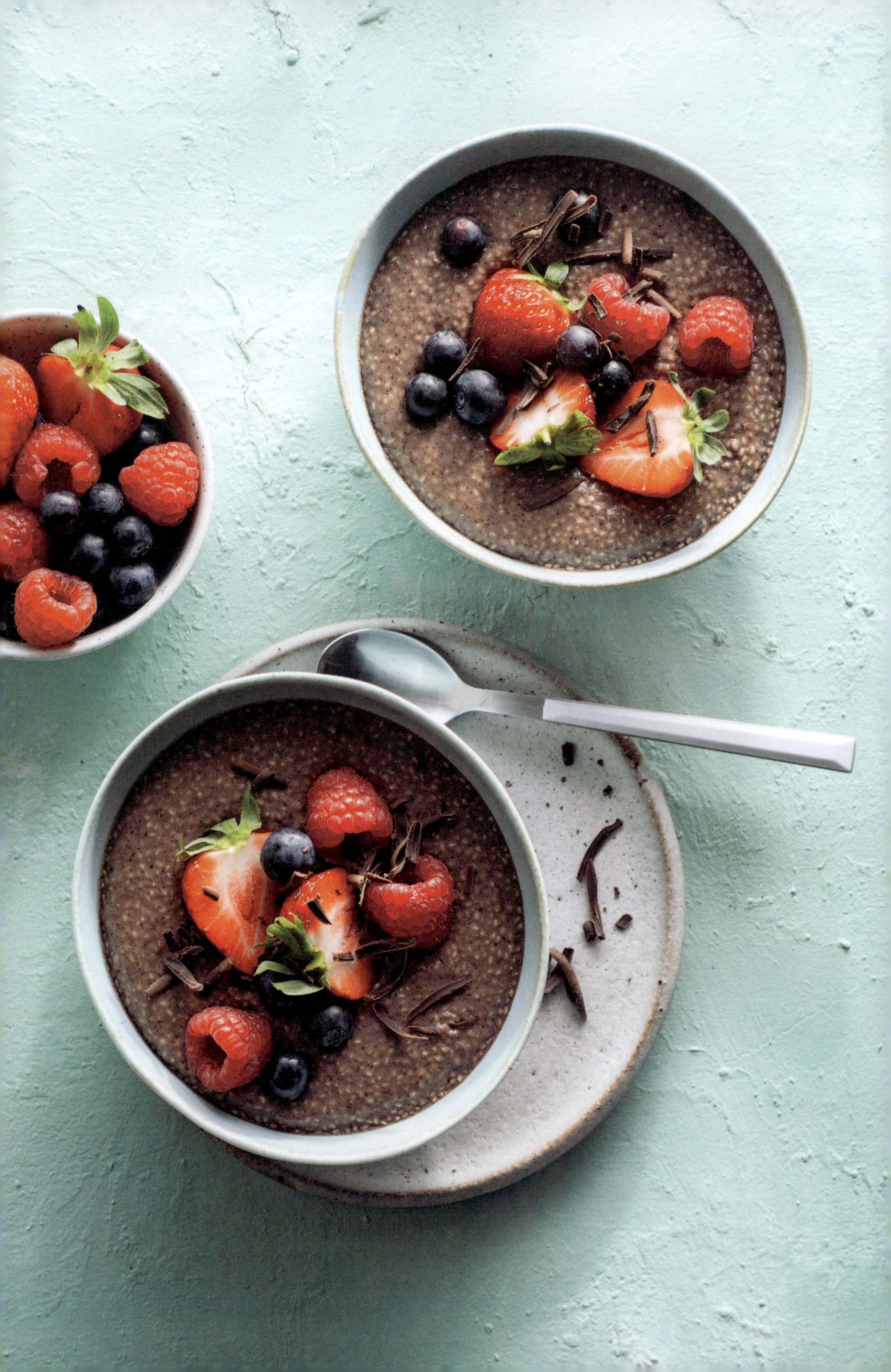

Makes 2

CHOCOLATE CHIA OVERNIGHT PUDDINGS

This already nutritious chia pudding recipe is boosted further with the addition of chocolate protein powder. It is also a great source of fibre. Prep the night before and take time to savour its gentle sweetness and rich cocoa flavour in the morning.

500 ml (2 cups) milk of your choice
2 tablespoons chocolate protein powder
1 teaspoon cacao powder (or good-quality cocoa powder)
2 tablespoons ground flaxseeds
2 teaspoons maple syrup
generous pinch of sea salt
4 tablespoons chia seeds

Toppings (optional)
2 teaspoons almond butter
plain Greek-style yoghurt
fresh berries
shavings of dark chocolate (70 per cent cocoa or higher)

Blend the milk, protein powder, cacoa or cocoa powder, flaxseeds, maple syrup and salt in a blender or food processor for 10 seconds, or until combined and smooth.

Transfer to a jug or bowl with the chia seeds and stir well, then leave for a minute. Stir again, then repeat one more time to ensure the chia seeds don't fall to the bottom and are evenly distributed.

Pour between two bowls, cover with plastic wrap and place in the fridge to set overnight.

Serve the following day with your favourite toppings.

02

LUNCH

When I take a diet history with my clients, I often notice that lunch is relegated to an afterthought or a grab-and-go – or it's skipped completely and replaced by an afternoon of grazing. But our mid-point meal is so important because a good one will get us through to dinner without reaching for a sugary snack. Lunch does not need to be complicated, but it does need to be balanced and satisfying. With just a little effort the night before or in the morning, you can enjoy a delicious and nourishing meal come lunchtime.

LUNCHBOXES

In my mind, there's no easier way to make a packed lunch than taking a bento box approach. Dedicating each section of the bento box to one food group speaks to my dietitian brain, and it's so easy to put together, especially early in the mornings when I'm not feeling particularly inspired! I open the fridge and pantry, and then it's just a matter of filling the compartments with whatever we have available and whatever I feel like eating that day. If you're also packing a lunchbox for kids, you can line and load them up assembly-style. I often pack myself many of the same foods as my kids, but I might do an adult variation depending on what I have on hand. The bento-style lunch is also great if you're working from home. The same principles apply, just arrange the various items on a large plate for a grazing experience and enjoy! Here are some combinations I come back to again and again.

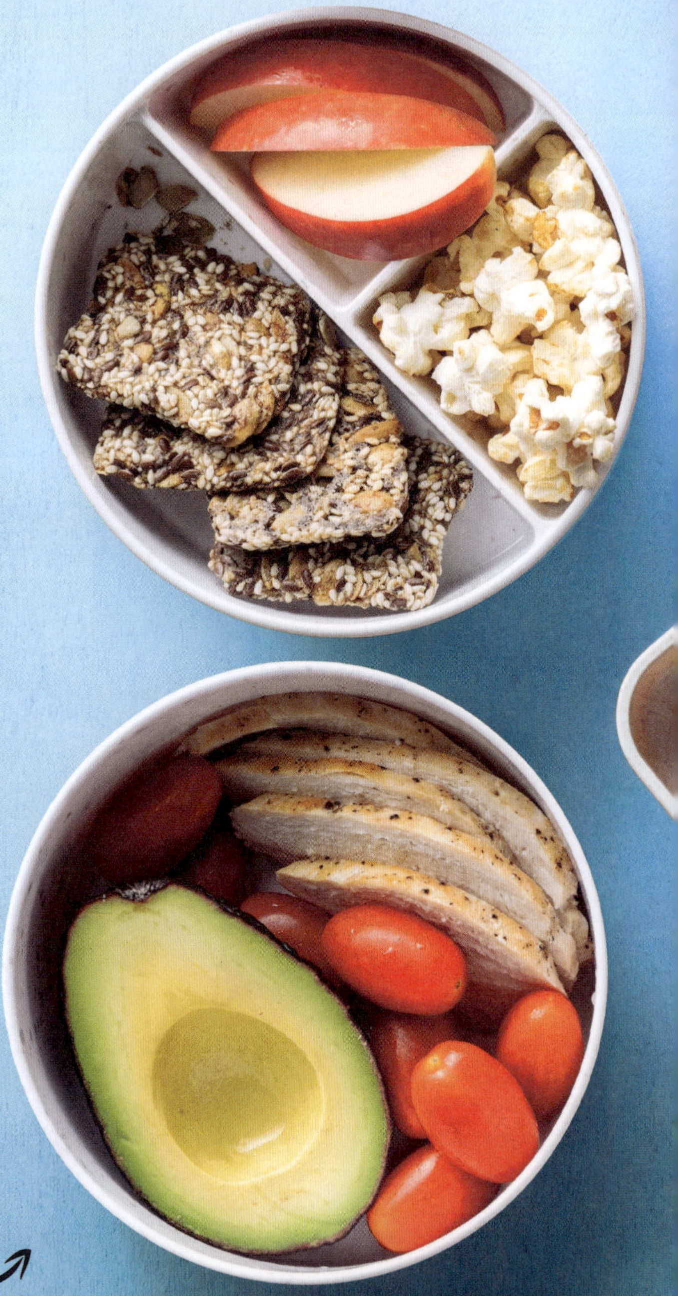

Compartment 2:

Healthy fats

CHOOSE: ½ small avocado, olives, nuts, seeds, natural peanut butter or other nut spread. Extra-virgin olive oil in a dressing also checks this box.

Compartment 1: Protein

TRY: 2 boiled eggs, leftover protein from dinner such as grilled chicken or tofu, a can of tuna, a packet of roast fava beans, edamame, yoghurt or hummus.

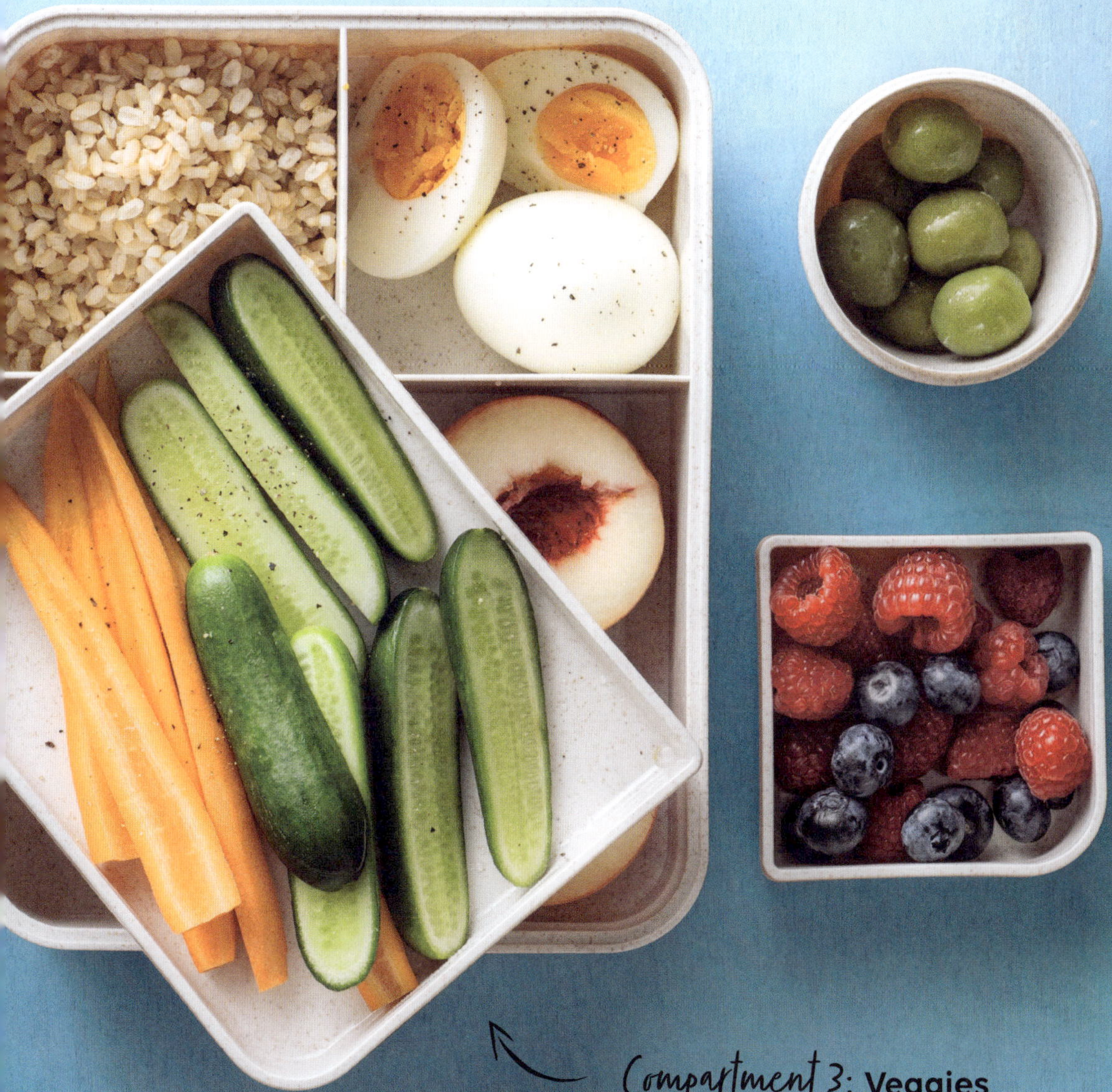

Compartment 3: Veggies

GO FOR: vegetables that travel well in a lunchbox. My favourites are cucumber, carrot, capsicum, radish, cherry tomatoes, fennel, celery and pickles.

Compartment 4: Good-quality carbohydrate

TRY: roast sweet potato, wholegrain crackers, sandwich made with wholegrain bread, brown rice, quinoa or a high-fibre wrap.

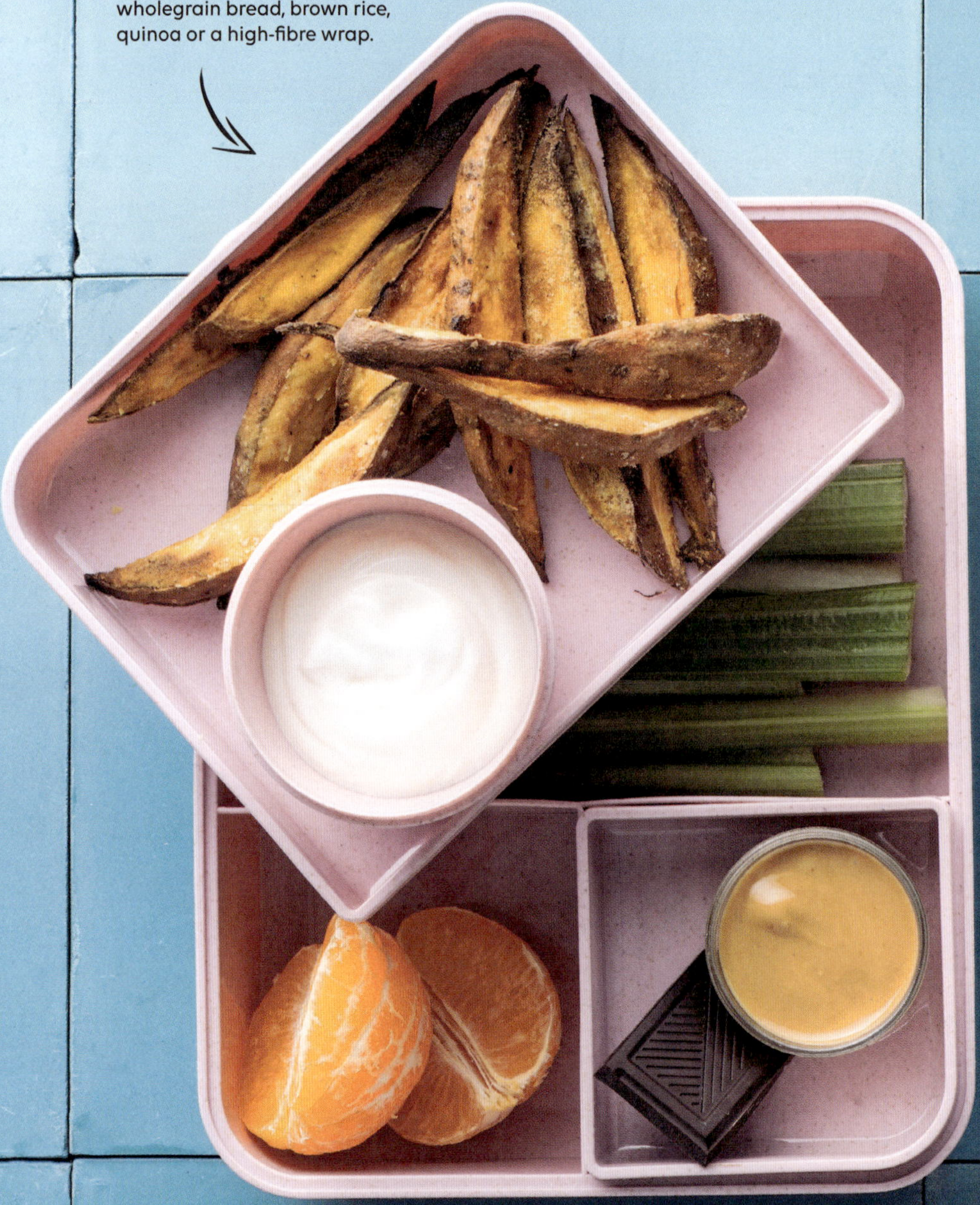

Compartment 5: Fruit

GO FOR: fruits that travel well and don't require a lot of prep. Mandarin, berries, apple, pear, kiwifruit, papaya or grapes are all good options. Steer clear of fruit that's likely to leak through the lunchbox, like watermelon.

Compartment 6: Something fun!

CHOOSE: a treat for you, such as a small chocolate, homemade cake, a muffin or a portion of one of the healthy treats in this book (see pages 202–219). If you prefer savoury snacks, then treats like pretzels or popcorn are good options.

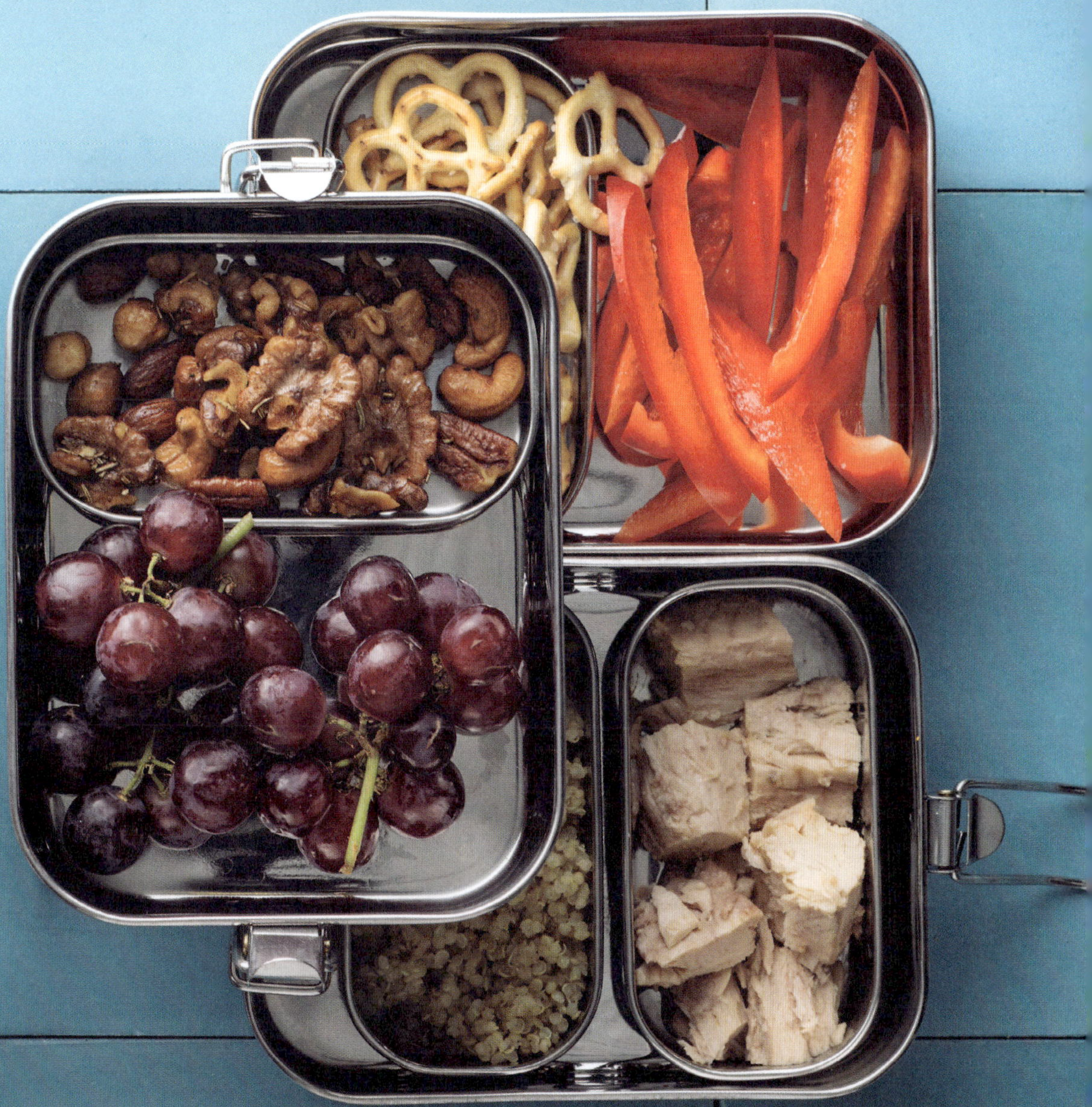

LEFTOVERS FOR LUNCH

One of my favourite lunchbox additions is leftovers from the night before. It doesn't have to be the whole dish, but rather an element of the meal, or a small spoonful of it with other snacks. Most of the dinners in the next chapter make for brilliant leftovers – the zucchini falafels and green mac and cheese are two of my favourites. Choose wisely and dinner leftovers will tick all the nutrition boxes for protein, healthy fats and veggies in your bento box. Throw in a piece of fruit and something fun, and you're good to go!

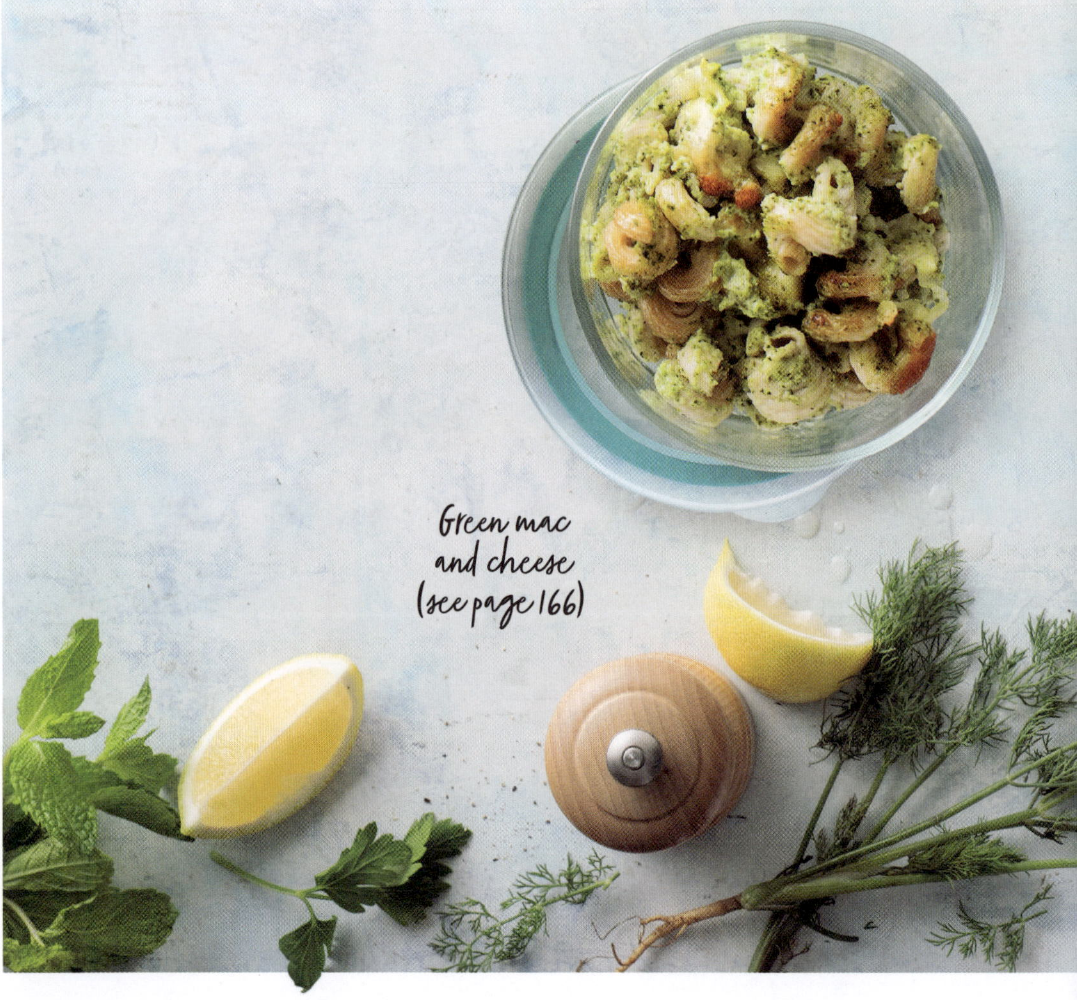

Green mac and cheese (see page 166)

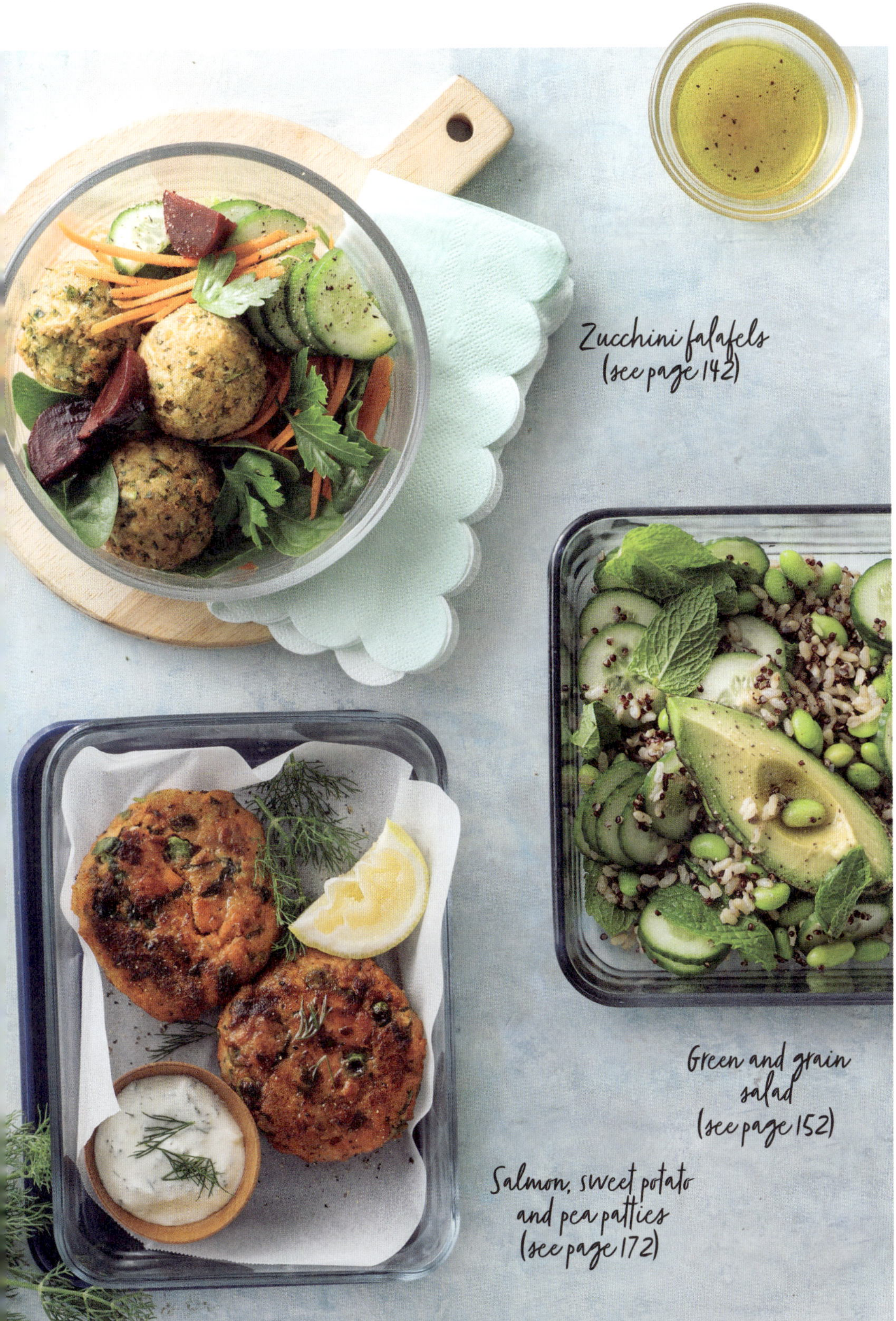

Zucchini falafels (see page 142)

Green and grain salad (see page 152)

Salmon, sweet potato and pea patties (see page 172)

03

DINNER

Most of us want to end our day sitting down to a delicious and nutritious home-cooked dinner with our loved ones. However, when we're busy, we often end up with a disappointing throw-together meal or an expensive takeaway. These recipes are here to help! They'll inspire you to incorporate some key power peri foods into your weekly repertoire, satisfying you as well as your family.

THE LADY DINNER

This style of eating has always been popular, but it's made a resurgence online in recent years under the guise of the 'girl dinner'. But for the sake of my lovely, accomplished readers (and myself!), I'm going to name it the 'lady dinner.' Essentially, it consists of bits and bobs from the fridge and pantry arranged on a plate and usually eaten in front of the TV or while reading a good book. I've always loved this way of eating so I'm happy to see it getting some time in the spotlight. It removes the pressure of 'cooking' a meal on those nights you're either not terribly hungry, late home from work or just can't be bothered! Choose your bits and bobs wisely and it ticks all the nutrition boxes, too.

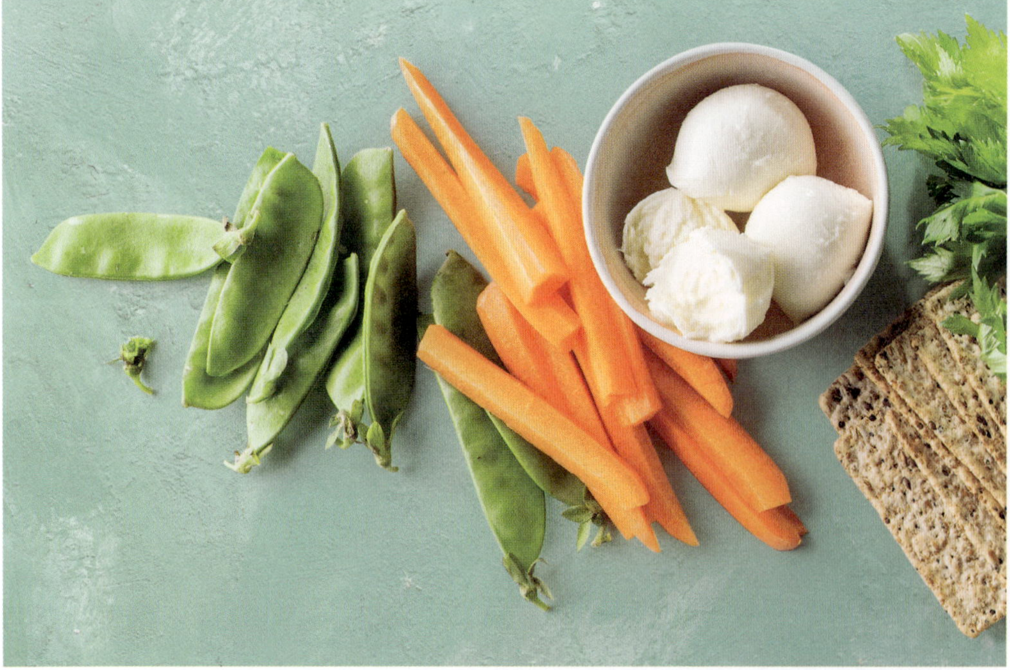

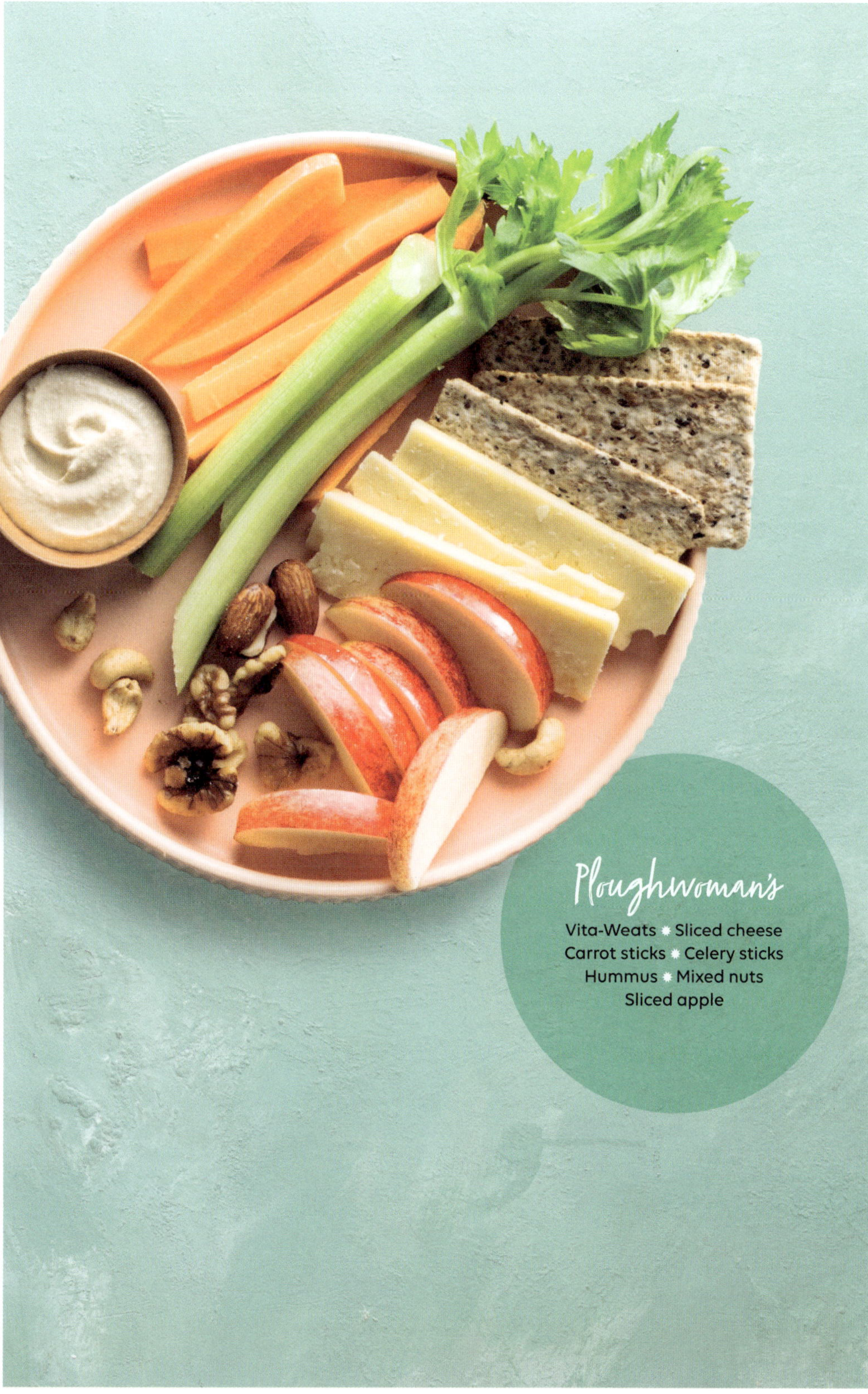

Ploughwoman's

Vita-Weats * Sliced cheese
Carrot sticks * Celery sticks
Hummus * Mixed nuts
Sliced apple

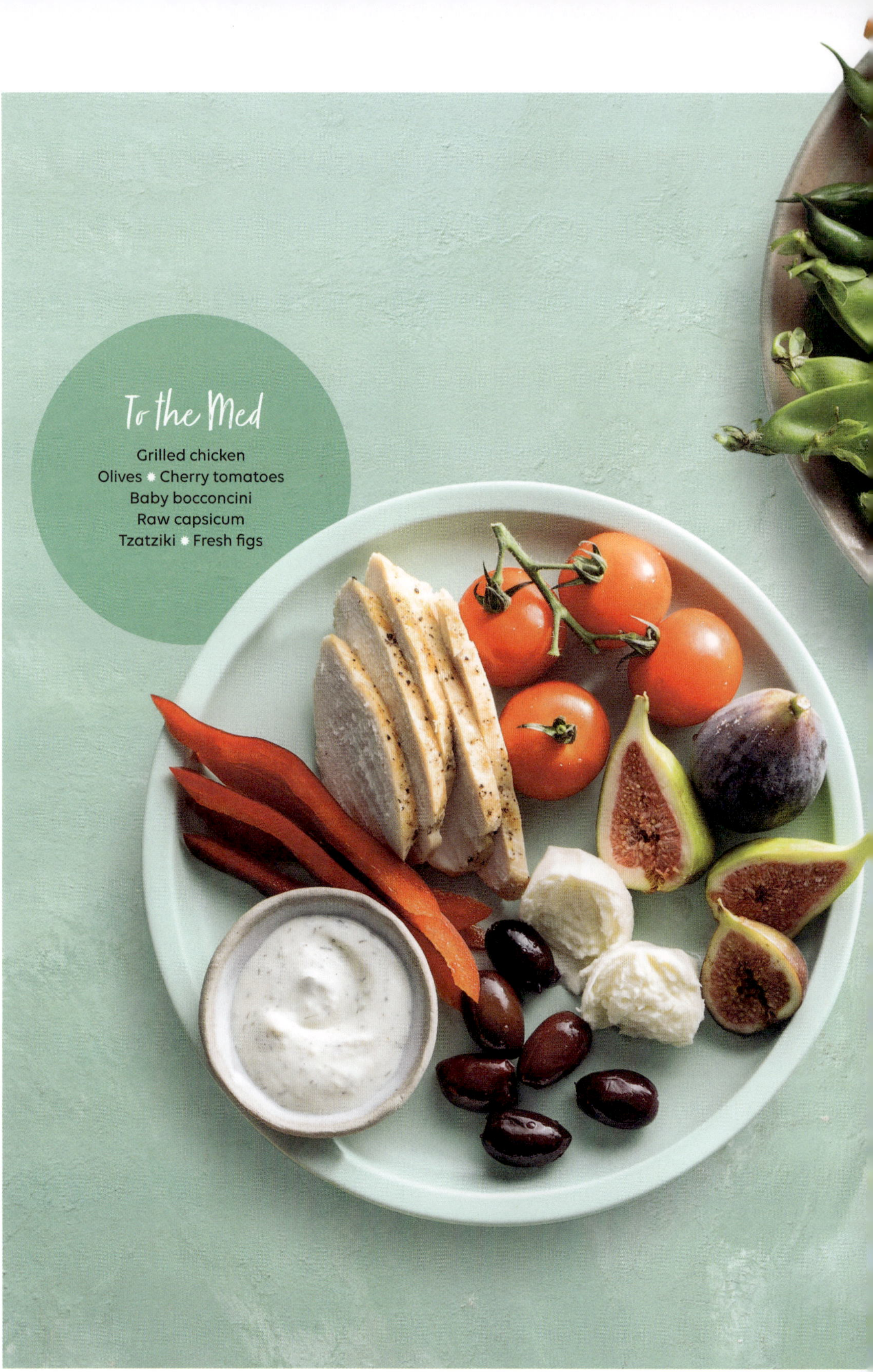
To the Med
Grilled chicken
Olives • Cherry tomatoes
Baby bocconcini
Raw capsicum
Tzatziki • Fresh figs

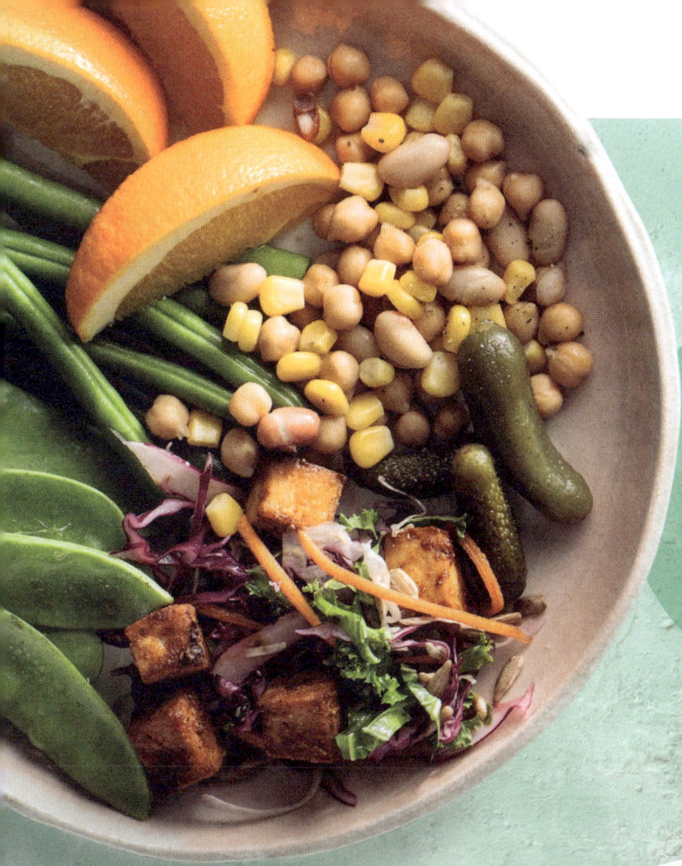

Crisp and zesty

Leftover Crispy barbecue tofu (see page 145)
Pickles • Raw snow peas and green beans
Mini can four-bean mix
Mini can corn kernels
Orange

The Scandi

Grainy crackers
Avocado
Smoked salmon
Broccoli sprouts
Boiled egg
Berries

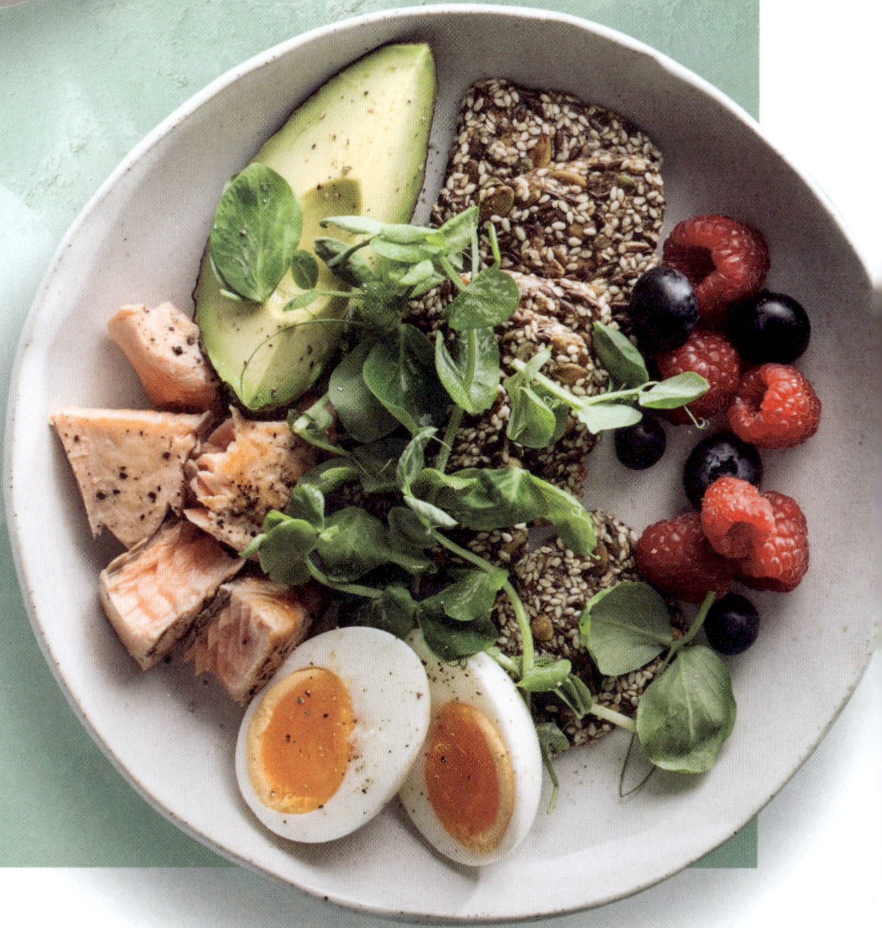

Serves 2
Vegetarian

SESAME-CRUSTED TOFU WEDGES

500 g very firm tofu
⅓ cup (80 ml) extra-virgin olive oil

Marinade
3 tablespoons tamari or soy sauce
2 tablespoons rice wine vinegar
1 tablespoon sesame oil
1 garlic clove, minced

Dipping sauce
3 tablespoons lime juice
2 tablespoons tamari or soy sauce
1 tablespoon honey or maple syrup
1 garlic clove, minced

Sesame crumb
30 g (¼ cup) cornflour
sea salt and freshly ground black pepper
2 eggs, whisked
60 g (1 cup) panko crumbs
80 g (½ cup) black/white sesame seeds

To serve (optional)
1 spring onion, green ends finely sliced
coriander leaves
dried chilli flakes or chilli oil
brown rice

If you're on the fence about tofu, I reckon this recipe will get you over the line! Tofu has very little flavour on its own – it is all about the preparation. Here we marinate it in Asian flavours before crumbing with panko and sesame. That's what elevates this amazing protein to star status.

Pat the block of tofu with paper towel, pressing down on each side to make sure it's as dry as possible (see Tip).

Cut the tofu in half, then cut each half into thirds. Cut each of these thirds on the diagonal so you end up with 12 small wedges.

Mix the marinade ingredients together in a large bowl, then add the tofu wedges and ensure they are well coated. Cover the bowl and place in the fridge for at least 1 hour. Turn the tofu over after 30 minutes.

While the tofu marinates, put all the ingredients for the dipping sauce in a small bowl and stir until combined.

Prepare three wide, shallow bowls with the sesame crumb ingredients: cornflour seasoned with salt and pepper in the first, whisked egg in the next and panko crumbs and sesame seeds in the third bowl.

Remove a piece of tofu from the marinade and press it into the cornflour until evenly coated. Shake off any excess and dip into the egg, then toss in the panko and sesame seed mixture until evenly coated. Set on a plate and repeat this process with the rest of the wedges.

Heat the olive oil in a frying pan over medium–high heat and place half the wedges in the pan. Cook for 2–3 minutes, or until the tofu is turning golden and crispy underneath. Turn over and cook for another few minutes, then transfer to a plate lined with paper towel. Repeat with the remaining wedges.

Enjoy with the dipping sauce and any or all of the suggested serving options.

TIP FOR CRISPY TOFU

The drier you can get your tofu, the more flavourful and crispy it will be. To really get the moisture out of it, press it dry with a few pieces of paper towel, then wrap it in a few new pieces of paper towel, pop it on a plate and set a heavy saucepan on top of it. After 5 minutes, it should be nice and dry.

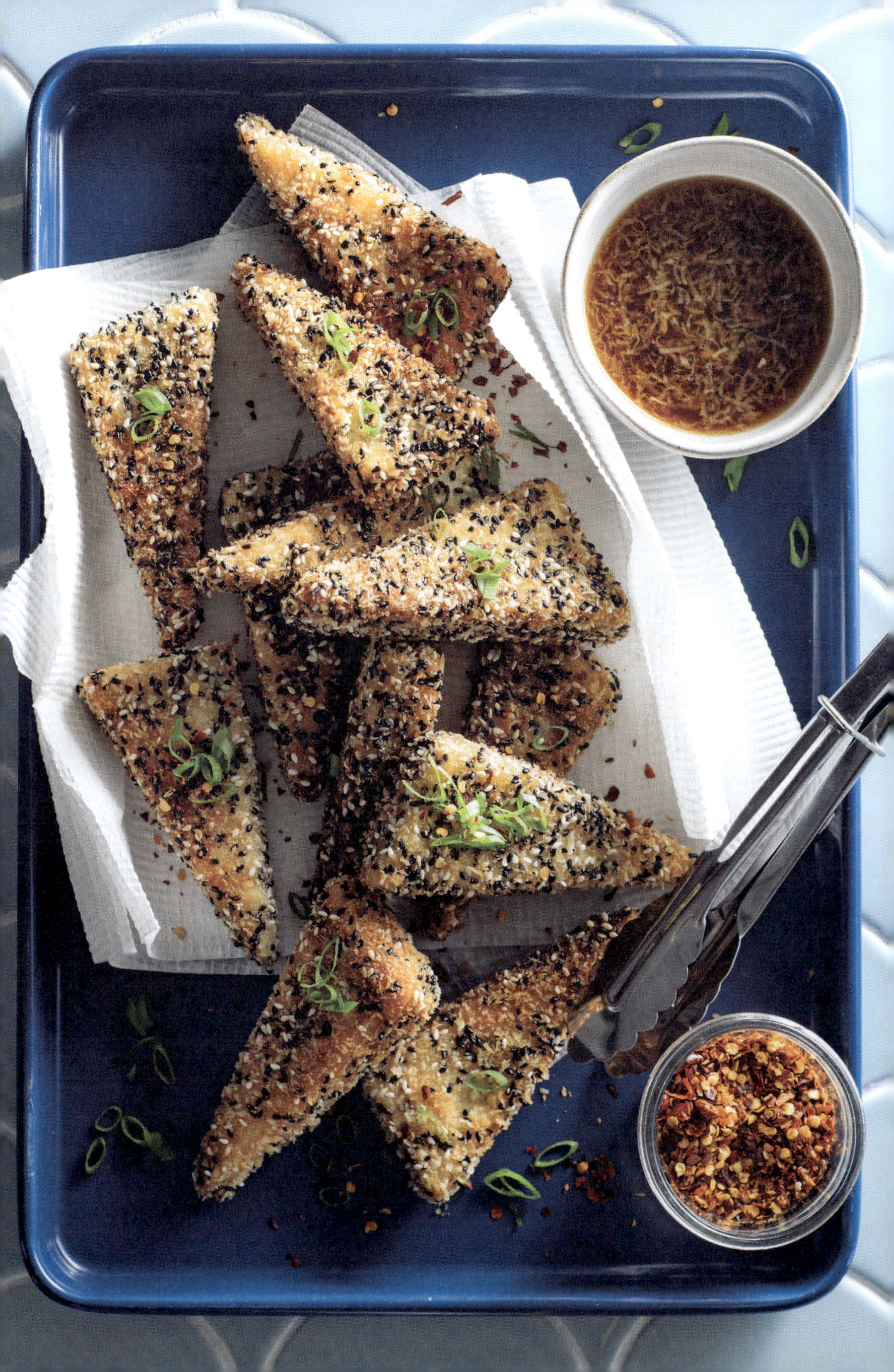

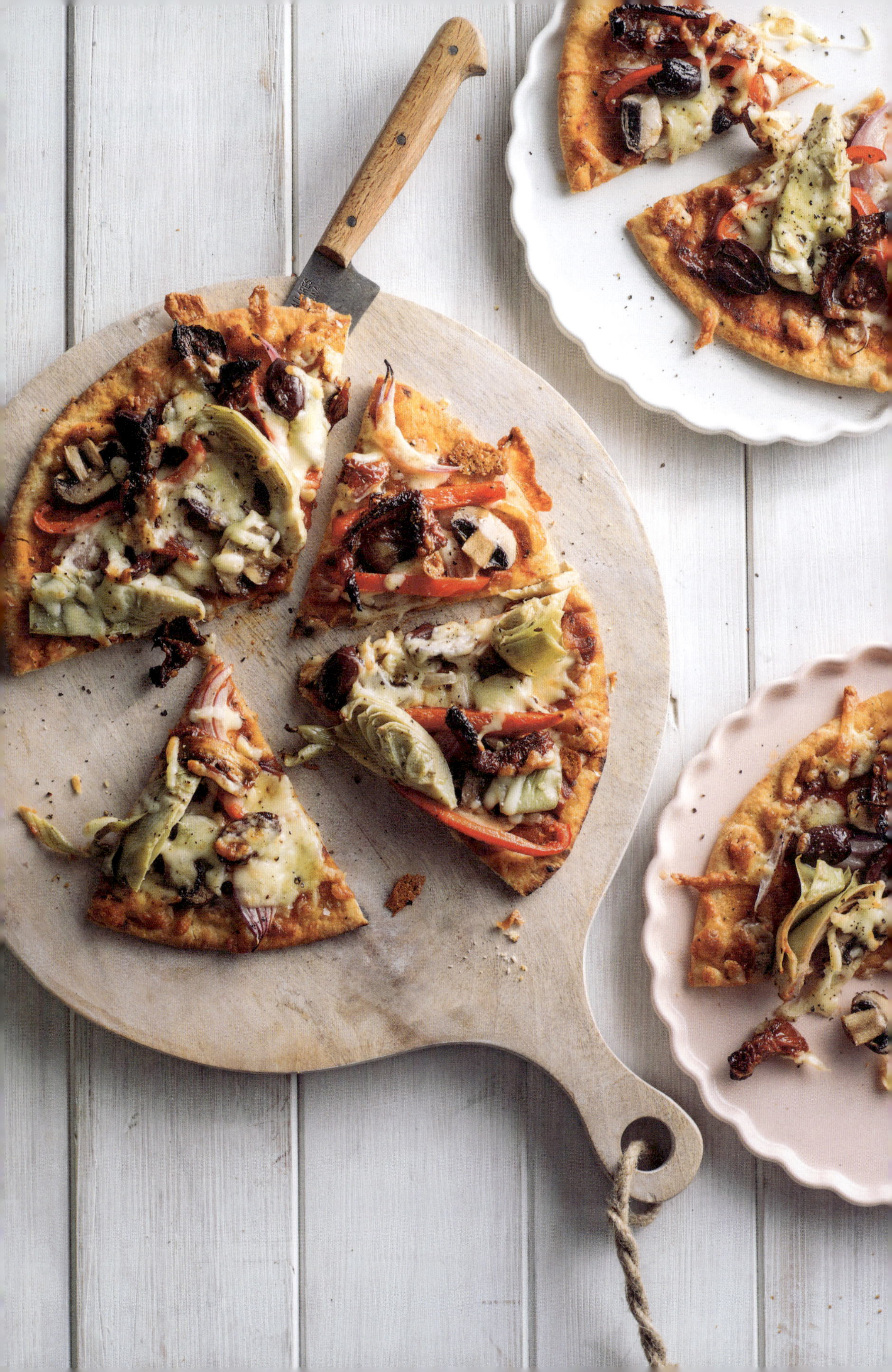

Serves 2
Vegetarian

THE EASIEST ANTIPASTI PIZZA

We make homemade pizzas every other week at our house because they're such an easy dinner – and not to mention a popular choice with every family member. The difference in flavour and nutrition between these pizzas and the ones my husband occasionally orders for himself is like chalk and cheese! These use a high-protein and lower-carbohydrate base, which all major supermarkets stock. Look for a brand containing less than 30 g of carbohydrate per base. Then, it's all about the toppings! I go for a very simple store-bought pizza sauce – just tomato puree, garlic and herbs, and then top each pizza with all the veggies I can possibly squeeze on.

- 2 lower-carbohydrate, high-protein pizza bases
- 3 tablespoons pizza sauce
- ½ small red onion, finely sliced
- 50 g (½ cup) mushrooms, finely sliced
- ¼ red capsicum, finely sliced
- 8 pitted olives, sliced
- 1 x 200 g jar marinated artichokes, drained well
- 2 tablespoons sundried tomatoes, finely chopped
- 50 g (⅓ cup) shredded pizza cheese or mozzarella

Preheat the oven to 200°C and place your pizza trays or stones in there to get really hot (this will help to make the base crispy).

Top the pizza bases with the pizza sauce, leaving a 1–2 cm border around the edge of each pizza.

Top each pizza with all the remaining ingredients, finishing with the shredded cheese.

Place on the hot trays or stones and bake for 15 minutes, or until golden and crispy around the edges and the cheese is melted and golden. Allow to cool for a minute or two, then eat right away.

Serves 2
Vegetarian

TOFU AND SHIITAKE MUSHROOM RAMEN

Ramen is one of my favourite comfort foods: the rich broth and slurpy noodles are just so delicious. However, it can be very high in carbohydrates and salt, and very light on protein and veggies. My recipe is a lovely balanced version that gives the best of the comforting ramen, boosted with peri-power ingredients for a gorgeous and nutritious meal.

200 g very firm tofu (see Tip on page 136)
sea salt and freshly ground black pepper
2 tablespoons extra-virgin olive oil
180 g soba (buckwheat) noodles
80 g (1 cup) snow peas
45 g (1 cup) baby spinach leaves
1 spring onion, sliced

Broth

750 ml (3 cups) vegetable or chicken stock, or bone broth
2 teaspoons minced ginger
1 tablespoon miso paste
2 teaspoons tamari or soy sauce
1 teaspoon sesame oil
6 dried shiitake mushrooms

To serve (optional)

sesame seeds
chilli oil or Sriracha sauce

Pat the block of tofu dry with paper towel, then cut into 2 cm cubes. Season with salt and pepper.

Heat the olive oil in a frying pan over medium–high heat, then add the tofu and cook for 3–4 minutes, stirring regularly, until golden and crispy. Transfer to paper towel.

Put all the broth ingredients into a saucepan and bring to a gentle simmer.

Add the noodles to the broth and simmer for 2 minutes (or follow the packet instructions). Turn off the heat, add the snow peas and baby spinach, then place the lid on the pan for a minute.

Divide the ramen between bowls. Serve topped with the crispy tofu and spring onion. Sprinkle over some sesame seeds and add a drizzle of chilli sauce, if you like.

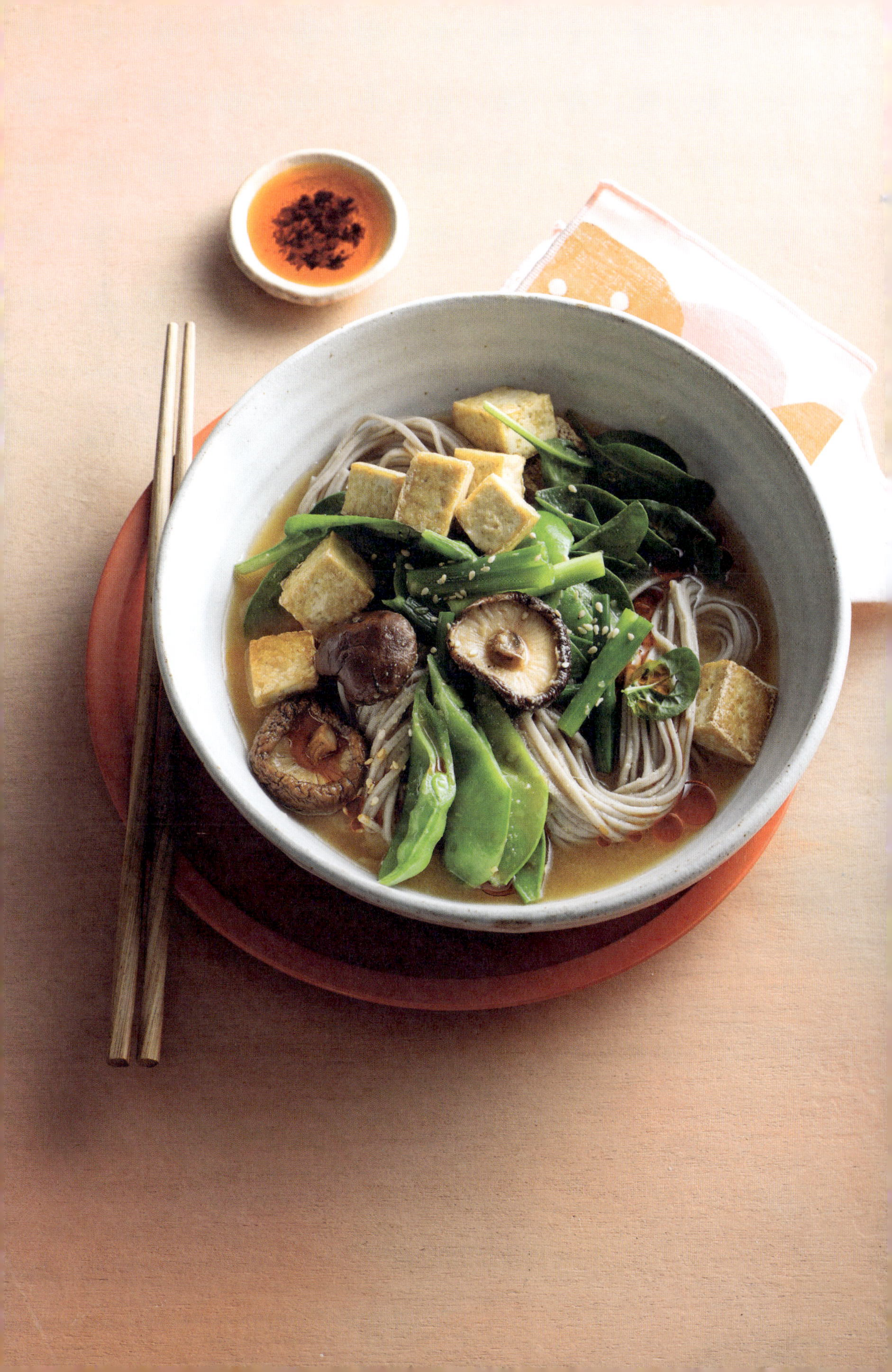

Serves 4
Vegetarian

ZUCCHINI FALAFEL KEBABS

Kebabs may be beloved, but they're also notorious for being very calorific because takeaway portions tend to be huge and include fatty cuts of meat. This version is much lighter and so much better for the body, thanks to the high-fibre wraps, lots of lovely salad and these tasty zucchini falafels.

125 ml (½ cup) extra-virgin olive oil

Zucchini falafel
320 g (2 cups) cooked or canned chickpeas, drained and rinsed
1 small onion, quartered
2 garlic cloves, minced
10 g (½ cup) flat-leaf parsley leaves
1 zucchini, coarsely grated (squeeze out as much liquid as possible)
50 g (⅓ cup) wholemeal or chickpea (besan) flour
1 teaspoon sea salt
freshly ground black pepper
1 teaspoon ground cumin
1 teaspoon ground coriander
juice of ½ lemon

To serve
4 wholegrain high-fibre wraps
4 heaped tablespoons hummus
1 avocado, quartered
1 large carrot, grated
120 g (2 cups) finely shredded iceberg lettuce
1 Lebanese cucumber, diced
45 g (1 cup) baby spinach leaves
160 g (1 cup) cooked beetroot (if canned, whole beets, pat dry with paper towel and roughly sliced)
your favourite sauces (optional)

To make the falafel, pulse the chickpeas, onion, garlic and parsley in a food processor until well combined. Spoon the mixture into a large bowl and add the zucchini, flour, salt, a generous pinch of pepper, the spices and lemon juice. Mix together gently with a spoon. Using damp hands, roll about 2 heaped tablespoons of falafel mixture into a small ball, then set on a plate. Repeat until the mixture is used up. You should end up with around 24 small falafel.

Heat the olive oil in a heavy-based frying pan and cook the falafel in batches, using a slotted spoon to gently turn each one until golden all over. Once cooked, transfer to a plate lined with paper towel to drain. Repeat until all the falafel mixture has been cooked.

Lay out the wraps. Dollop a tablespoon of hummus onto the centre of each wrap and use the back of a spoon to spread it. Place the avocado slices on top of the hummus, then top with the other salad ingredients.

Add 4–6 falafel to each wrap, breaking them up a little on top of the salad.

Top with your favourite sauces, if you like, then roll the wraps up tightly and enjoy. Have napkins on hand because it may get messy, but that's part of the fun!

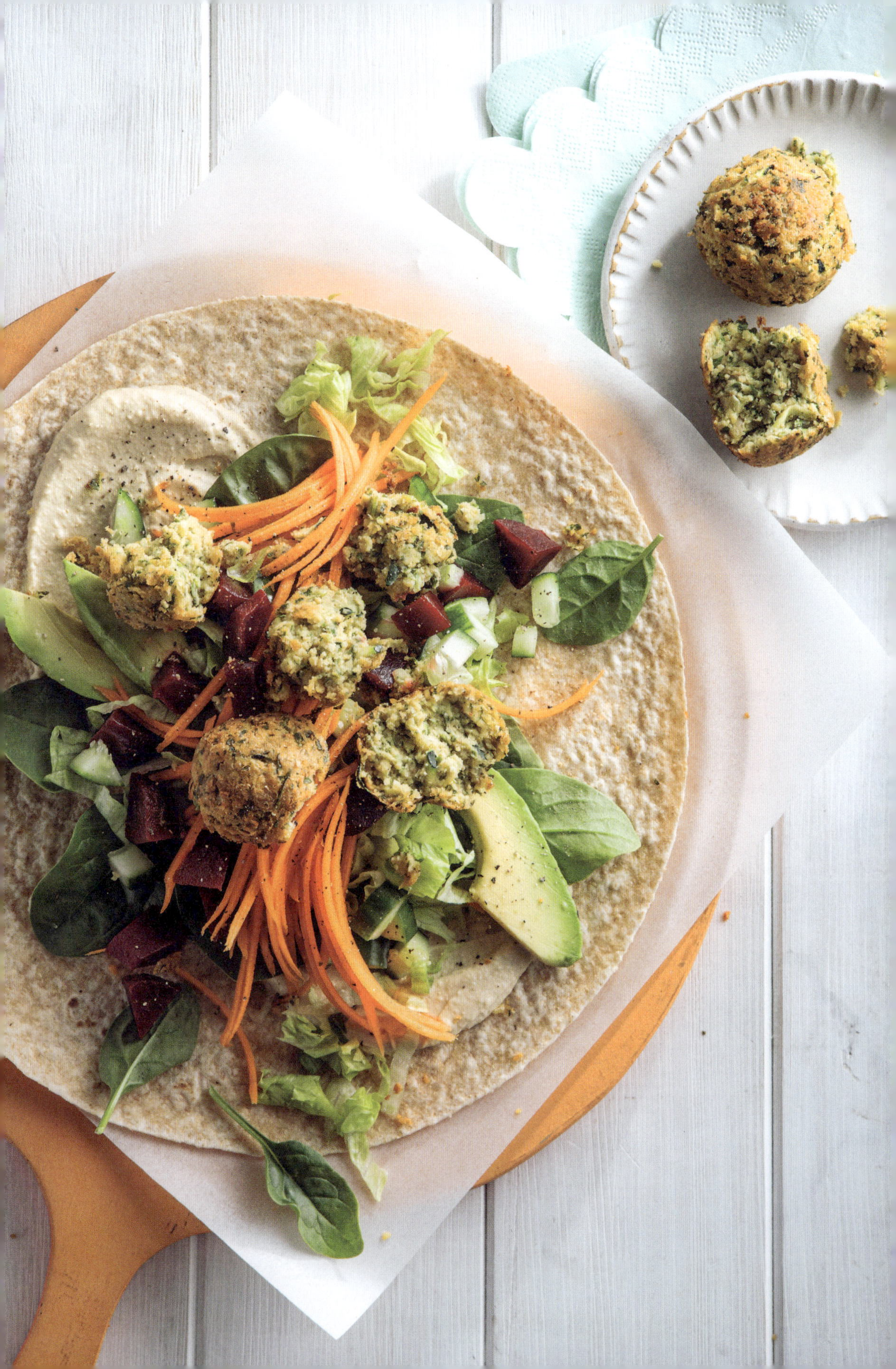

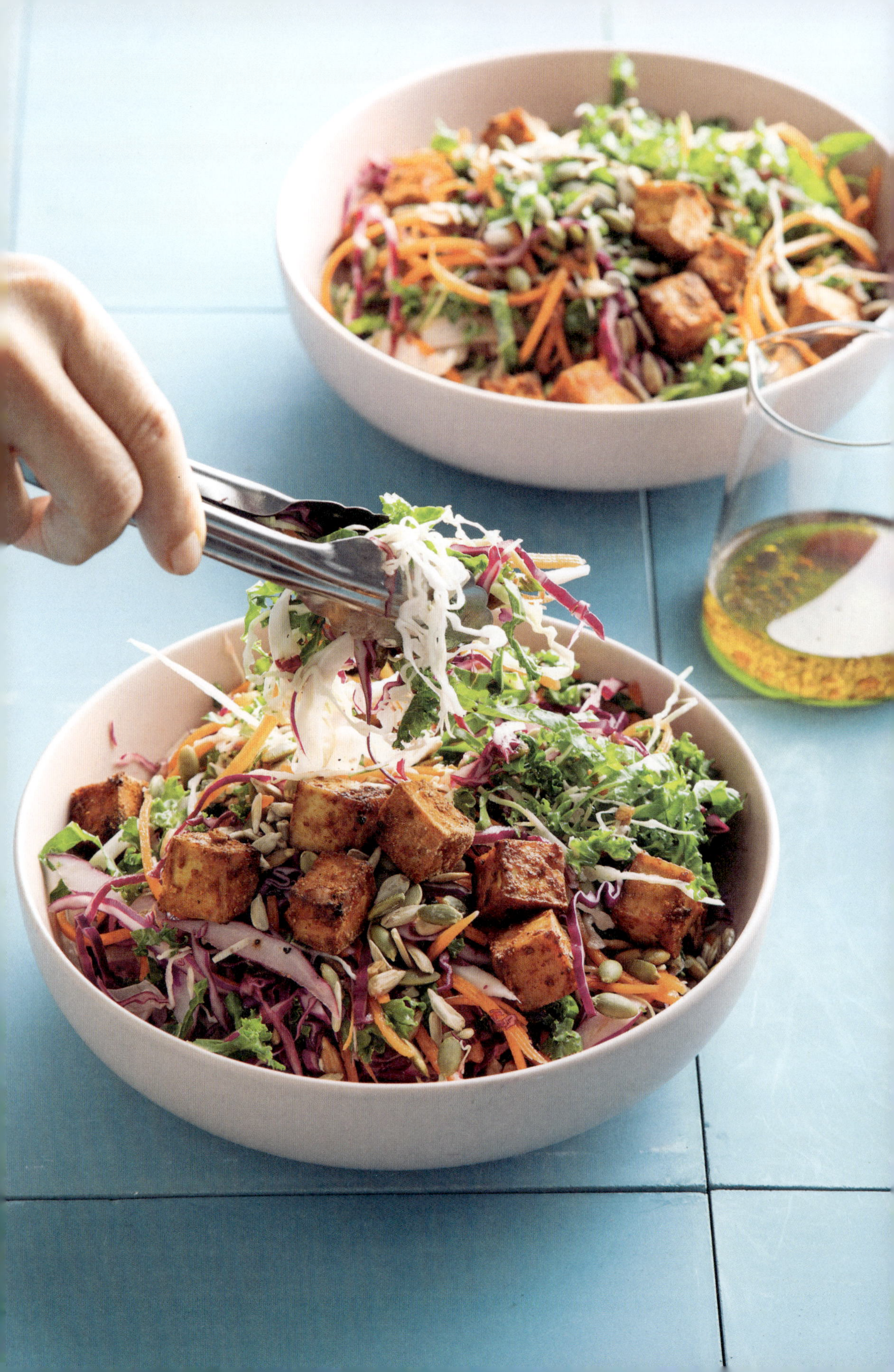

Serves 4
Vegetarian

CRISPY BARBECUE TOFU WITH KALE SLAW

The air fryer has to be one of the handiest kitchen tools around. I love making protein super-crunchy using minimal or even zero oil. This recipe illustrates how easy it is to achieve amazing flavour and texture with tofu. It pairs brilliantly with the slaw, but I've also served it as part of a poke or buddha bowl, with a leafy salad or brown rice and veggies – it's lovely and versatile.

extra-virgin olive oil spray

Crispy barbecue-flavoured tofu

- 500 g very firm tofu (see Tip on page 136)
- 2 teaspoons tamari or soy sauce
- 1 teaspoon garlic powder
- 1 teaspoon onion powder
- 1 teaspoon smoked or sweet paprika
- 1 teaspoon brown sugar
- 2 teaspoons cornflour
- 1 teaspoon extra-virgin olive oil
- pinch of freshly ground black pepper

Dressing

- 3 tablespoons extra-virgin olive oil
- 3 tablespoons red wine vinegar
- 1 garlic clove, minced
- sea salt and freshly ground pepper

Kale slaw

- 70 g (1 cup) finely sliced kale leaves
- 150 g (2 cups) finely sliced red cabbage
- 150 g (2 cups) finely sliced white cabbage
- 2 large carrots, grated
- 2 spring onions, finely sliced
- 3 tablespoons toasted pumpkin seeds or sunflower seeds

Dice the tofu into 2 cm pieces, then place on paper towel and press down gently with more paper towel to remove as much liquid as possible.

Put the tofu in a container with the tamari or soy sauce and toss until well coated.

Put the remaining ingredients for the crispy tofu in a large container and mix well. Add the tofu, cover with a lid or plate and toss together well until the tofu is completely coated in all the flavours.

Heat the air-fryer to 200°C. Arrange the tofu around the base of the air-fryer basket so it's well spread out, then spray lightly with the olive oil. Cook for 10 minutes, then open the lid and give the tofu a shake around. Cook for another 5 minutes, then turn off the air-fryer. The tofu should be golden and crunchy by this point.

While the tofu cooks, make a dressing for the slaw by whisking all of the dressing ingredients in a salad bowl.

For the slaw, add the kale to the dressing and massage with your hands for a few minutes (this softens the texture and flavour of the leaves). Add the cabbage, carrot and spring onion, then toss together to coat in the dressing. Top the kale slaw with the toasted seeds and the hot, crispy tofu.

Serves 6
Vegetarian

LENTIL RAGU

As you can see from the photo opposite, the sauce for this beautiful pasta dish closely resembles a traditional bolognese. However, it's entirely plant-based. Red lentils, which form the base of the sauce, are high in peri-friendly nutrients such as fibre and protein. Another bonus is that they are much more cost-effective than meat, meaning you can enjoy bolognese more often!

- 250 g (1 cup) dried red lentils
- 2 tablespoons extra-virgin olive oil
- 1 small red onion, finely diced
- 2 garlic cloves, minced
- sea salt and freshly ground black pepper
- 3 tablespoons tomato paste
- 1 tablespoon tomato sauce
- 1 x 400 g can crushed tomatoes
- 1 vegetable stock cube

To serve

- 500 g wholemeal or spelt spaghetti
- grated parmesan
- flat-leaf parsley leaves, roughly chopped (optional)
- dried chilli flakes or chilli oil (optional)

Soak the lentils in a bowl of water for 15 minutes, then drain.

Heat the olive oil in a large frying pan or saucepan over medium–high heat. Add the onion and garlic, then season with salt and pepper. Cook for around 3 minutes, or until the onion begins to soften and turn translucent. Stir in the tomato paste and cook for another minute.

Add the lentils to the pan with the tomato sauce, the can of tomatoes and a full can's worth of water. Crumble in the stock cube, then stir and bring to a simmer. Once simmering, reduce the heat to low and partially cover the pan as the ragu cooks for another 15 minutes.

Meanwhile, cook the pasta according to the packet instructions, then drain, saving a cup of the pasta water.

Add the pasta to the sauce, and if the sauce needs loosening, add a splash or two of reserved pasta water as needed. Divide between serving bowls and top with grated parmesan, plus parsley and chilli if you wish.

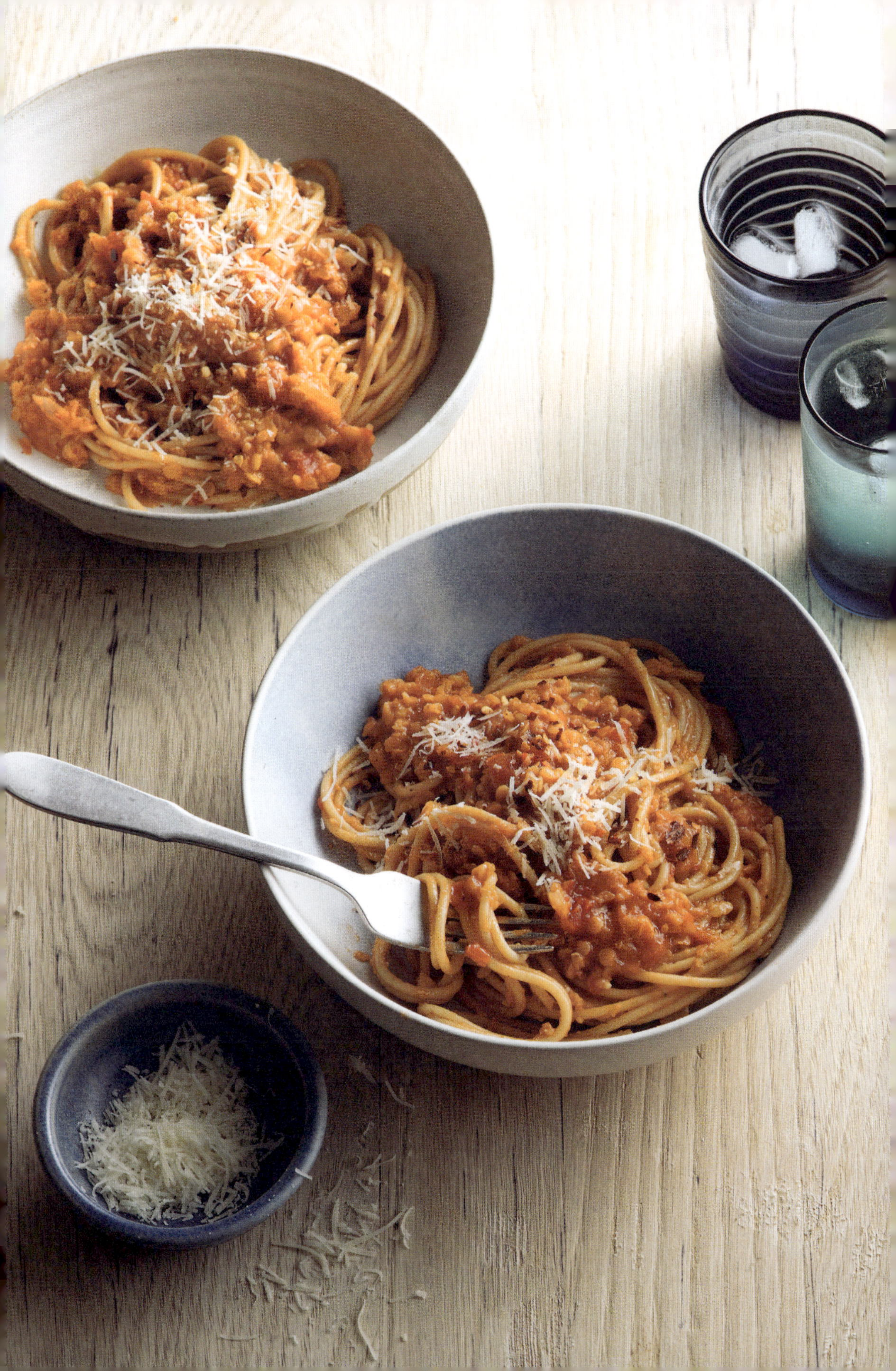

Serves 4–6
Vegetarian

PROTEIN-PACKED PERI CURRY

A precious ingredient during peri and beyond, tofu is also an inexpensive source of protein when compared to animal proteins, plus it's better for the environment. But many of us are still not sure how to make it tasty! As I've mentioned, the key is a delicious sauce or marinade. This curry is a case in point: it's so good, my husband eats it and barely registers it's tofu!

1 tablespoon extra-virgin olive oil
1 onion, roughly diced
2 teaspoons minced garlic
2 teaspoons minced ginger
2 teaspoons curry powder
1 teaspoon ground cumin
½ teaspoon ground turmeric
¼ teaspoon ground cinnamon
sea salt and freshly ground black pepper
500 g very firm tofu, diced into 1–2 cm pieces
1 x 400 g can chickpeas, drained and rinsed
375 ml (1½ cups) tomato passata
125 ml (½ cup) vegetable or chicken stock
1–2 handfuls of baby spinach leaves
125 g (½ cup) plain yoghurt

To serve
brown rice
coriander leaves (optional)
pappadums (optional)

Heat the olive oil in a large frying pan over medium–high heat and add the onion. Cook for a few minutes, or until the onion softens and becomes translucent.

Add the garlic, ginger and spices, then season well with salt and pepper. Stir together well until fragrant.

Add the diced tofu and chickpeas to the pan, then stir in the passata and stock. Bring to a simmer, then lower the heat and cook for another 10 minutes, or until the sauce has thickened a little. Stir through the spinach.

Serve the curry spooned over rice, with a dollop of yoghurt, and some coriander and poppadums, if you like.

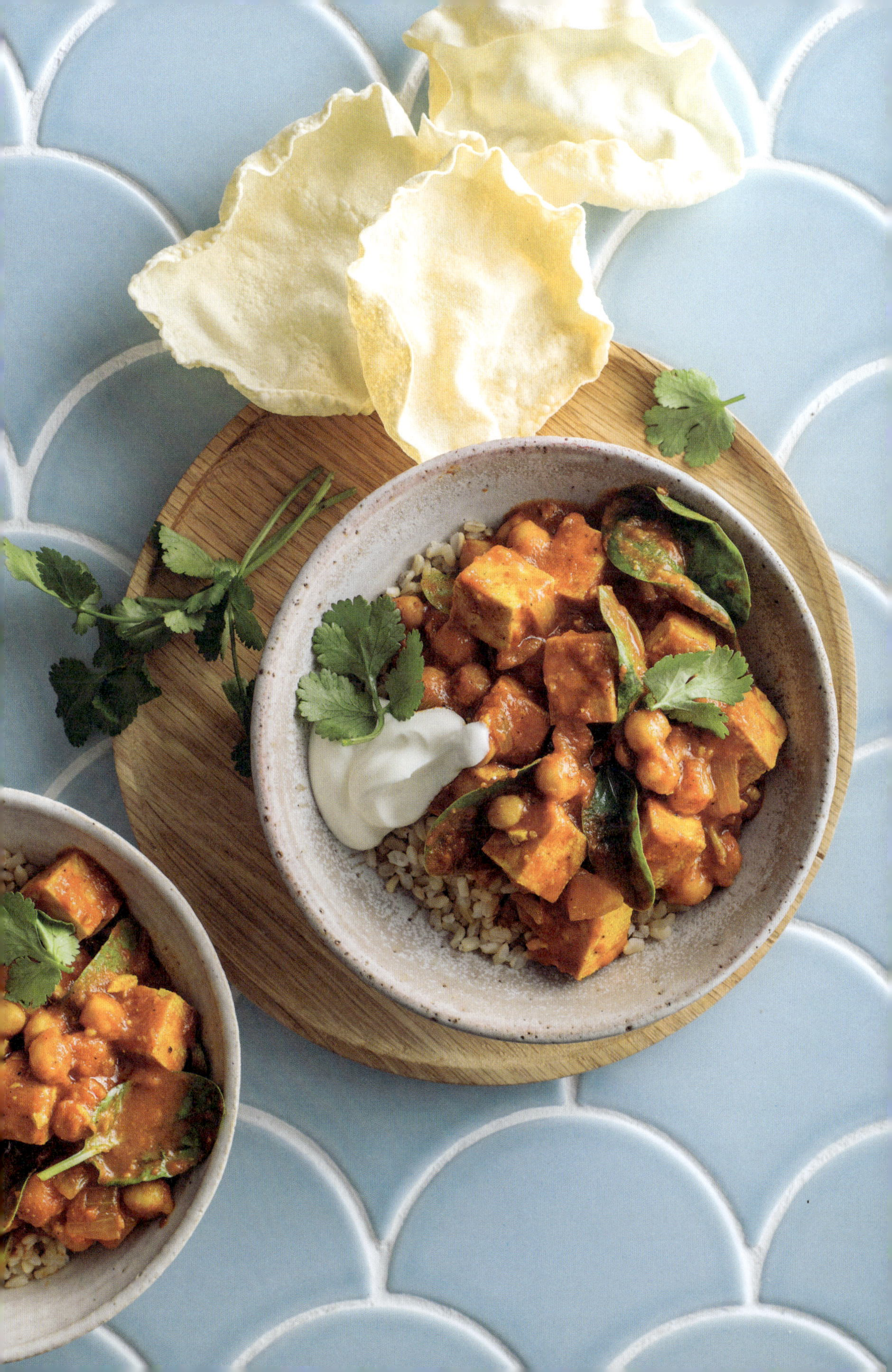

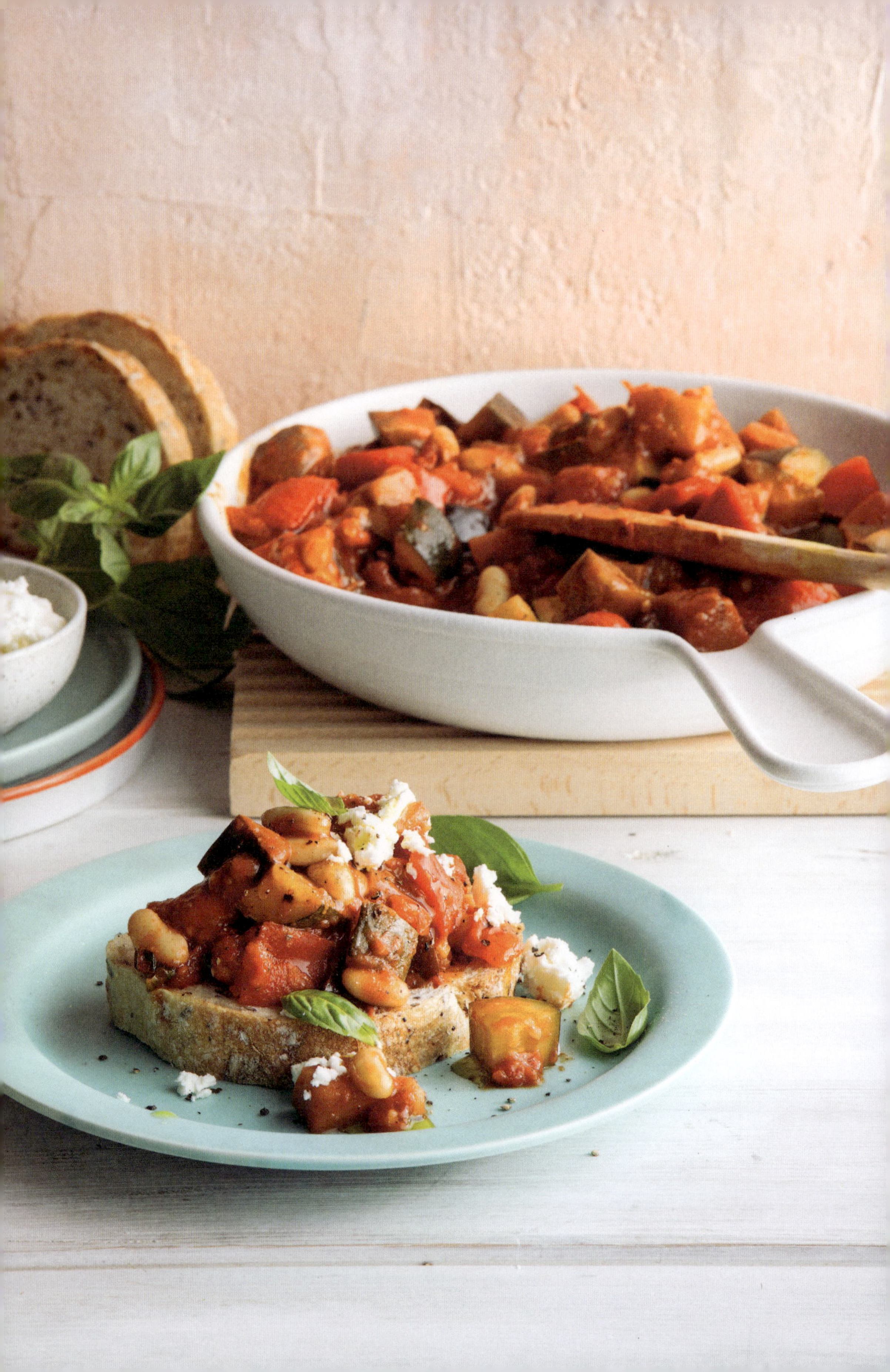

BEAN RATATOUILLE

Serves 4–6 as a main, 6–8 as a side
Vegetarian

I'll often eat this protein-boosted ratatouille on its own, or with a slice of sourdough, but it also makes a beautiful accompaniment to white fish or chicken. Save any leftovers for quick lunches or the amazing breakfast shakshuka on page 111.

- 1 large eggplant, diced into 1 cm pieces
- sea salt
- 3 tablespoons extra-virgin olive oil
- 1 red onion, roughly chopped
- 2 zucchini, trimmed and diced into 1 cm pieces
- 1 red capsicum, deseeded and diced into 1 cm pieces
- freshly ground black pepper
- 4 garlic cloves, finely chopped
- 2 tablespoons tomato paste
- ½ teaspoon dried oregano
- 1 teaspoon smoked or sweet paprika
- 2 x 400 g cans crushed or diced tomatoes
- 1 teaspoon sugar (or tomato sauce)
- 1 x 400 g can butter or cannellini beans, drained and rinsed
- small handful of basil leaves, roughly torn
- crumbled feta, to serve (optional)
- good bread, to serve

Place the diced eggplant in a colander and sprinkle over a couple of generous pinches of salt. Leave for 5 minutes so the salt has time to draw out the liquid.

Heat the olive oil in a large, heavy-based frying pan over medium–high heat, then add the onion and cook for 2–3 minutes, or until translucent.

Add the eggplant, zucchini and capsicum to the pan and season with salt and pepper. Cook for another 5 minutes until the vegetables have softened. Add the garlic, tomato paste, oregano and paprika. Stir to combine, then add the canned tomatoes, sugar or sauce and beans.

Stir well, then bring to a simmer and lower the heat. Cover and cook for around 10 minutes, then remove the lid and continue cooking for another 5 minutes, or until most of the liquid has cooked away and the vegetables have broken down.

Serve the ratatouille sprinkled with basil and crumbled feta, if you like, with a slice of bread to mop up the sauce.

Serves 2
Vegetarian

GREEN AND GRAIN SALAD

This beautiful green, grainy salad is so satisfying and wholesome. It will keep you feeling full for hours and is jam-packed with goodness. Keep leftovers in an airtight container in the fridge without the avocado (because it will go brown), then dice fresh avocado before you serve.

- 200 g (1 cup) brown rice and quinoa (see Notes)
- 135 g (¾ cup) shelled edamame, thawed (See Notes)
- 1 small cucumber, thinly sliced
- 1 tablespoon finely chopped mint, plus extra leaves to serve
- 1 small avocado, sliced
- 2 tablespoons pumpkin seeds

Dressing

- zest and juice of 1 lemon
- 1 teaspoon honey
- 1 tablespoon extra-virgin olive oil
- sea salt and freshly ground black pepper

Cook the rice and quinoa according to the packet instructions.

Meanwhile, bring a small saucepan of water to the boil and fill another bowl with cold water. Add the edamame to the boiling water, cook for 3 minutes, then drain and plunge straight into the cold water to stop them cooking further. Drain again, then set aside to dry on a clean tea towel or paper towel.

Add the dressing ingredients to a small bowl or jar with a lid and mix or shake together well.

Use a fork to fluff up the cooked rice and quinoa, then transfer to a bowl with the edamame, cucumber and mint. Drizzle the dressing on top, then toss together.

Divide the salad between two bowls and top with avocado and pumpkin seeds, to serve.

NOTES

Mixed grains: Several brands make brown rice and quinoa mixtures these days, but if you prefer to make your own blend, cook ¾ brown rice with ¼ quinoa, using the instructions on the rice packet for guidance. Alternatively, you can also use just brown rice or just quinoa rather than a mix.

Edamame: You'll find edamame in the frozen section of most supermarkets these days, as well as in specialist or Asian grocers. They come whole, in their pods, or podded. Whole edamame are great steamed for a snack or as part of a dinner, while podded edamame are more convenient for recipes like this one.

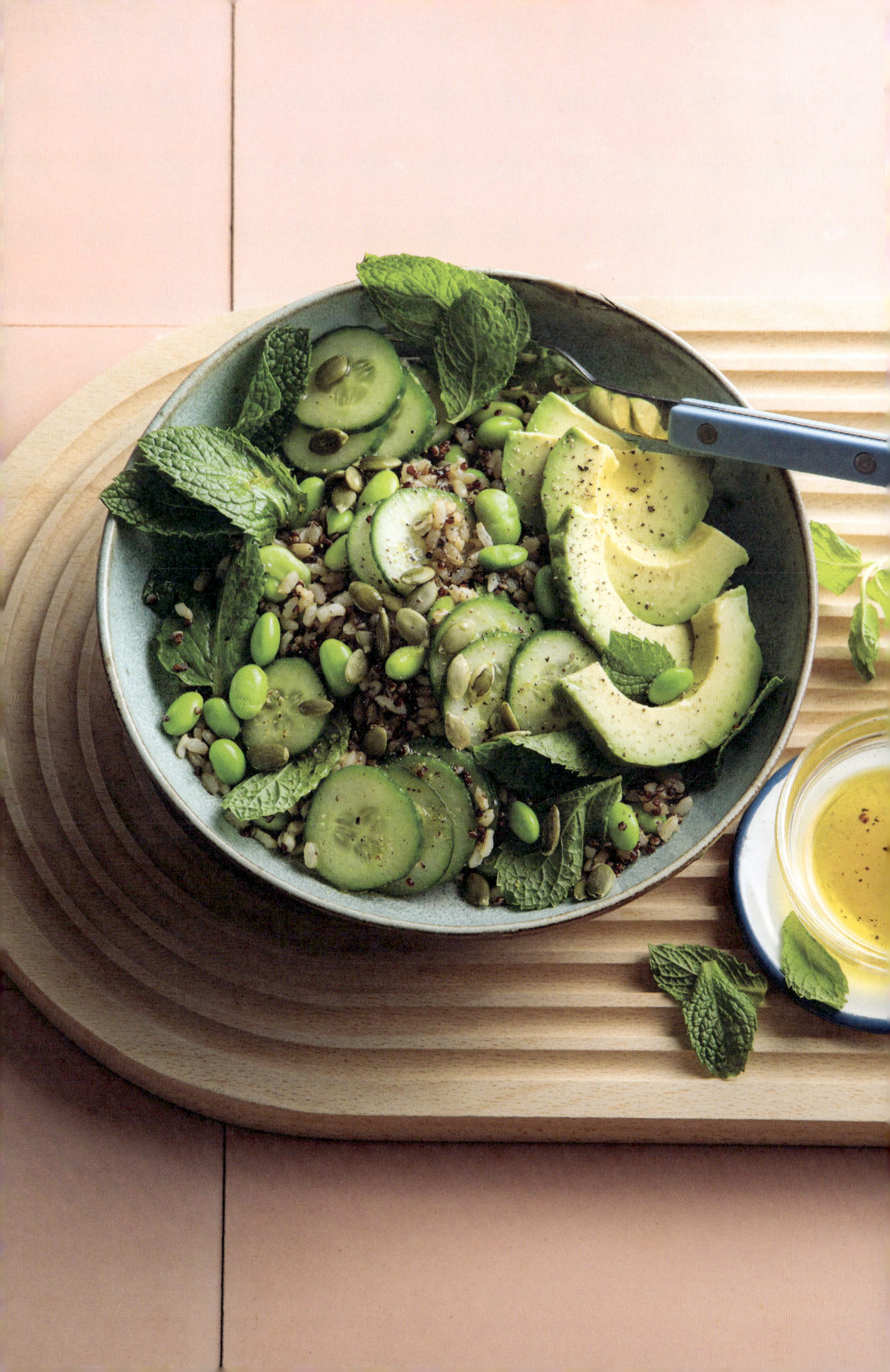

Serves 4–6
Vegetarian

TUSCAN WHITE BEAN SOUP

I'm always looking for ways to incorporate legumes into our family meals. They are true nutrition powerhouses, very cost-effective and great for make-ahead meals. This soup ticks all the boxes. It is full of protein and fibre, and a perfect light dish for weight management as it's high volume but low in energy or calories. It also comes in at less than $1 per serve.

- extra-virgin olive oil
- 1 large onion, roughly chopped
- 4 garlic cloves, finely chopped
- 3 large carrots, roughly diced
- 4 celery stalks, roughly diced
- 1 large zucchini, roughly diced
- sea salt and freshly ground black pepper
- 3 tablespoons tomato paste
- 750 ml (3 cups) chicken or vegetable stock
- 1 x 400 g can butter or cannellini beans, drained and rinsed
- 1 teaspoon dried Italian herbs
- 100 g baby spinach leaves or frozen spinach
- roughly chopped flat-leaf parsley, to serve
- 1 slice of crusty, wholegrain bread per person (optional)

Heat the olive oil in a large saucepan over medium–high heat. Add all the diced vegetables and season well with salt and pepper. Cook, stirring often, for 5–7 minutes, or until the vegetables are soft.

Stir the tomato paste into the vegetable mixture and cook for a minute. Stir in the stock, beans and dried herbs, and bring to a simmer. Reduce the heat to low, cover with a lid and cook for 10–15 minutes.

Remove the pan from the heat. Add the spinach, cover with the lid and give the spinach a minute or two to wilt down (longer, if using frozen).

Serve the soup topped with parsley and with a slice of crusty bread on the side.

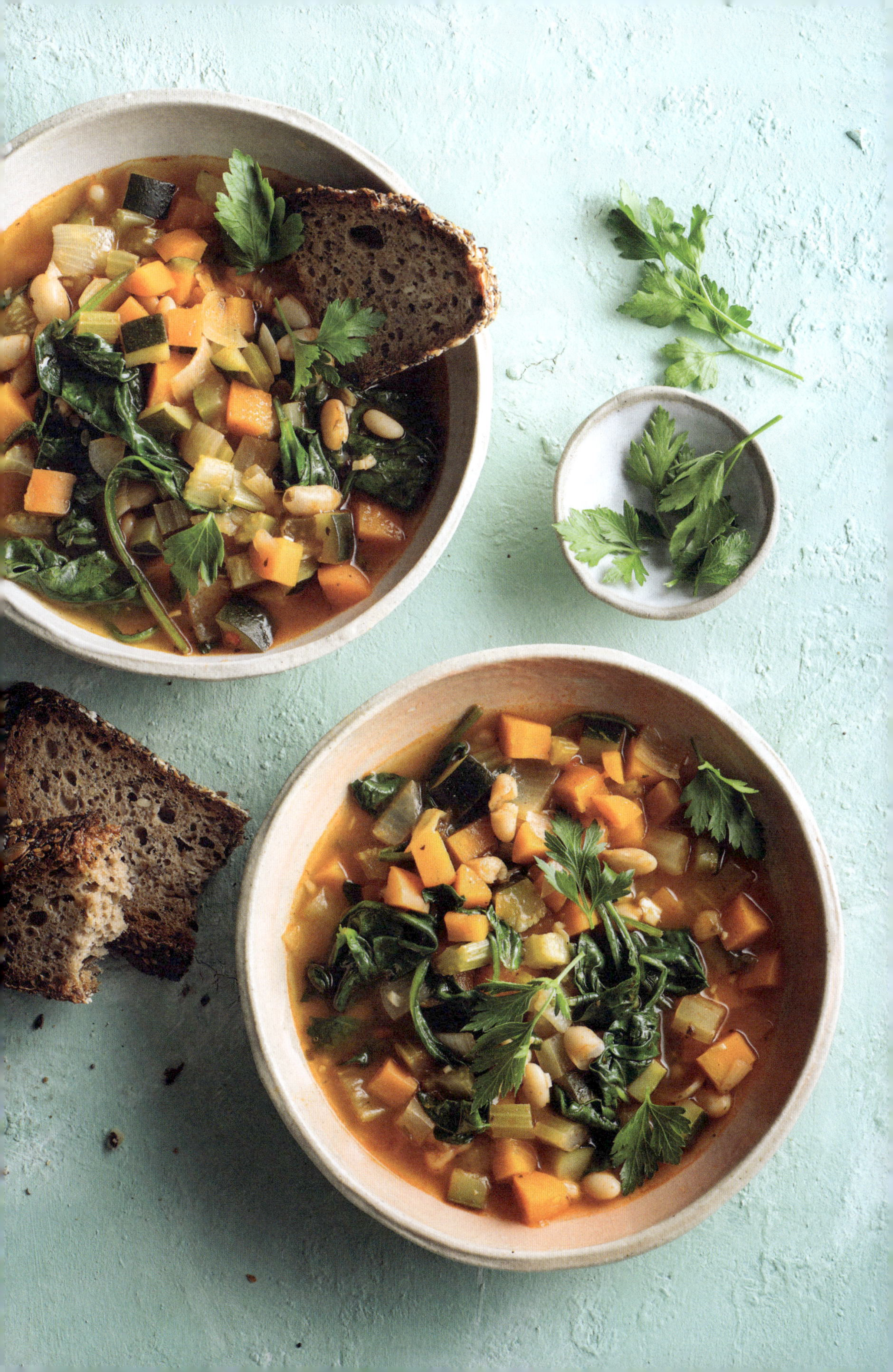

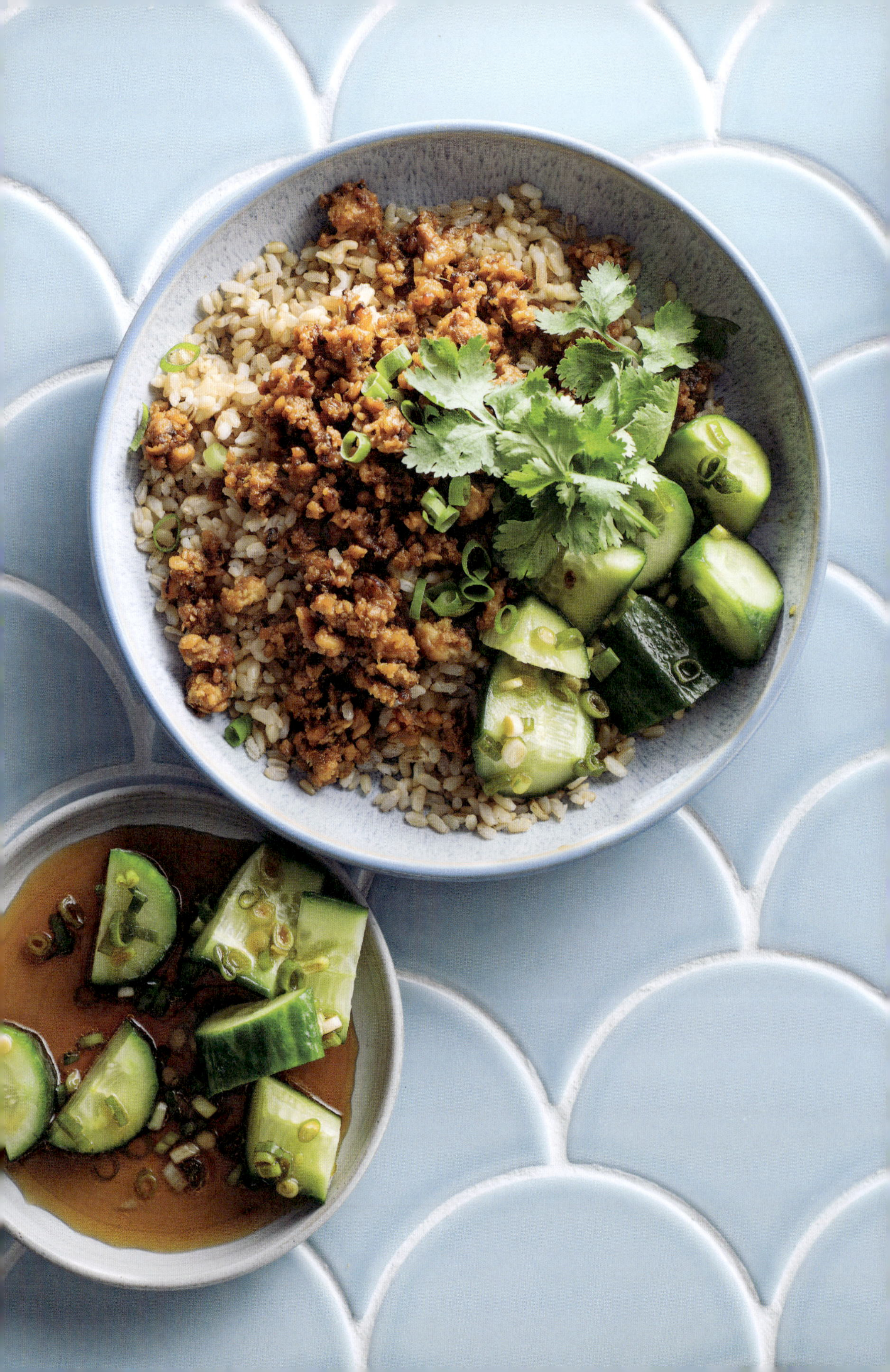

Serves 2
Vegetarian

STICKY GOLDEN TEMPEH WITH CUCUMBER SALAD

Did you look at the photo opposite and assume it was a minced meat dish? If so, good! That's sort of the idea here. Like tofu, tempeh is made from soy and is a brilliant source of plant protein packed with nutrition. However, while tofu is made from soy milk, tempeh is made from whole soybeans that are cooked and fermented together into a block. This gives it a meatier consistency and a wonderful nutty taste that makes it a great plant-based option for those wanting to swap out the meat in dishes like this one. If you're unsure where to start with tempeh, this recipe showcases it in one of the most delicious ways.

Cucumber salad

½ spring onion, finely chopped (save a little for garnish)
1 tablespoon tamari or soy sauce
2 teaspoons rice wine vinegar
½ teaspoon sesame oil
1 cucumber, roughly chopped

Sticky tempeh

250 g tempeh
1 tablespoon kecap manis (see Note)
1 tablespoon tamari or soy sauce
1 tablespoon sesame oil
1 tablespoon rice wine vinegar
2 garlic cloves, minced
1 tablespoon minced ginger
2 tablespoons extra-virgin olive oil

To serve

brown or basmati rice
toasted sesame seeds
coriander, roughly chopped
chilli sauce, Sriracha or dried chilli flakes

To make the cucumber salad, whisk the spring onion, tamari or soy sauce, vinegar and sesame oil together in a large bowl. Add the cucumber and toss it in the dressing, then cover and place in the fridge.

For the sticky tempeh, crumble the tempeh into a large bowl until it looks like minced meat.

In a small bowl, whisk the kecap manis, tamari or soy sauce, sesame oil, vinegar, garlic and ginger together.

Heat the olive oil in a large frying pan over medium heat, then add the tempeh. Stirring regularly, fry until the tempeh is golden – this should take 5–8 minutes.

Pour the sauce over the tempeh and cook for another 30 seconds or so until the tempeh is covered in sauce.

Serve the tempeh on a bed of rice with the cucumber salad and a sprinkle of toasted sesame seeds. Garnish with the reserved spring onion, the coriander and chilli.

NOTE

Kecap manis is a thick and sweet Indonesian soy sauce that is widely available at supermarkets.

SPICY ROAST VEG WITH TOFU 'RICOTTA'

Serves 2 as a main or 4 as a side
Vegetarian

This is a truly beautiful way to enjoy tofu. It's blended to make a sort of ricotta or hummus, then served with sweet roast vegetables. It is just packed with goodness. Like the whipped ricotta on page 114, it's also very versatile. Try it spread on seeded crackers alongside sliced raw veggies.

- 1 small sweet potato, very thinly sliced
- 4 large carrots, thinly sliced on an angle
- 1 x 400 g can chickpeas, drained, rinsed well and patted dry
- 1 tablespoon harissa paste (see Note)
- 2 tablespoons extra-virgin olive oil
- sea salt and freshly ground black pepper
- flat-leaf parsley, roughly chopped, to serve

Tofu 'ricotta'

- 250 g very firm tofu
- juice of 1 lemon
- ½ teaspoon garlic powder
- ½ teaspoon onion powder
- sea salt and freshly ground black pepper

Dressing

- 2 tablespoons extra-virgin olive oil
- 2 teaspoons harissa paste (see Note)
- 1 teaspoon maple syrup
- 2 tablespoons lemon juice

Preheat the oven to 180°C. Line two baking trays with baking paper.

Put the sweet potato in a large bowl with the carrot, chickpeas, harissa paste and olive oil and toss together well. Spread the mixture evenly over the baking trays and season with salt and pepper. Roast for 30–35 minutes, or until the vegetables are soft and turning golden.

Meanwhile, make the tofu 'ricotta'. Break the tofu up into chunks and put it in a food processor with the lemon juice, garlic and onion powders, and a good pinch of salt and pepper. Process until smooth and creamy. You may need to add a couple of teaspoons of water as you go to loosen the consistency (you're looking for a hummus-like consistency).

Mix the dressing ingredients in a small bowl or jar with a lid and mix or shake well to combine.

To serve, spread a few heaped tablespoons of the tofu ricotta over a large serving platter. Pile the roasted vegetables and chickpeas on top, drizzle over the spicy dressing and garnish with parsley.

NOTE

Harissa can be very spicy, so if you aren't big on heat you can use less so it's not too firey. You can always add more to the dressing if needed.

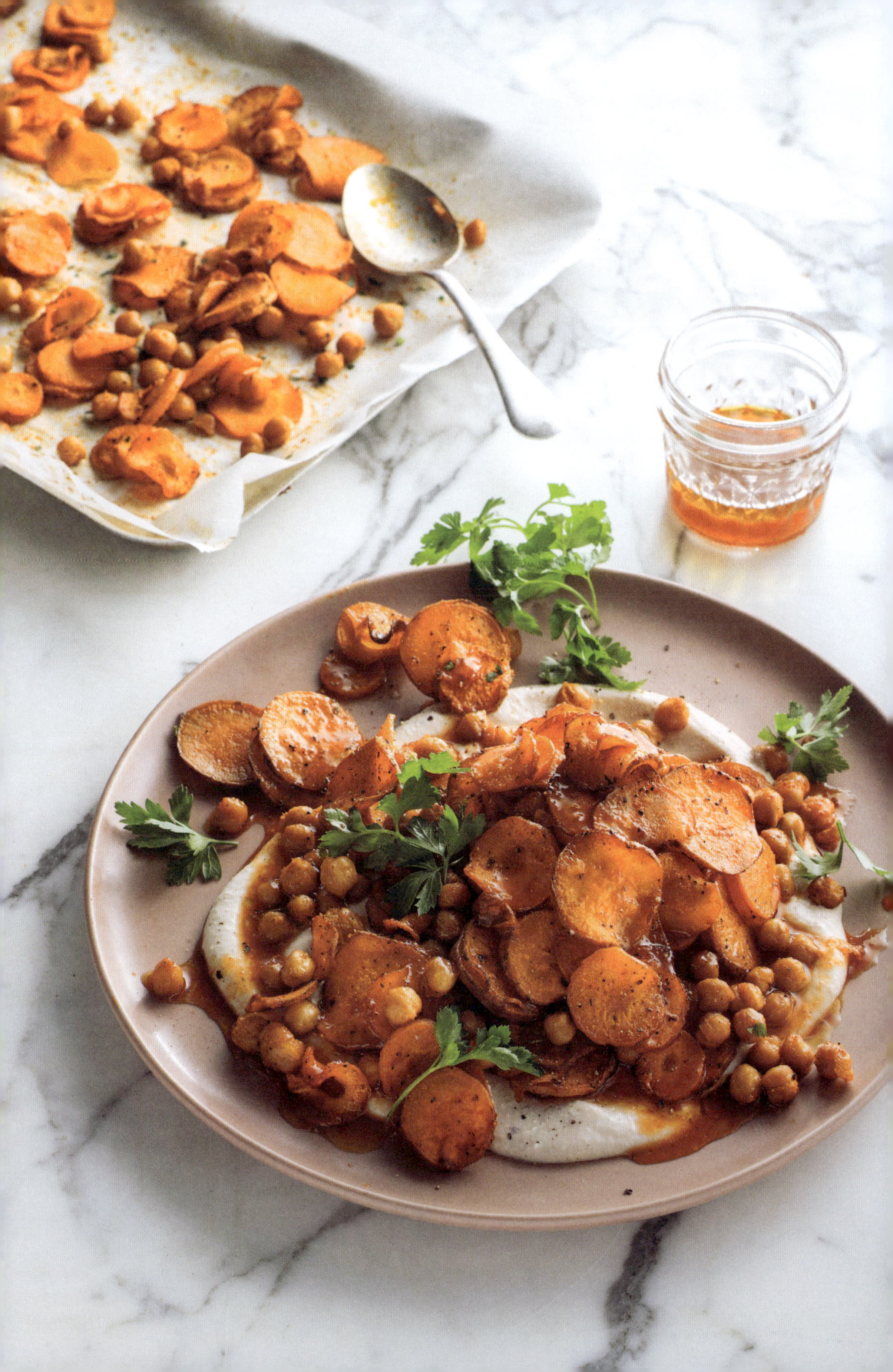

Serves 2
Vegetarian

OLD-SCHOOL SALAD SANDWICH

It's time we bring back the salad sandwich! It was everywhere when I was a child but seems to have fallen off the radar a bit. This is a shame because a good salad sandwich can be one of the healthiest and most satisfying meals around when you use a good-quality bread and a decent meat-free protein. An excellent lunch option, it's also an easy dinner, especially in those hotter months.

½ small red onion, thinly sliced
1 tablespoon red, white or apple cider vinegar
sea salt
4 x 40 g slices of grainy sourdough bread
½ small avocado, mashed
4 tablespoons hummus
2 x 40 g slices low-fat hard cheese of your choice (tasty cheddar, jarlsberg, colby)
4 thick slices canned beetroot, drained and patted dry
1 tomato, sliced (see Note)
½ cucumber, thinly sliced
1 small carrot, grated
30 g (½ cup) alfalfa sprouts
25 g (½ cup) baby spinach leaves
pinch of freshly ground black pepper

Put the onion and vinegar in a small bowl with a good pinch of salt. Mix together and then set aside to pickle while you make the sandwich.

Lay out your four slices of bread. Top two of them with the avocado. Spread hummus on the other two slices and lay the cheese over the hummus. Arrange the remaining ingredients on top. Finish by adding some pickled onion (allow any excess vinegar to drain off first) and the avocado-topped sandwich lid. Slice in half and devour!

NOTE

It pays to buy the nicest, ripest tomatoes you can get your hands on. Vine-ripened tomatoes are in most grocery stores these days, and they're generally tastier, with better flavour than most of the rock-hard barely ripe alternatives.

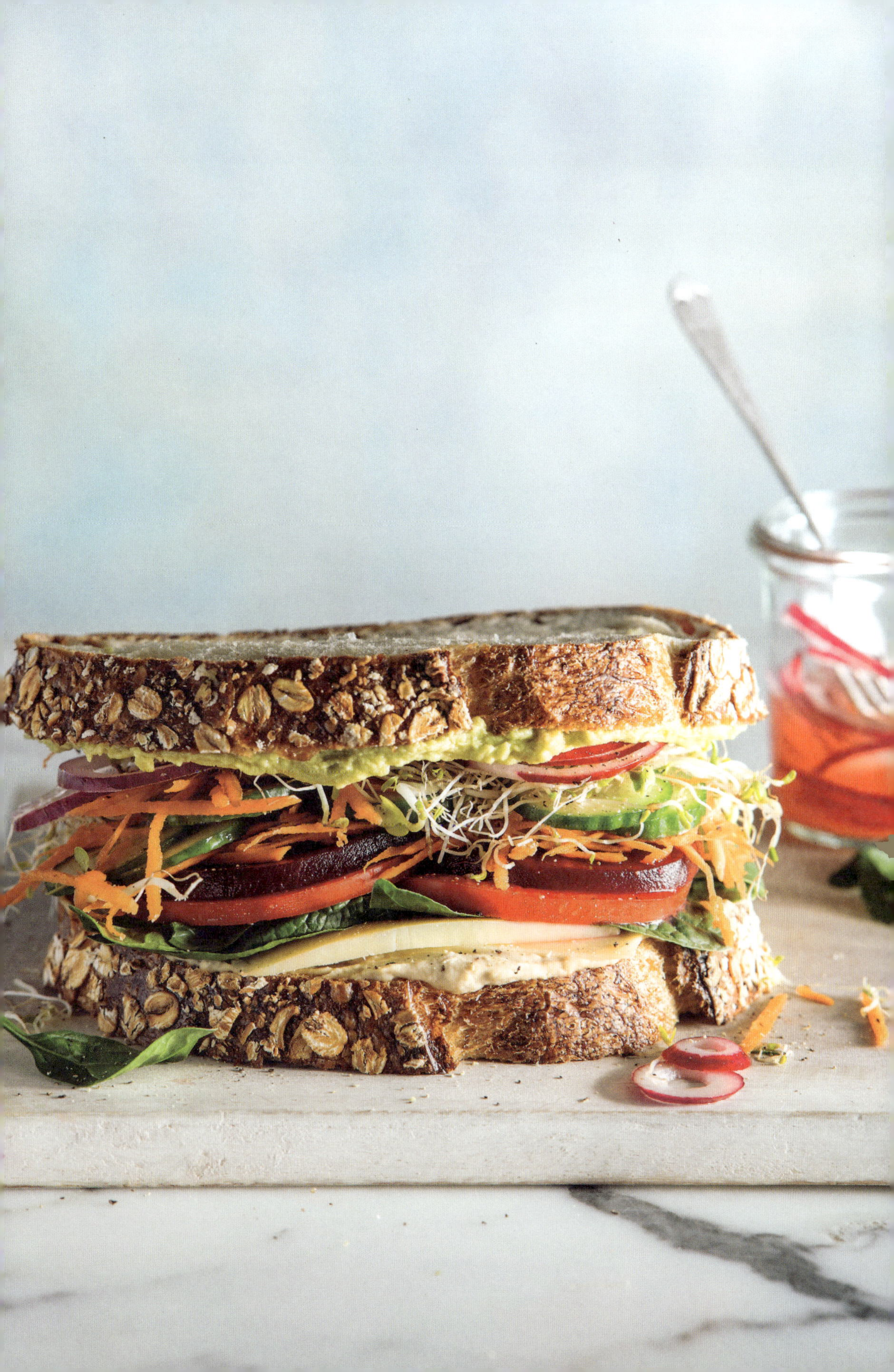

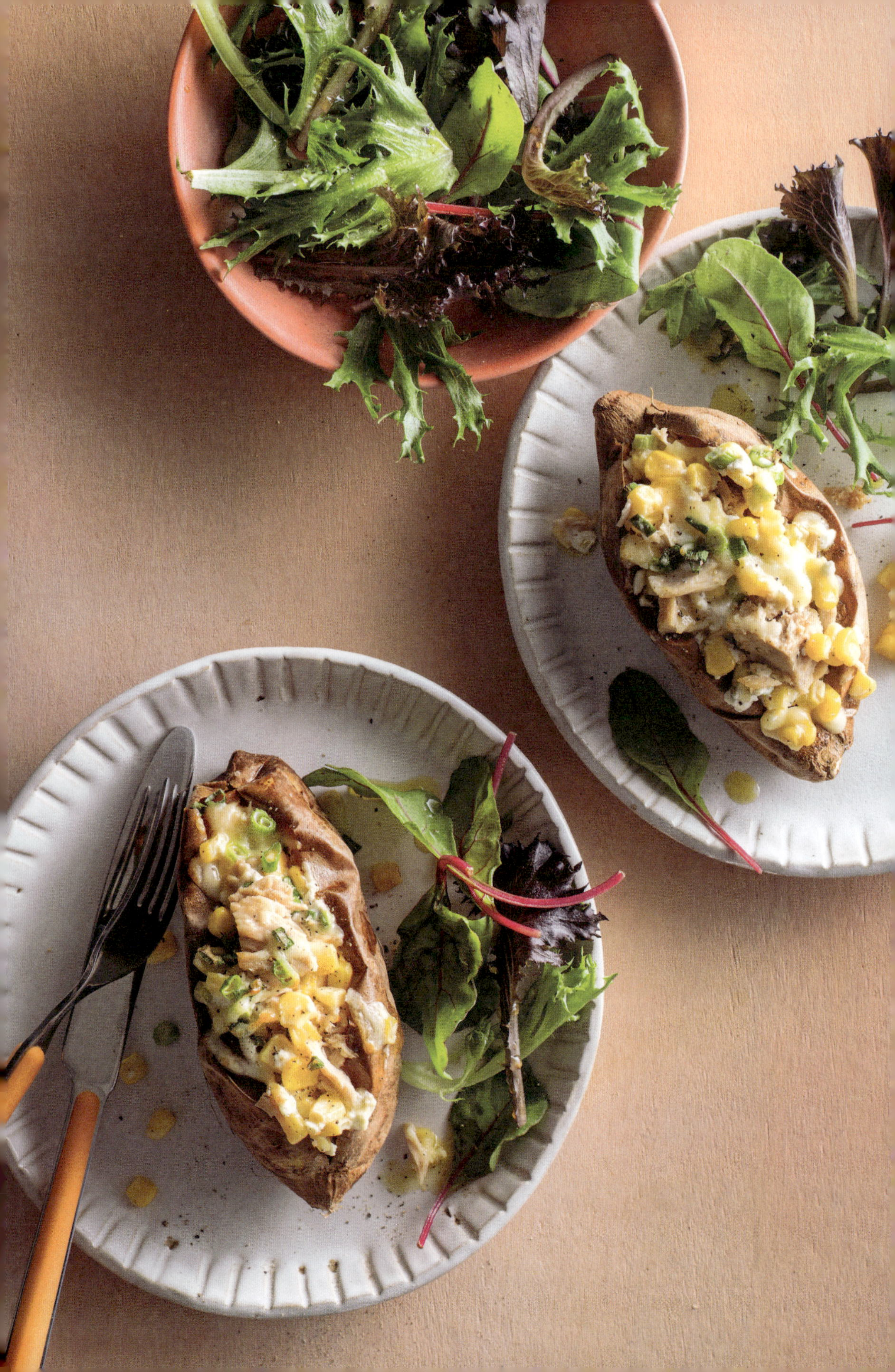

Serves 2

LOADED SWEET POTATOES

One of my favourite comfort foods is a loaded baked potato, but a really nice alternative is the sweet potato, its nutritionally superior cousin. I've used a delicious tuna and corn mix here, but you can load yours up with any protein-rich fillings of your choice – try Mexican beans, chickpea curry, mince, hummus, melty cheese . . .

2 small sweet potatoes, skins on
mixed leaves, to serve

Filling

1 x 95 g can tuna in oil, drained
1 x 125 g can corn kernels, drained
60 g (¼ cup) cottage cheese
25 g (¼ cup) low-fat grated cheese
1 spring onion, finely sliced
sea salt and freshly ground black pepper

Preheat the oven to 200°C.

Place the sweet potatoes on a baking tray lined with baking paper. Bake for 50–60 minutes, or until soft all the way through.

Cut the sweet potato down the centre lengthway, but only halfway through so it still holds together.

Place the filling ingredients in a bowl, season with salt and pepper, and mix together well.

Heat the grill to medium. Spoon generous amounts of the filling into each sweet potato, then place them under the grill for another 5 minutes, or until a bit melty on top.

Serve with mixed leaves.

Serves 2
Vegetarian

NASI GORENG WITH SESAME-FRIED EGGS

A traditional Indonesian dish, nasi goreng is a delicious take on fried rice. I love the fried egg on top, and the contrast of the fresh, cold tomato and cucumber.

Nasi goreng
extra-virgin olive oil, for cooking
2 shallots, thinly sliced
2 teaspoons minced garlic
550 g (3 cups) cooked and cooled brown rice
2 tablespoons kecap manis (see Note on page 157)
90 g (½ cup) shelled edamame
2 eggs
2 tablespoons sesame seeds

To serve
1 large tomato, cut into wedges
½ cucumber, sliced on an angle
2 lime wedges
chilli sauce (optional)

Heat 1 tablespoon of olive oil in a wok or large frying pan over high heat, then add the shallot and garlic. Fry quickly, moving them around the pan.

Add the rice and kecap manis and stir-fry for a few minutes, or until the rice begins to caramelise. Add the edamame, continuing to toss together for another 20 seconds. Divide the rice between two bowls.

Place the pan back on the heat and add 1 teaspoon of olive oil and 1 tablespoon of sesame seeds. Crack an egg over the seeds and cook to your liking, then slide on top of the rice. Repeat with the remaining sesame seeds and the second egg.

Top each portion with the tomato and cucumber, a squeeze of lime and a drizzle of chilli sauce, if you like.

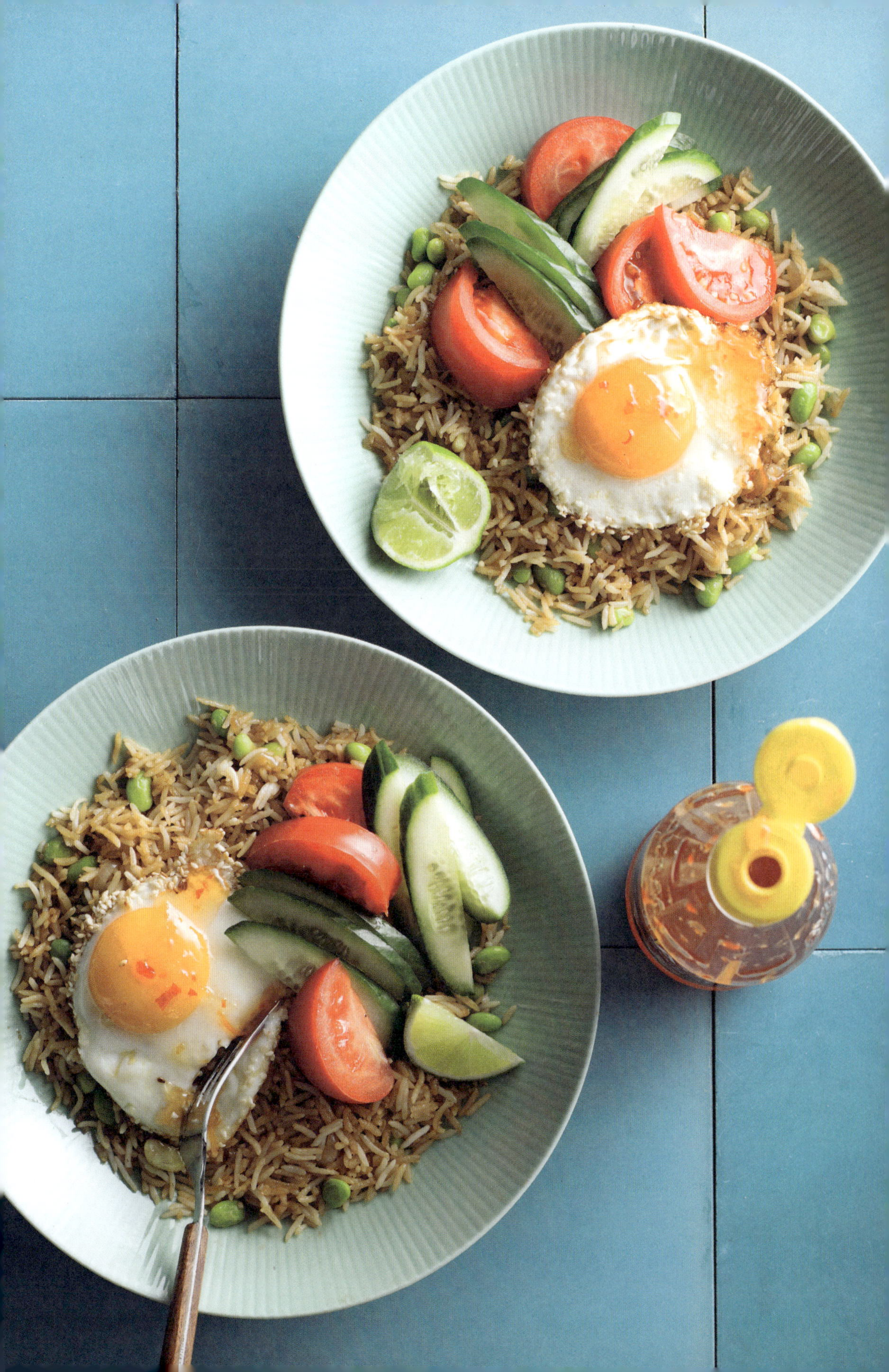

Serves 6–8
Vegetarian

GREEN MAC AND CHEESE

This green, healthy twist on traditional mac and cheese is an oozy delight and I guarantee you'll be both comforted and deeply satisfied after eating it. Wholemeal macaroni is ideal here, but don't worry too much if you can't get it. You can use any spiral wholemeal pasta, or a regular macaroni – the fibre in the green veg will ensure this is still a much leaner option than the traditional dish.

- 500 g wholemeal macaroni or spiral pasta
- 1 small head of broccoli, cut into small florets
- 130 g (1 cup) frozen peas
- 2 tablespoons extra-virgin olive oil
- 1 small onion, finely diced
- 2 garlic cloves, minced
- 2 tablespoons plain flour
- 500 ml (2 cups) milk of your choice
- sea salt and freshly ground black pepper
- 300 g (3 cups) grated cheddar
- 45 g (1 cup) baby spinach leaves

Preheat the oven to 180°C.

Cook the pasta for 2 minutes less than the packet instructions (it will continue to cook in the oven). Drain, then set aside.

In a small saucepan or steamer, steam the broccoli and peas for 4–5 minutes, or until the broccoli is tender.

Meanwhile, heat the olive oil in a large frying pan over medium heat and add the onion and garlic. Cook for 2–3 minutes, or until the onion softens and becomes translucent. Sprinkle the flour over the onion and stir for around 30 seconds – the mixture should become lumpy and dry.

Gradually add 125 ml (½ cup) of milk at a time, whisking as you go to break up any lumps. Once all of the milk is added, season well with salt and pepper and simmer over low heat, stirring occasionally, until it thickens enough to coat the back of the spoon. Add 200 g (2 cups) of cheddar and stir until completely melted.

Transfer the cheese sauce to a blender or food processor with the cooked greens and the spinach leaves and blend until smooth.

Pour the green sauce over the cooked pasta, stir together well, then transfer to a deep baking tray or casserole dish and scatter over the remaining cheese.

Bake for around 20 minutes, or until golden and bubbly. Serve in a bowl with a grind of pepper, then hop on the couch and enjoy your easy, cosy dinner!

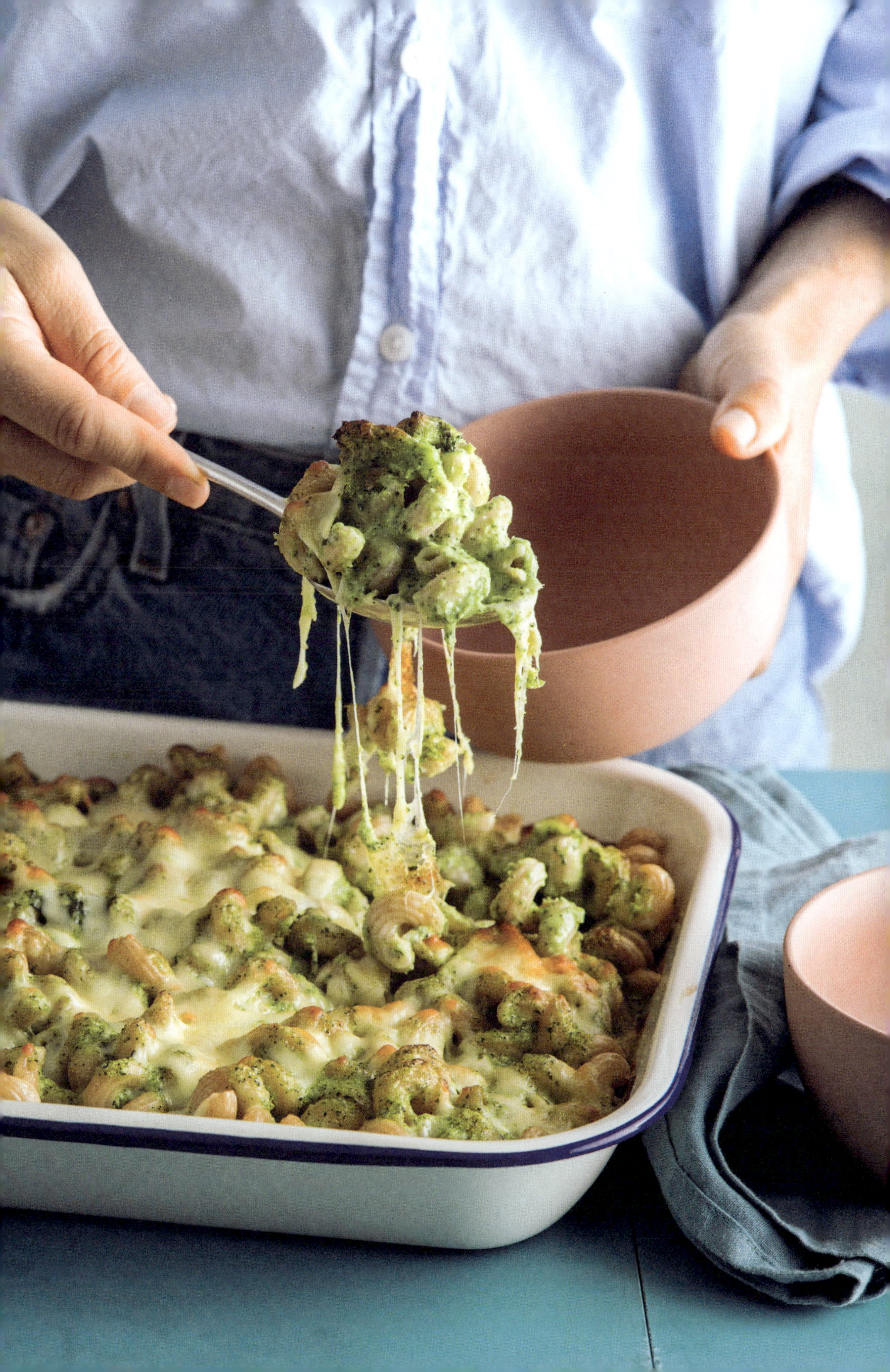

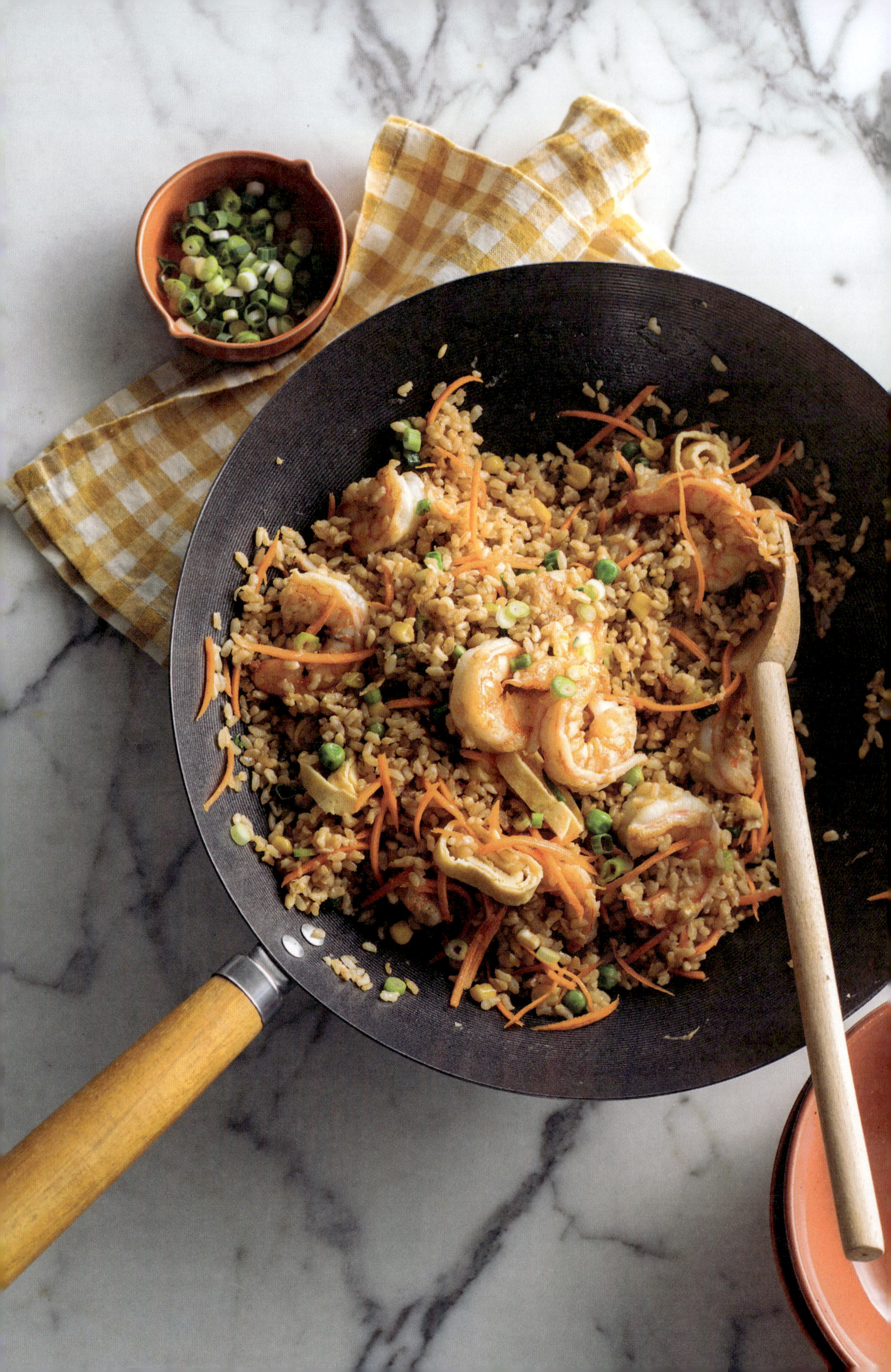

Serves 2

PRAWN AND EGG VERY SPECIAL FRIED RICE

Cooked and cooled rice contains resistant starch, a type of fibre our gut loves. This quick and easy midweek meal is a delicious way to use up leftovers.

200 g raw prawns, peeled and deveined
sea salt and freshly ground white pepper
extra-virgin olive oil, for frying
2 eggs, whisked
2 spring onions, whites finely sliced, greens finely diced
1 tablespoon minced garlic
1 carrot, shredded
550 g (3 cups) cooked and cooled brown rice
70 g (½ cup) frozen peas and corn
3 tablespoons tamari or soy sauce
1 teaspoon sesame oil

Pat the prawns dry with paper towel, then season with a pinch of salt and white pepper.

Heat 2 teaspoons of olive oil in a wok or large frying pan over high heat. Add the prawns and cook for 1–2 minutes, or until they turn pink. Once cooked, transfer to a plate.

Return the wok to the heat and heat another 2 teaspoons of olive oil, swirling the wok to coat evenly. Pour in the egg and swirl immediately to create a thin layer. As it begins to cook and crisp up at the edges, use tongs or a spatula to roll it into a cigar shape. Transfer to a chopping board and slice thinly.

Return the wok to the heat, add 1 tablespoon of olive oil, the spring onion whites, garlic and carrot. Cook for 30 seconds or so before adding the rice, peas and corn, tamari or soy sauce and sesame oil. Stir-fry and toss together for 1–2 minutes, then return the prawns and sliced egg to the wok and toss to combine.

Divide the fried rice between bowls and serve topped with the green spring onion.

Serves 2

HOT-SMOKED SALMON AND FREEKEH SALAD

When people think of smoked salmon, it's often cold-smoked salmon, which is sold thinly sliced and has a soft, almost raw texture. Hot-smoked salmon has a very different flavour profile and personality; its texture is much closer to that of cooked fish. It's usually sold as a whole fillet, and is a really easy, hassle-free way to add oily fish to your diet. If you like, you can also use regular cooked salmon in place of the smoked salmon here.

Salad

- 200 g (1 cup) freekeh
- 1 bunch broccolini, stalks trimmed, cut into 3 cm pieces
- 1 bunch asparagus, woody ends trimmed, cut into 3 cm pieces
- 3 tablespoons pumpkin seeds
- small handful of flat-leaf parsley, leaves roughly chopped
- 150 g hot-smoked salmon

Dressing

- 2 tablespoons extra-virgin olive oil
- 1 teaspoon minced garlic
- juice of 1 large lemon
- 1 teaspoon dijon mustard
- sea salt and freshly ground black pepper

Bring a large saucepan of water to the boil and add the freekeh. Reduce the heat and cook according to the packet instructions. Drain well, then set aside to cool.

Bring another large saucepan of water to the boil and cook the broccolini for around 2 minutes. Add the asparagus and cook for another minute, then drain and plunge the greens into a bowl of iced water for 1 minute. Drain again and pat dry with a clean tea towel.

Heat a small frying pan over medium–high heat and toast the pumpkin seeds, tossing regularly, until they begin to turn golden. Remove from the heat.

Mix the dressing ingredients in a small bowl or jar with a lid, season with salt and pepper and mix or shake well.

Use a fork to fluff up the freekeh, then spoon it into a large serving bowl and add the cooked greens and parsley. Drizzle the dressing on top and toss together gently before dividing between bowls. Top each portion with generous flakes of salmon and toasted pumpkin seeds.

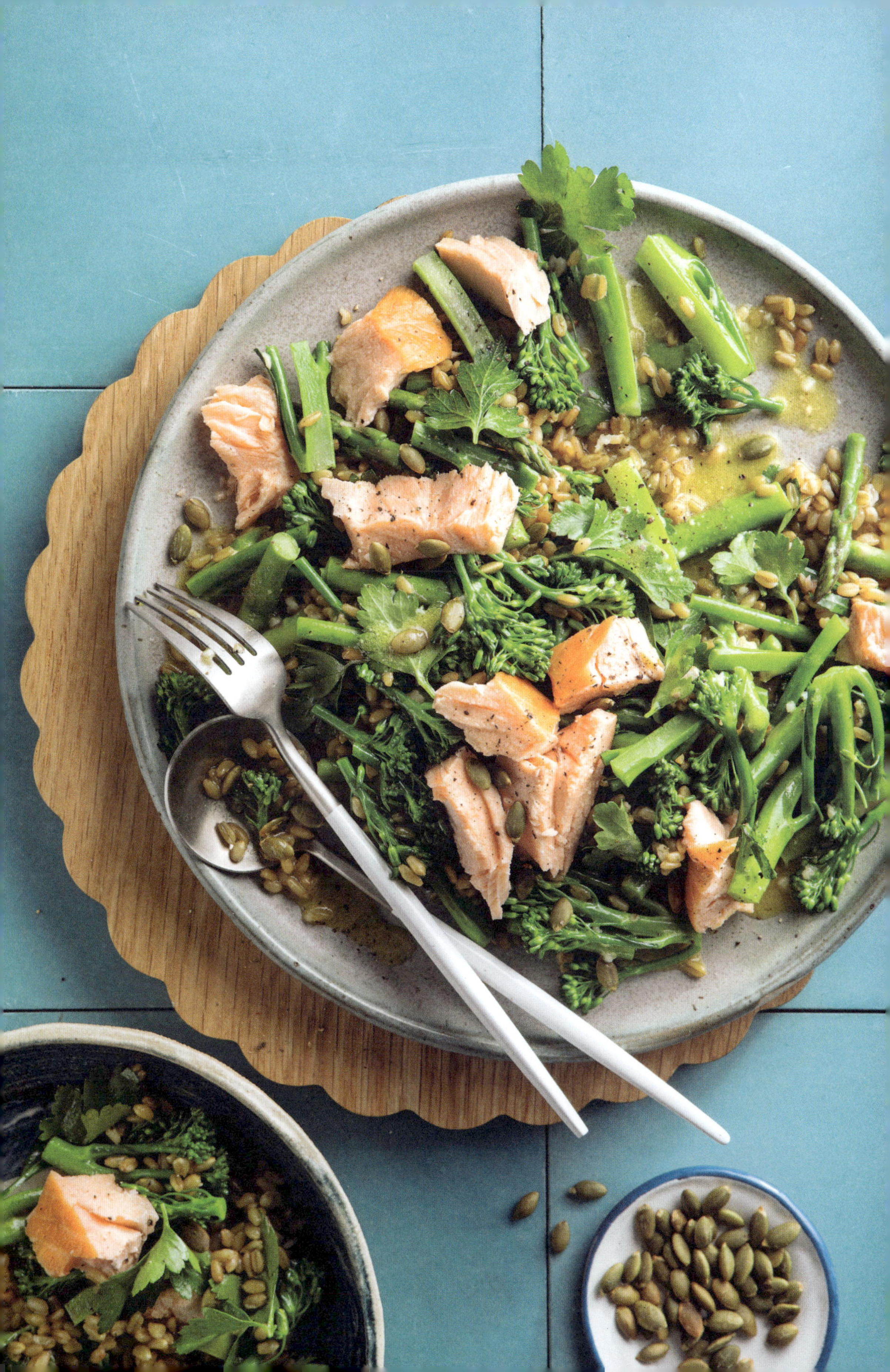

Serves 4

SALMON, SWEET POTATO AND PEA PATTIES

This dish is full of nostalgia for me – I remember eating it a lot as a kid! It was an easy, family-friendly way for my parents to incorporate oily fish into our diet and now it's a favourite with my kids, too. While they're delicious served warm for dinner, I'd argue these patties are even better cold in a lunchbox the next day.

750 g sweet potato, peeled and diced into 2–3 cm pieces
155 g (1 cup) frozen peas
1 x 400 g can red salmon (see Note)
60 g (1 cup) wholemeal breadcrumbs, plus extra if needed
1 egg, lightly beaten
a few flat-leaf parsley sprigs, finely chopped
sea salt and freshly ground black pepper
3 tablespoons olive oil
lemon wedges and mixed leaves, to serve

Yoghurt sauce
250 g (1 cup) plain Greek-style yoghurt
zest and juice of 1 lemon
a few dill fronds, finely chopped
sea salt and freshly ground black pepper

Line a large tray with baking paper.

Bring a large saucepan of water to the boil and add the sweet potato. Boil for 10–12 minutes, or until a knife slides through the largest piece easily. Add the peas and cook for another 30 seconds before draining. Set aside to cool slightly.

Flake the salmon into a large bowl with the breadcrumbs, egg and parsley. Add the cooled sweet potato and peas, season with salt and pepper, then mash together roughly. Add more breadcrumbs if the mixture seems too wet.

With damp hands, form the salmon mixture into around 10–12 patties. Place these on the lined tray as you go, then cover and place in the fridge for around 30 minutes so the patties firm up.

Meanwhile, mix the ingredients for the yoghurt sauce together in a bowl and season with salt and pepper. Mix again, then put in the fridge until you're ready to serve.

Heat the olive oil in a large frying pan over medium–high heat. Cook the patties in batches for around 3 minutes on each side until they are golden and crunchy. Set aside on a plate lined with paper towel.

Serve two or three patties per person with a dollop of the yoghurt sauce, lemon wedges and mixed leaves.

NOTE
When it comes to canned fish such as salmon or sardines, you can remove the bones if you wish but they are a great source of calcium.

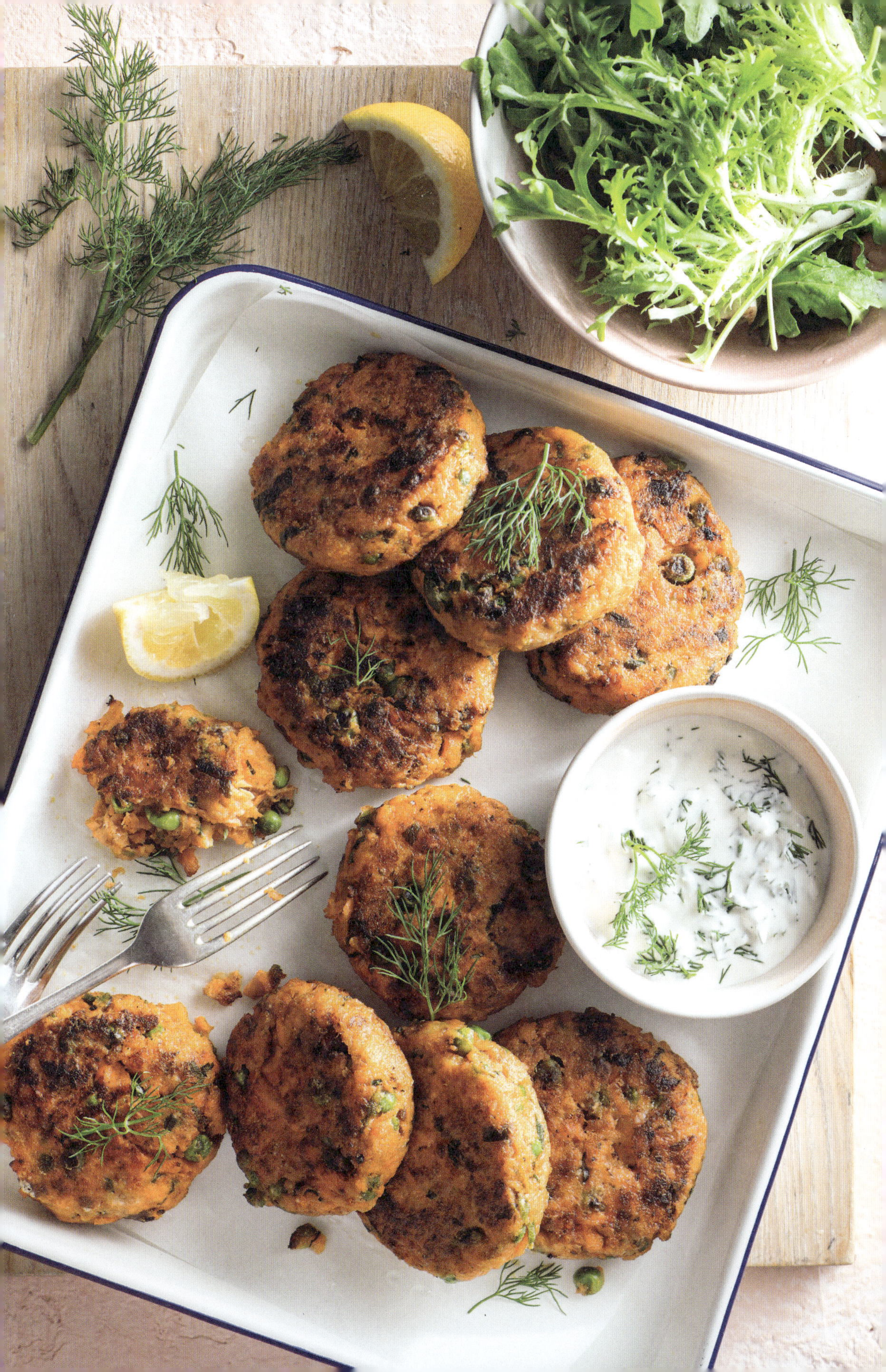

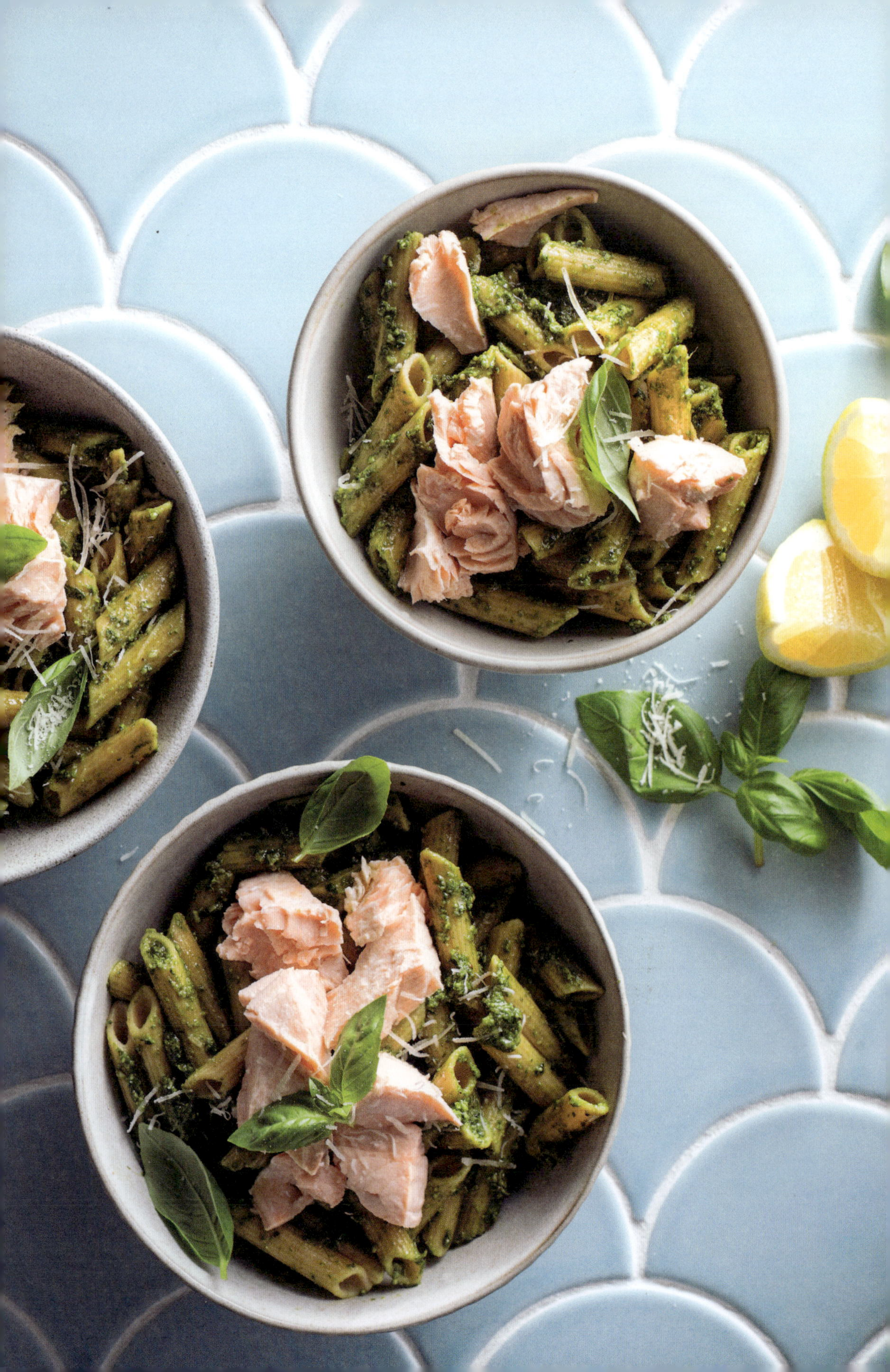

Serves 6

SPINACH AND WALNUT PESTO PASTA WITH POACHED SALMON

I created this pesto to make the most of the fragrant basil that was going nuts in my garden. Walnuts are such a fabulous nutrient-dense nut and a perfect pairing for the basil. Add some oily fish and it's an all-round winner.

3 x 150 g salmon fillets, skin removed
sea salt and freshly ground black pepper
juice of ½ lemon
500 g wholemeal, spelt or pulse pasta
grated parmesan and lemon wedges, for serving

Pesto
60 g (½ cup) walnuts
2 garlic cloves
200 g (4 cups densely packed) baby spinach
25 g (½ cup densely packed) basil leaves
25 g (¼ cup) grated parmesan
3 tablespoons extra-virgin olive oil, plus extra if required
sea salt and freshly ground black pepper

Place the salmon in a large saucepan over medium heat and just cover with water. Season with salt and pepper and squeeze in the juice of ½ lemon. Bring to a simmer, then turn off the heat. Turn the salmon fillets over, cover the saucepan with a lid and leave the salmon to continue poaching for another 10 minutes or so.

For the pesto, toast the walnuts in a hot frying pan over medium heat, tossing regularly, for around 4–5 minutes, or until they become fragrant and begin to darken. Set aside to cool.

Once the walnuts have cooled a little, put them in a food processor with the rest of the pesto ingredients. Blitz until combined. If the pesto looks a bit dry, you can add an extra tablespoon of olive oil.

Cook the pasta according to the packet instructions. Drain, reserving a cup of the cooking water, then return the pasta to its saucepan and add half the pesto. Toss together gently until combined and add more pesto if you want a stronger flavour.

Use a slotted spoon to transfer the poached salmon to a plate lined with paper towel.

Divide the pasta between serving dishes and top each portion with the flaked poached salmon. Serve with a sprinkle of grated parmesan and a wedge of lemon.

Serves 4

THAI RED FISH CURRY

Look for a good-quality red curry paste for this end-of-the-week favourite. Asian grocery stores are always the best bet, but you can also find some tasty and authentic brands in the international food section of the major supermarkets.

- 200 g (1 cup) brown or basmati rice
- 1 tablespoon extra-virgin olive oil
- 1 onion, thinly sliced
- 4 garlic cloves, thinly sliced
- 1 tablespoon minced ginger
- 3 heaped tablespoons good-quality red curry paste
- 310 g (2 cups) peeled, diced pumpkin
- 2 Lebanese eggplants, sliced into 2 cm rounds
- 250 ml (1 cup) fish or chicken stock
- 1 x 400 ml can light coconut milk
- 400 g firm white fish, cut into 3–4 cm pieces
- 100 g green beans, trimmed
- 150 g (1 cup) cherry tomatoes
- juice of ½ lime
- small handful of Thai basil or basil leaves

Cook the rice according to the packet instructions. Once cooked, set aside with the lid on to keep warm.

Meanwhile, heat the olive oil in a large wok or frying pan over high heat, then add the onion and stir-fry for 2–3 minutes, or until the onion is soft and translucent. Stir in the garlic and ginger, then add the curry paste and cook for around a minute.

Add the pumpkin and eggplant, cook for another minute, then pour in the stock and coconut milk. Bring to a simmer, then reduce the heat to low and cook for another 10 minutes, or until the curry thickens.

Add the fish, green beans and cherry tomatoes, and cook for 5 more minutes. Remove from the heat and finish with a good squeeze of lime.

To serve, spoon the curry over the rice and top with the basil leaves.

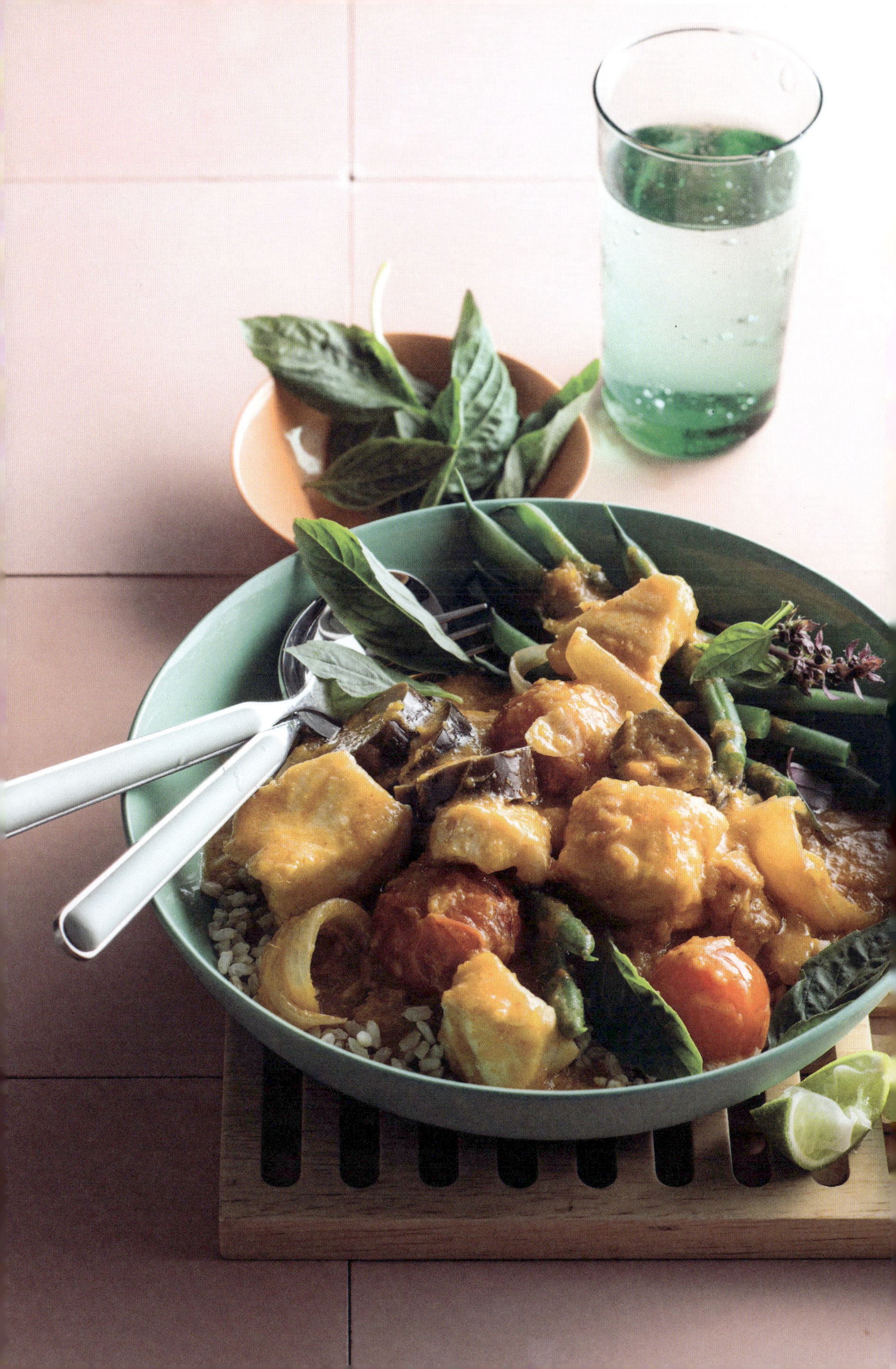

Serves 4

QUINOA, LENTIL AND SALMON SALAD

I like to use hot smoked salmon fillets in salads because they're an easy-to-use source of protein and omega-3, plus they're generally less expensive than a fresh fillet. But, if you prefer, you can also use cooked salmon in place of the smoked salmon here.

200 g (1 cup) quinoa
1 x 400 g can brown lentils, drained and rinsed
45 g (1 cup) rocket leaves
1 bunch asparagus, woody ends trimmed, stalks halved
1 avocado, finely sliced
300 g hot-smoked salmon, in flakes or chunks
3 tablespoons extra-virgin olive oil
freshly ground black pepper

Quick pickled onion

½ red onion, finely sliced
3 tablespoons red wine vinegar
sea salt

Cook the quinoa according to the packet instructions, then allow to cool slightly.

For the quick pickled onion, place the onion in a small bowl with the vinegar and a good pinch of salt. Allow to pickle for 5–10 minutes while you prepare the rest of the salad.

Put the cooked quinoa in a large bowl with the lentils and rocket and toss to combine. Divide among bowls.

Blanch the asparagus in boiling water for 1 minute, then drain and rinse under cold water. Arrange on top of the quinoa, lentil and rocket mix, along with the avocado slices and the salmon.

Lift the pickled onion out of the vinegar and add to the salad. Add the olive oil and a good grind of pepper to the remaining pickling vinegar, then whisk together and drizzle over the salad to finish.

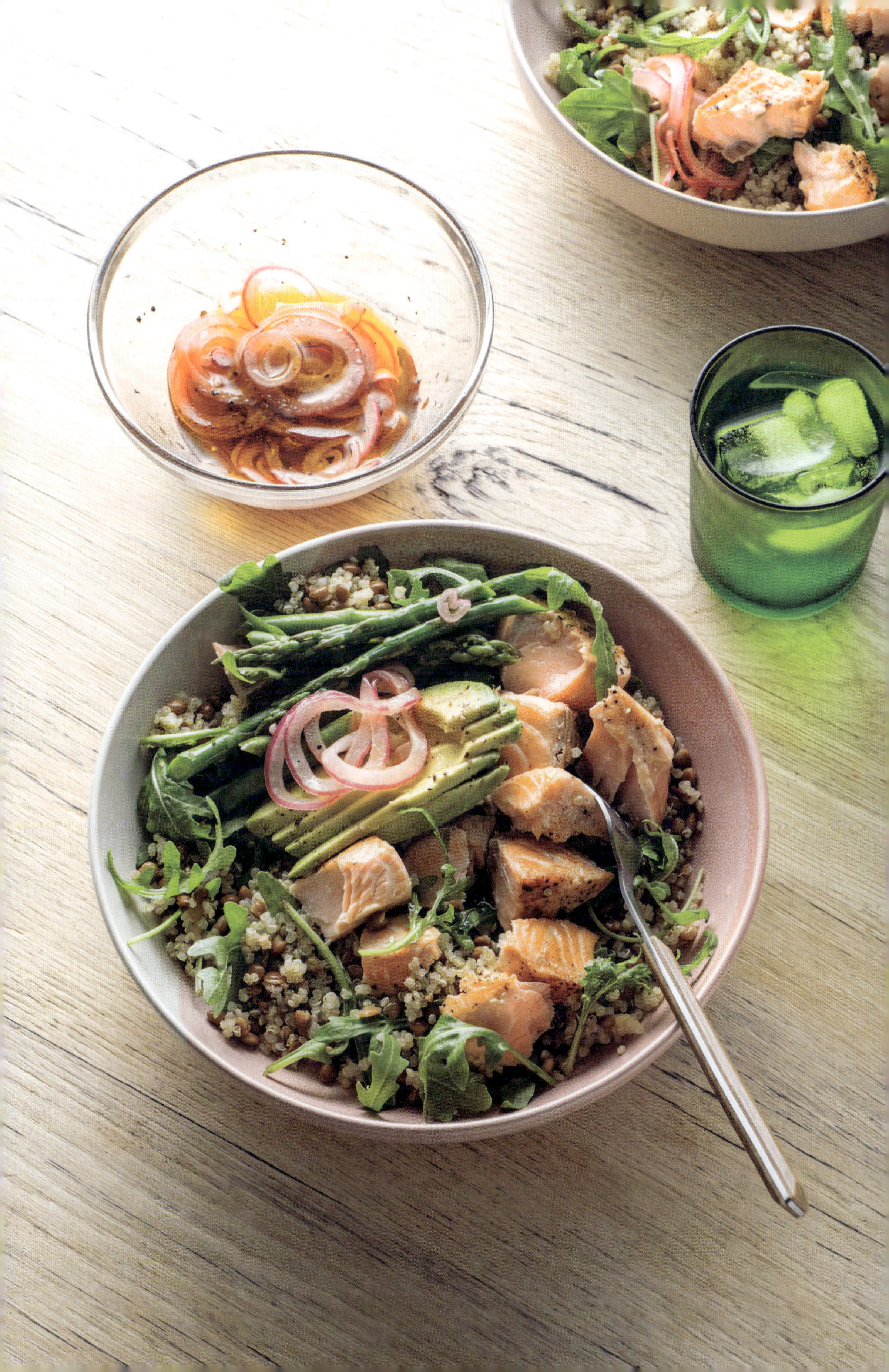

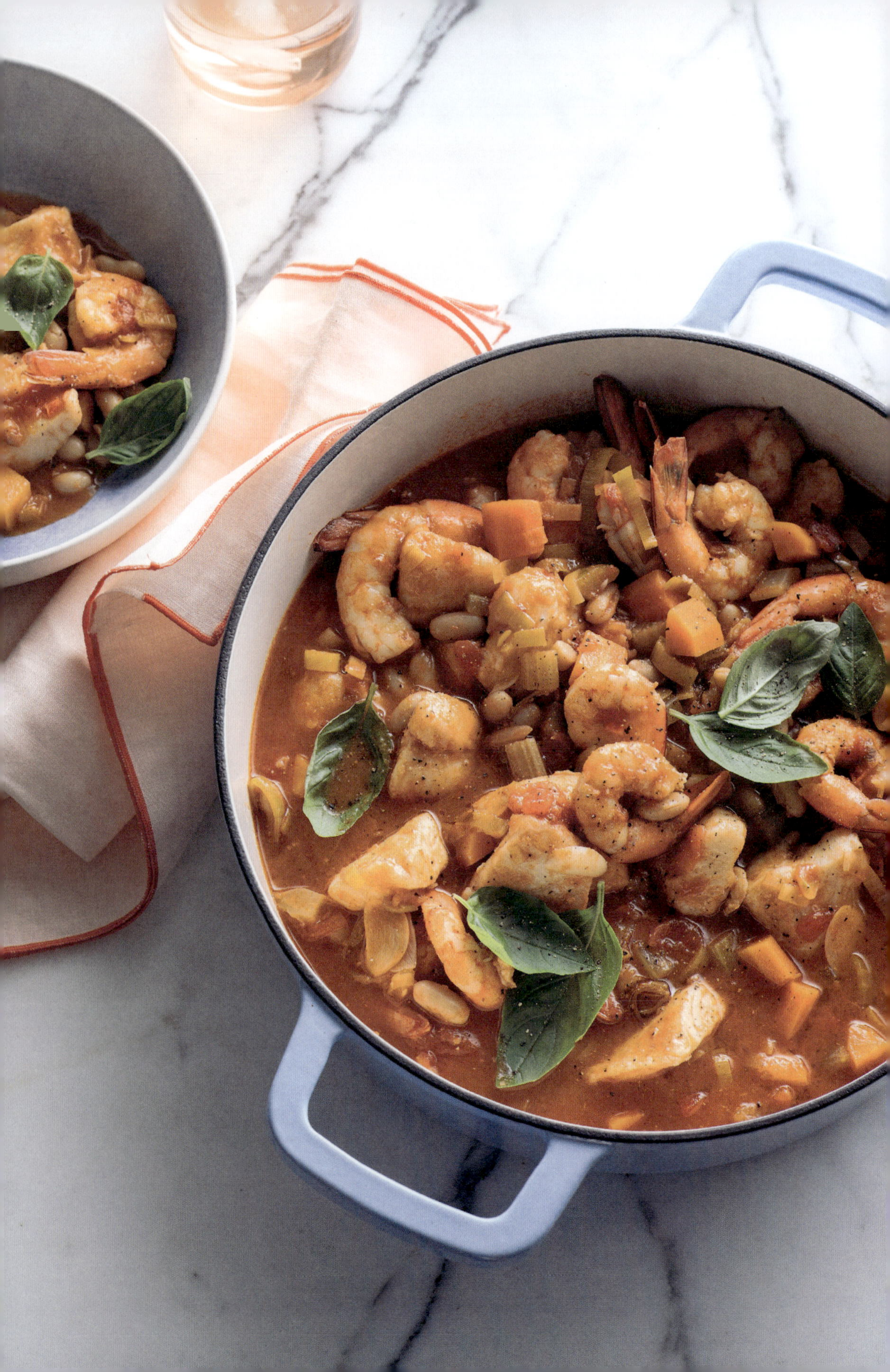

Serves 4

SEAFOOD STEW

I like to keep fish and prawns in the freezer for dishes such as this wholesome stew. All I need to do is grab a few items from the pantry and chop up some veg and I've got a decadent seafood dish on the table in around 20 minutes.

- 2 tablespoons extra-virgin olive oil
- 1 leek, white part halved and finely sliced
- 1 carrot, finely chopped
- 2 celery stalks, finely chopped
- 3 garlic cloves, finely sliced
- sea salt
- 1 teaspoon smoked or sweet paprika
- 1 x 400 g can chopped tomatoes
- 750 ml (3 cups) chicken stock
- 1 x 400 g can butter or cannellini beans, drained and rinsed
- 500 g frozen skinless white fish, thawed
- 200 g frozen prawn meat, thawed
- freshly ground black pepper
- a few basil leaves, roughly chopped
- 4 slices of grainy or rye sourdough

Heat a large saucepan over low–medium heat. Add 1 tablespoon of olive oil, the leek, carrot, celery and garlic and a pinch of salt and cook slowly for 7–8 minutes, or until the onion is translucent and the vegetables are softened but not browned.

Add the paprika, tomatoes and stock and bring to a simmer, then cover and cook for around 15 minutes until the sauce has thickened a little.

Add the beans, fish and prawns to the stew, along with a good grind of pepper. Cook for 2–3 minutes, or until the seafood has cooked through.

When the stew has nearly finished cooking, heat half of the remaining olive oil in a large frying pan over medium-high heat. Add two slices of sourdough and cook on both sides for around 2–3 minutes until golden. Repeat with the remaining olive oil and sourdough.

Divide the stew between bowls, scatter over some basil and serve with a slice of sourdough.

Serves 4

MOROCCAN-SPICED VEG, CHICKPEA AND TROUT TRAY BAKE

I love a one-tray bake. Throwing all the ingredients in together allows the flavours to meld beautifully – and of course it's so much easier to clean up afterwards.

1 x 400 g can chickpeas, drained and rinsed
1 small head of cauliflower, cut into small florets
2 large potatoes, diced into 2–3 cm pieces
1 red onion, cut into wedges
1 red capsicum, cut into 2–3 cm pieces
60 g (½ cup) pitted green olives
2 tablespoons harissa paste
2 tablespoons extra-virgin olive oil
juice of ½ lemon
sea salt and freshly ground black pepper
4 x 150 g trout or salmon fillets

To serve

a few flat-leaf parsley sprigs, roughly chopped
lemon wedges

Preheat the oven to 220°C. Line a large deep baking tray with baking paper.

Pat the chickpeas dry with paper towel and place in a large bowl with the vegetables and olives. Add 1 tablespoon harissa, 1 tablespoon olive oil and the lemon juice, then season well with salt and pepper. Toss until well coated, then tip onto the baking tray. Bake for 20–30 minutes, or until a knife slides easily into a potato. Remove from the oven.

Whisk the remaining harissa and olive oil in a small bowl. Place the trout on top of the vegetables, skin-side down. Spoon on the harissa mix, then season with salt and pepper. Return to the oven for 10–15 minutes, or until the trout is cooked and the vegetables are golden.

Divide the spiced chickpeas, veg and trout among plates. Top with parsley and a wedge of lemon, to serve.

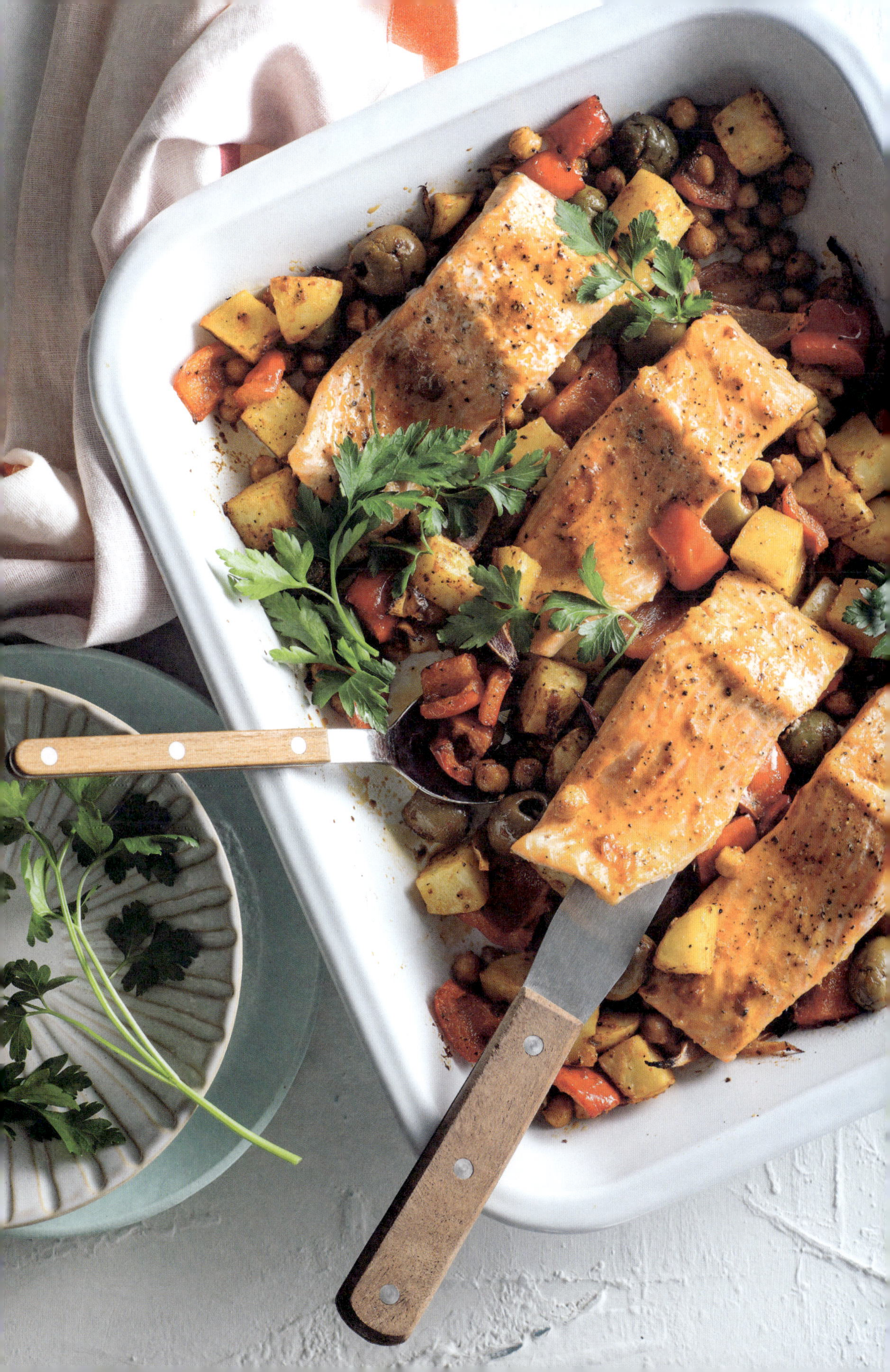

Serves 4

SUPREME GREEN GODDESS CHICKEN SALAD

This is my version of the finely chopped dip that recently went viral online. In the original recipe, the dip is served with corn chips – I mean, yum! – but I've elevated it to a nutritious main meal by adding a decent amount of protein.

2 x 200 g chicken breast fillets
sea salt and freshly ground black pepper
1 tablespoon extra-virgin olive oil

Dressing

250 g (1 cup) plain Greek-style yoghurt
generous handful of flat-leaf parsley
generous handful of other soft green herbs (e.g. dill, mint, coriander)
2 tablespoons finely chopped chives
1 tablespoon capers, drained
1 garlic clove
juice of 1 lemon
1 tablespoon extra-virgin olive oil
sea salt and freshly ground black pepper

Salad

240 g (6 cups) chopped cos lettuce
150 g (2 cups) chopped white cabbage
2 spring onions, finely sliced
1 Lebanese cucumber, diced
1 avocado, diced

Place all the dressing ingredients in a food processor with a generous pinch of salt and pepper and blitz until smooth and creamy.

Pat the chicken breasts dry with paper towel, then halve each breast lengthways so you end up with two strips of chicken per breast. Season both sides well with salt and pepper.

Heat the olive oil in a large frying pan over high heat and add the chicken. Cook each strip on both sides for 2–3 minutes per side, or until golden and cooked through. Transfer to a chopping board to rest for 5 minutes, then roughly dice.

Toss the salad ingredients in a large bowl with half the dressing. Divide the salad among bowls, then top with the diced chicken and an extra drizzle of dressing.

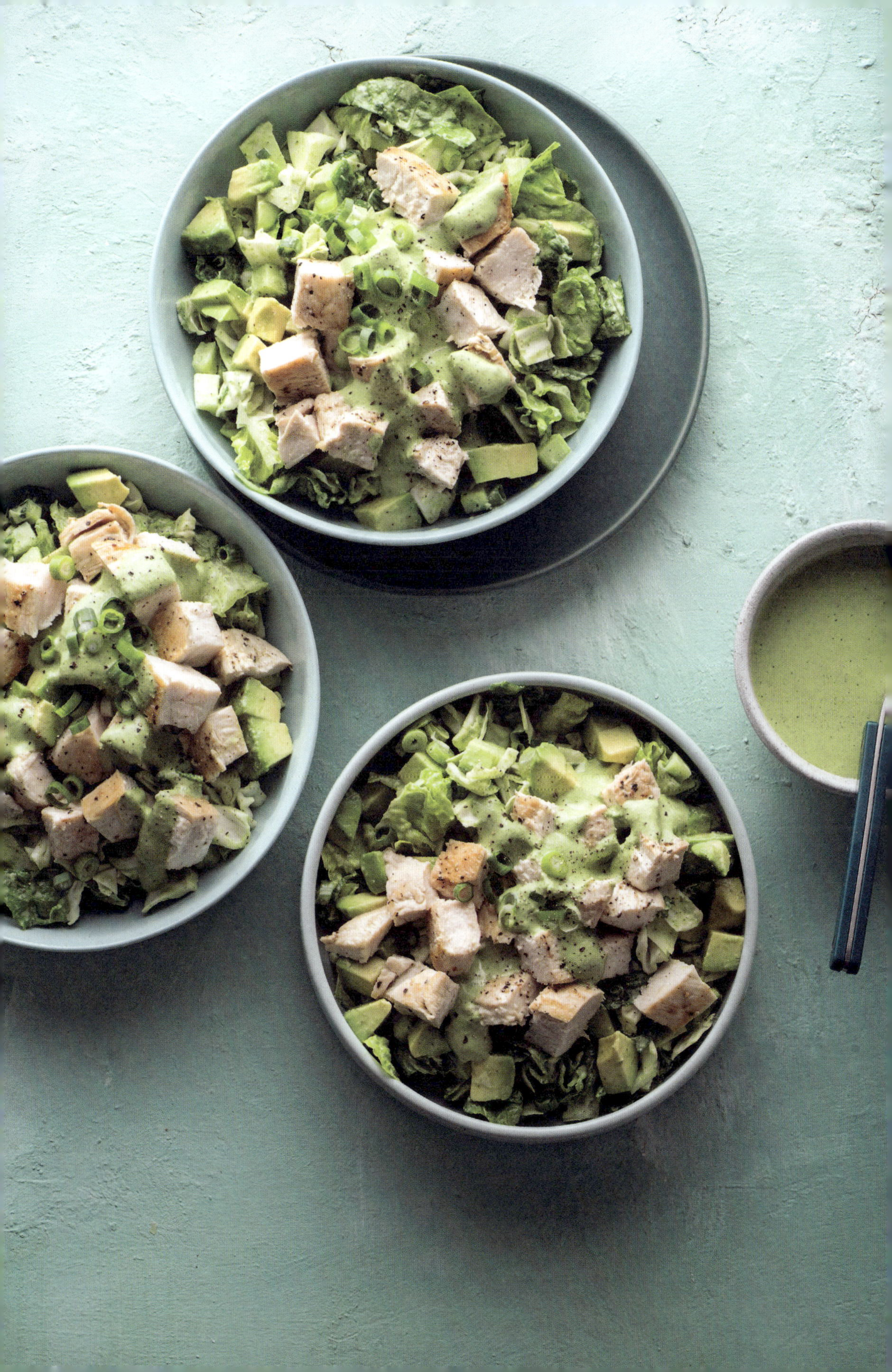

Serves 4

CHICKEN, SUNDRIED TOMATO AND BASIL MEATBALLS

I really dislike touching meat when I'm cooking, so any recipe where I can slide it into a processor to do the work for me, I'm in. I love how light and tasty these meatballs are. They also make for the best leftovers in a lunchbox the next day.

1 x 40 g slice wholegrain bread, toasted (or 3 tablespoons wholemeal breadcrumbs)
2 x 200 g chicken breast fillets, roughly chopped
4 large or 6 small sundried tomatoes
small handful of basil leaves
2 tablespoons crumbled feta
1 garlic clove
sea salt and freshly ground black pepper
260 g (2 cups) frozen peas
1 teaspoon extra-virgin olive oil
lemon wedges, to serve

Preheat the oven to 200°C. Line a baking tray with baking paper.

Pulse the toast in a food processor until it forms coarse breadcrumbs. Add the chopped chicken, sundried tomatoes, basil, feta and garlic to the processor with a good pinch of salt and pepper. Pulse until just combined – don't over-process.

Using damp hands, lightly roll a heaped tablespoon or ice-cream scoop's worth of mixture into balls and place these on the tray.

Bake for 20–25 minutes, or until golden and cooked through.

When the meatballs are nearly done, cook the peas in a small saucepan of boiling water for 2–3 minutes, then drain and toss them in the olive oil while still hot. Season with salt and pepper.

Divide the meatballs among bowls and serve with peas and a lemon wedge.

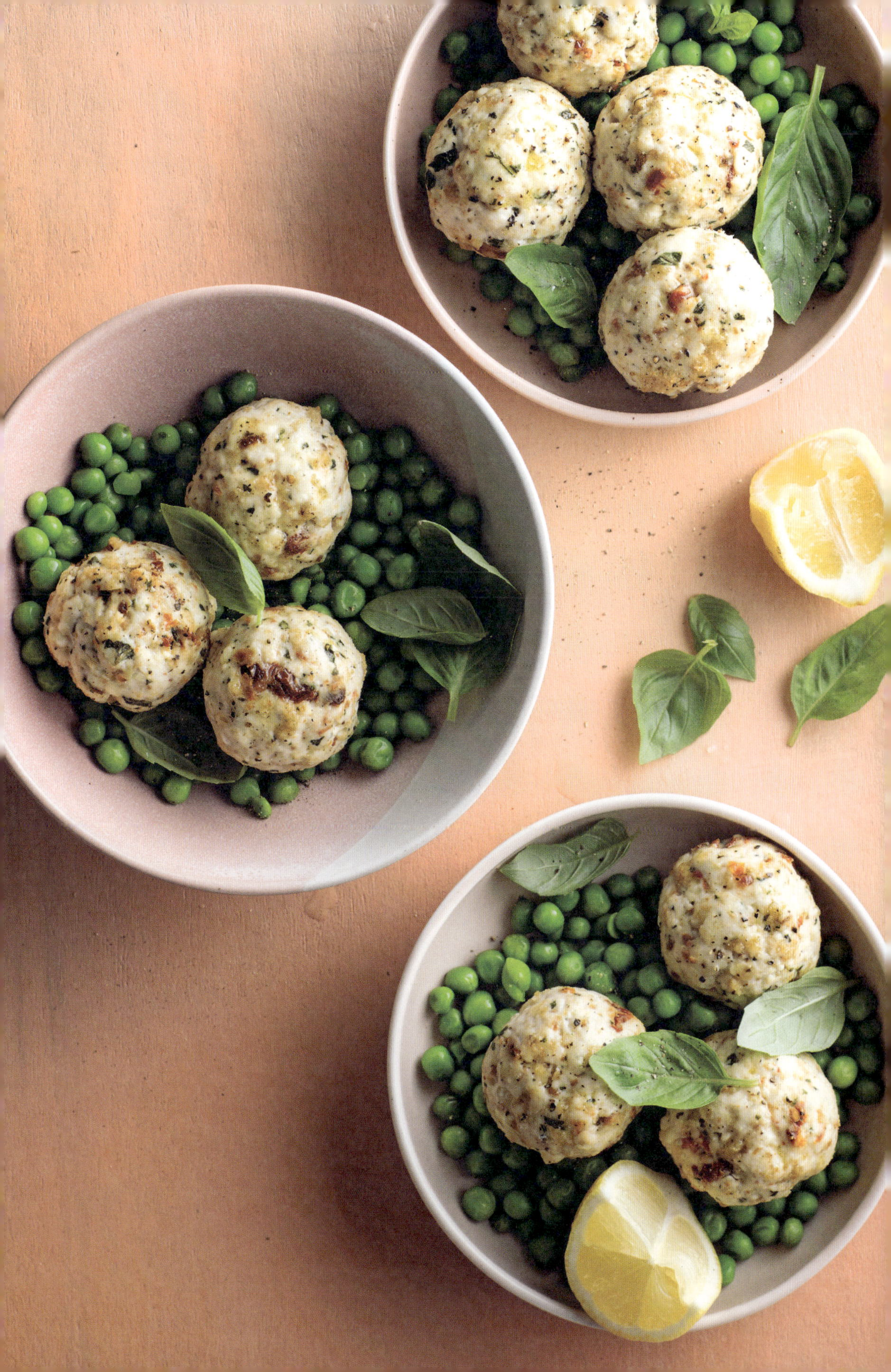

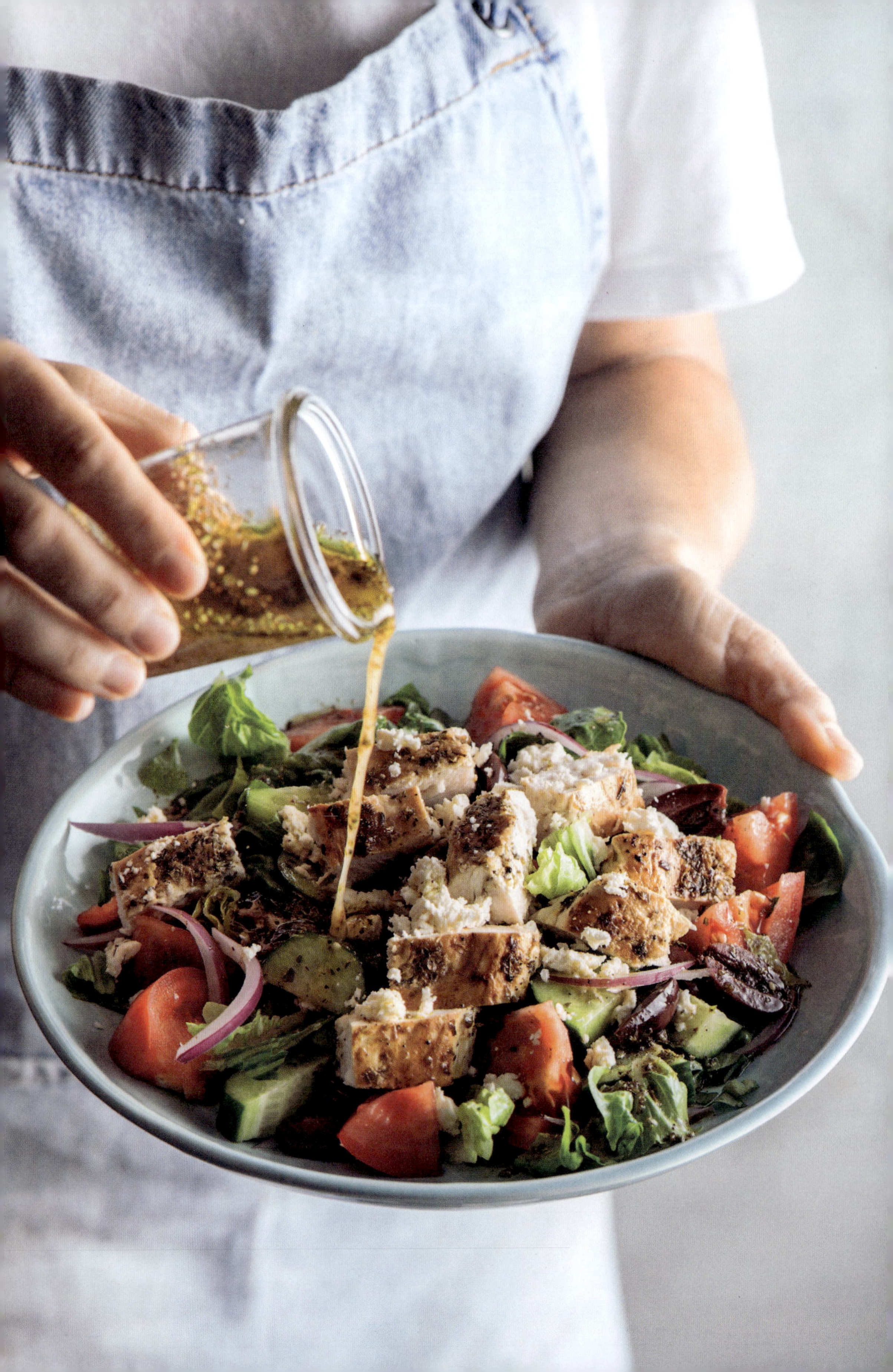

Serves 2

PERI CHICKEN SALAD

Not to be mistaken for peri peri chicken, which is exactly what my friend thought I was writing a book about when I first told her the title! This salad is really a mix of some of my favourite peri ingredients, tied together with a fabulous dressing. The perfect summer meal.

1 x 250 g chicken breast fillet
1 tablespoon extra-virgin olive oil
juice of ½ small lemon
1 garlic clove, minced
½ teaspoon dried oregano
sea salt and freshly ground black pepper

Dressing

3 tablespoons extra-virgin olive oil
3 tablespoons red wine vinegar
1 garlic clove, minced
1 teaspoon dried oregano
1 teaspoon honey
1 teaspoon dijon mustard

Salad

160 g (4 cups) chopped crunchy cos or iceberg lettuce
2 large tomatoes, roughly chopped
½ red or green capsicum, roughly chopped
1 Lebanese cucumber, roughly chopped
½ small red onion, finely sliced
small handful of flat-leaf parsley, roughly chopped
40 g (¼ cup) pitted kalamata olives
80 g feta cheese

Pat the chicken dry, then place it on a large piece of baking paper. Stab the chicken several times with a fork on both sides, then pull the baking paper over the top and pound it with a meat mallet or rolling pin to flatten the chicken a little.

Drizzle 1 teaspoon of olive oil and the lemon juice all over the chicken, then sprinkle with the garlic and oregano. Season with salt and pepper. Massage the ingredients into both sides of the chicken.

Heat the remaining olive oil in a frying pan over medium–high heat. Add the chicken and cook on both sides for 3–4 minutes, or until golden on the outside and cooked through. Transfer to a chopping board to rest for 5 minutes before slicing thinly.

Whisk all the dressing ingredients in a small bowl or shake in a jar with a lid until combined.

Put all the salad ingredients except the feta into a large bowl and toss together with most of the dressing.

To serve, divide the salad between bowls or plates, top with the chicken and crumble on the feta. Finish with another drizzle of dressing.

Serves 6–8

TURKEY MEATLOAF

Meatloaf makes an excellent high-protein dinner – and even better leftovers for lunch the next day. If you don't have a loaf tin or rectangular baking dish, you can always shape this by hand into a more rustic 'freestyle' loaf.

- extra-virgin olive oil
- 4 eggs
- 2 x 40 g slices of wholegrain bread, toasted (or 45 g/¾ cup wholemeal breadcrumbs)
- 1 onion, finely diced
- 1 garlic clove, minced
- 1 kg lean turkey mince (or chicken mince)
- 2 teaspoons smoked or sweet paprika
- 1 teaspoon dried oregano
- 2 tablespoons worcestershire sauce
- 1 heaped tablespoon dijon or American mustard
- sea salt and freshly ground black pepper
- green salad, to serve

Glaze

- 165 ml (⅔ cup) low-sugar barbecue sauce
- 2 tablespoons brown sugar
- 1 tablespoon apple cider vinegar
- ½ teaspoon dijon or American mustard

Preheat the oven to 180°C. Line a baking tray with baking paper and lightly grease a loaf tin or baking dish with olive oil.

Cook the eggs in boiling water for 5 minutes, then remove from the pan and set aside to cool slightly before peeling under cold, running water. Set aside.

Pulse the toast in a food processor until it forms coarse breadcrumbs.

Whisk all the ingredients for the glaze in a small bowl and set aside.

Heat 1 tablespoon of olive oil in a small frying pan over medium–high heat and add the onion and garlic. Cook for 3–5 minutes, or until the onion is soft and translucent. Remove the pan from the heat and tip the onion mixture into a large bowl along with the breadcrumbs, mince, paprika, oregano, worcestershire sauce and mustard. Add 2 tablespoons of the glaze. Season well with salt and pepper and use your hands to mix everything together.

Spoon half the meatloaf mixture into the tin or dish. Place the boiled eggs lengthways in a line down the centre of the meatloaf. Spoon over the remaining meatloaf mixture, then gently press to compress.

Drizzle the remaining glaze over the meatloaf and bake for around 45 minutes. Check to ensure it's cooked through, then slice and serve with a green salad.

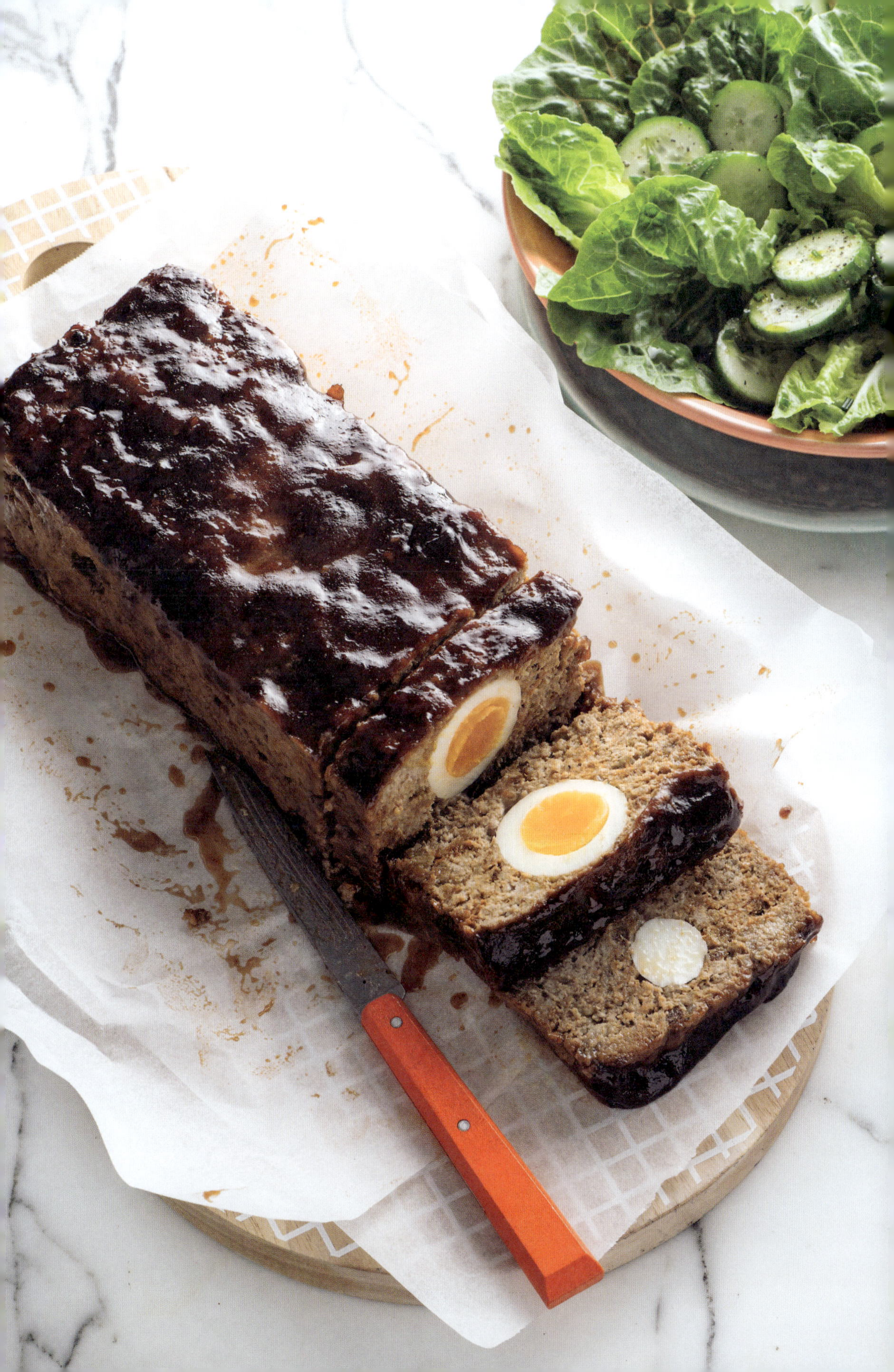

Serves 4

THE BEST (NO) BUTTER CHICKEN

One of my favourite parts of a curry dinner is the crunchy pappadums that go with it – and the great news is that they're actually pretty good for you! That's because they're made from urid flour, which is made from white lentils. The easiest way to make pappadums at home is to buy microwave ones from the supermarket. They only take 1 minute to cook, and because they're cooked in the microwave, they don't require extra cooking oil, which is even better.

500 g chicken breast fillets, diced into 2 cm pieces
2 tablespoons extra-virgin olive oil
370 g (2 cups) cooked basmati or brown rice
small handful of coriander leaves
12 pappadums

Marinade
125 g (½ cup) plain Greek-style yoghurt, plus extra to serve
1 teaspoon ground turmeric
2 teaspoons garam masala
1 teaspoon ground cumin
1 tablespoon minced ginger
2 garlic cloves, minced
juice of ½ lemon

Curry sauce
250 ml (1 cup) tomato passata
250 ml (1 cup) low-fat coconut milk
1 tablespoon honey
2 teaspoons salt

Combine all the ingredients for the marinade in a large bowl. Add the chicken and stir until completely coated. Cover and place in the fridge for at least 30 minutes, or overnight if you can.

Heat the olive oil in a large frying pan over medium–high heat and add the marinated chicken. Spoon in any leftover marinade from the bowl and cook for a few minutes, stirring regularly until the chicken has turned from pink to white.

Add the curry sauce ingredients to the pan and stir together well. Bring to a gentle simmer and cook uncovered for around 10 minutes, or until the sauce thickens slightly.

Spoon the rice into bowls, then place the curry on top. Add a dollop of yoghurt and some coriander leaves, then serve with crunchy pappadums.

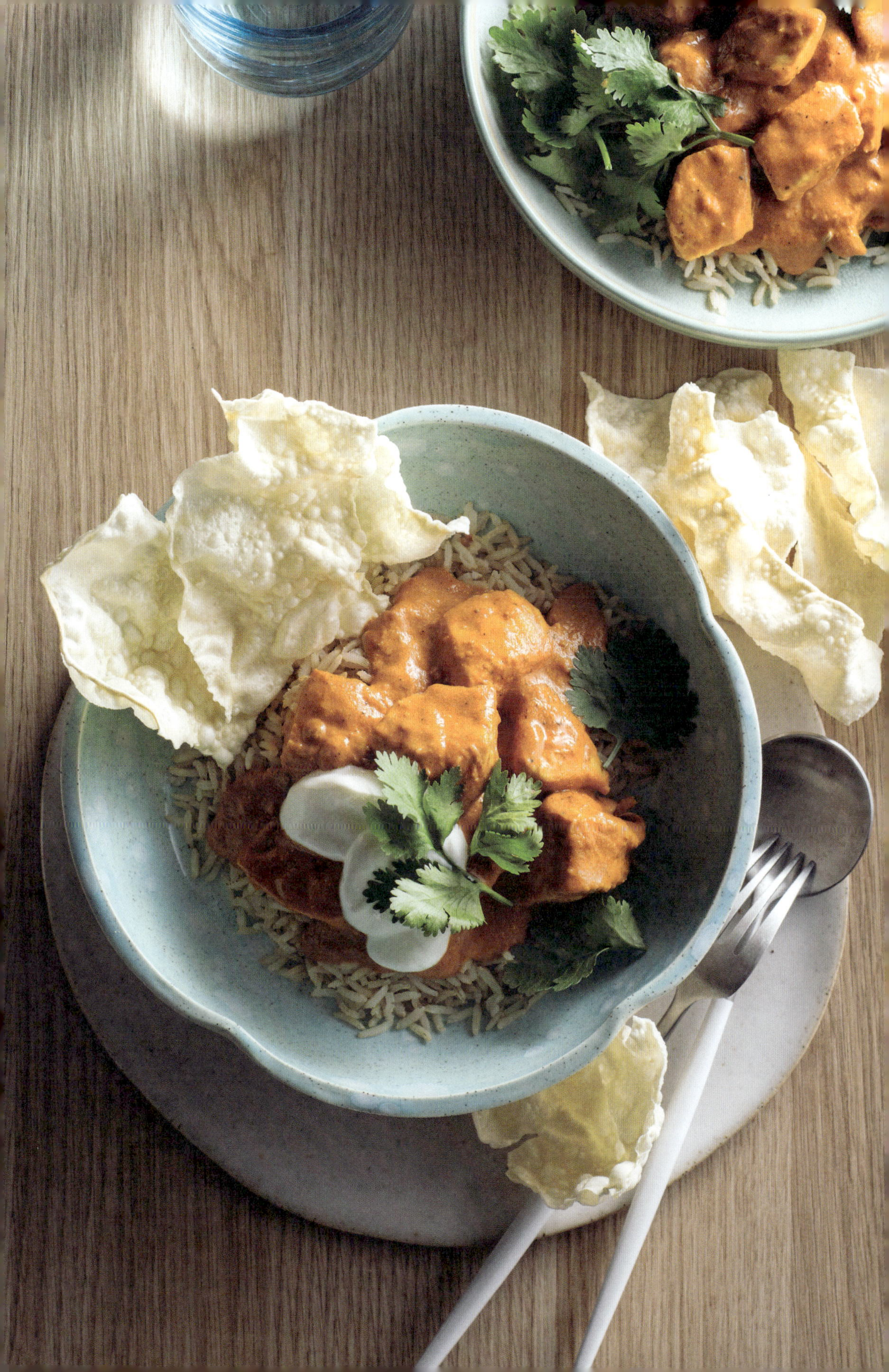

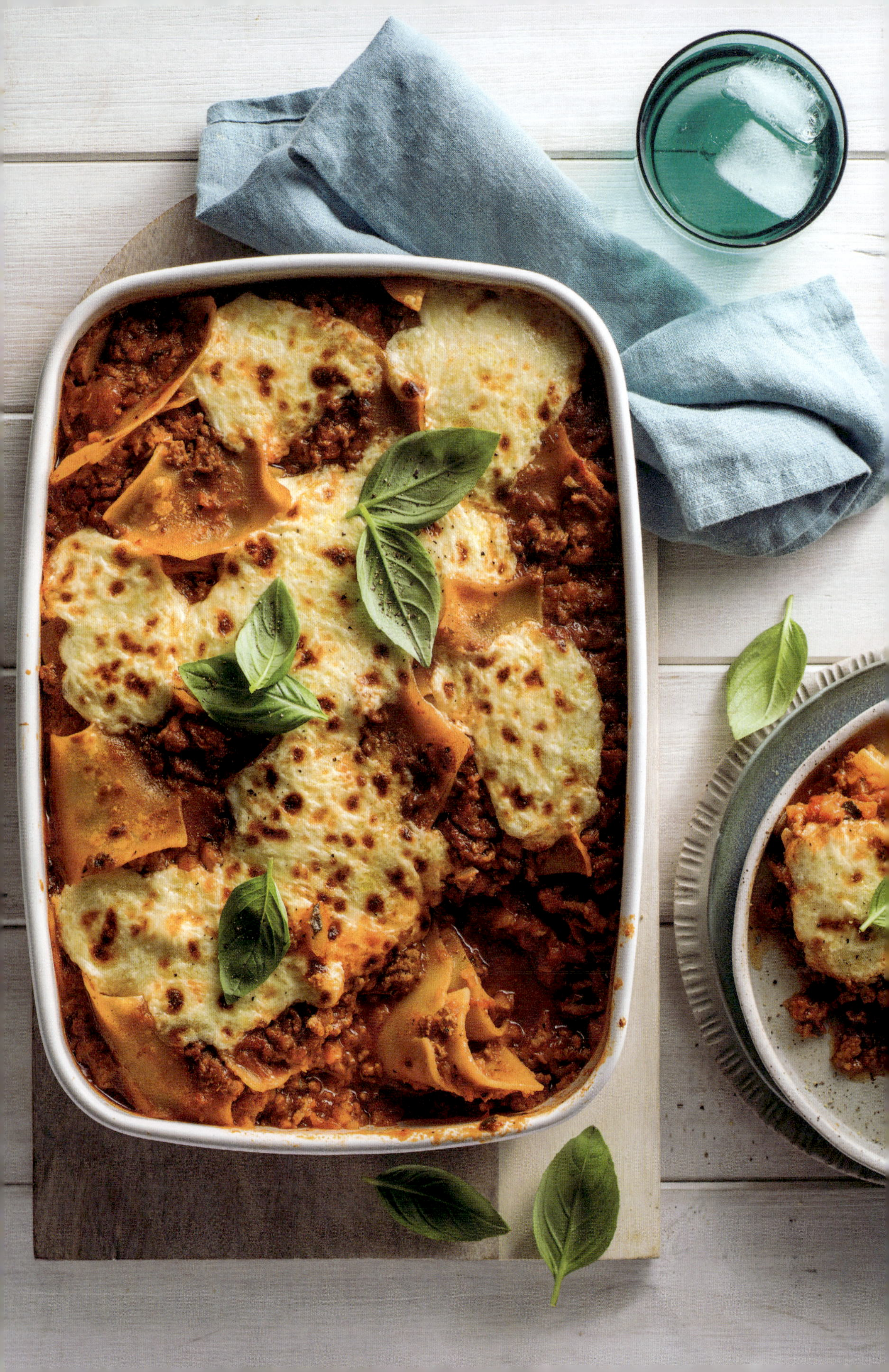

Serves 6

LAZY LASAGNE

Before any lasagne purists come for me, I want to point out that I do recognise this is not lasagne in the traditional form! I like to think of it as more of an homage: it is much faster and easier to put together, with a boost of veggies and minus that extra-creamy cheesy sauce.

- 1 onion, quartered
- 2 large carrots, chopped
- 3 celery stalks, chopped
- 1 zucchini, chopped
- 2 tablespoons extra-virgin olive oil
- sea salt and freshly ground black pepper
- 500 g extra-lean beef mince (go for grass-fed and organic, if you can)
- 2 tablespoons minced garlic
- 2 tablespoons tomato paste
- 2 x 400 g cans crushed tomatoes
- 2 teaspoons Italian seasoning or herb mix
- 1 litre (4 cups) chicken stock
- 6 lasagne sheets (wholemeal if you can get them)
- small handful of basil leaves, roughly chopped

Cheese topping

- 200 g fresh ricotta
- 150 g (1 cup) grated mozzarella
- 50 g (½ cup) grated parmesan

Pulse the onion, carrot, celery and zucchini in a food processor until finely chopped.

Heat the olive oil in a large saucepan over medium heat and add the chopped vegetables. Season well with salt and pepper and cook for 10 minutes, stirring occasionally, until the vegetables have softened. Add the mince and garlic and use a spoon or spatula to break the mince up. Stir regularly until the mince is browned.

Add the tomato paste and stir through for 1 minute, then add the crushed tomatoes, Italian herbs and stock and stir well. Bring to a gentle simmer, then place the lid on top and cook for around 20 minutes.

Meanwhile, combine all the ingredients for the cheese topping.

Remove the lid from the pan and break the lasagne sheets into the mince mix, stirring occasionally to prevent them from sticking together. Cook the pasta to al dente according to the packet instructions – by this point, most of the liquid will have cooked away.

Preheat the grill to medium–high. Transfer the lasagne to a baking dish and dollop on the cheese topping. Grill for 10 minutes, or until golden. Spoon onto serving plates and serve topped with basil.

RED MEAT

At home, extra-lean beef mince is our primary source of red meat as it's cost-effective, very low in fat and goes a long way, which means we can bulk sauces out with veggies and beans. A bonus of this is that we're eating smaller portions of red meat overall, which isn't a bad thing.

When shopping, I look for the heart-smart label or 'extra-lean' so I know it has the lowest amount of saturated fat. Lamb mince is also a great source of protein and iron, but is generally higher in fat and not available in extra-lean or heart-smart varieties.

Serves 4–6

BROWN RICE BURRITO BOWL

When patients ask me to suggest some healthy takeaway meals they can have when they're out and about, one of the options I usually recommend is a Mexican brown rice burrito bowl. Nutritionally, these can be beautifully balanced, and they taste so delicious I like to replicate them at home. You can swap the meat for the same quantity of black beans, four-bean mix or red kidney beans.

300 g (1½ cups) brown rice
80 g (2 cups) shredded iceberg lettuce
1 batch meat sauce from the Upside-down nachos (see page 198), reheated
1 cup (100 g) grated tasty cheddar

Corn salsa
150 g (1 cup) cherry tomatoes, quartered
1 x 400 g can corn kernels
1 small cucumber, roughly chopped
1 large avocado, roughly diced
½ small red onion, finely diced
sea salt and freshly ground black pepper

To serve (optional)
plain Greek-style yoghurt
pickled jalapeños

Cook the rice according to the packet instructions.

Place the corn salsa ingredients in a bowl and toss together with a good seasoning of salt and pepper. Set aside.

Divide the rice, shredded lettuce and meat sauce among serving bowls. Top each portion with corn salsa and grated cheese. Serve with dollops of yoghurt and jalapeños, if you like.

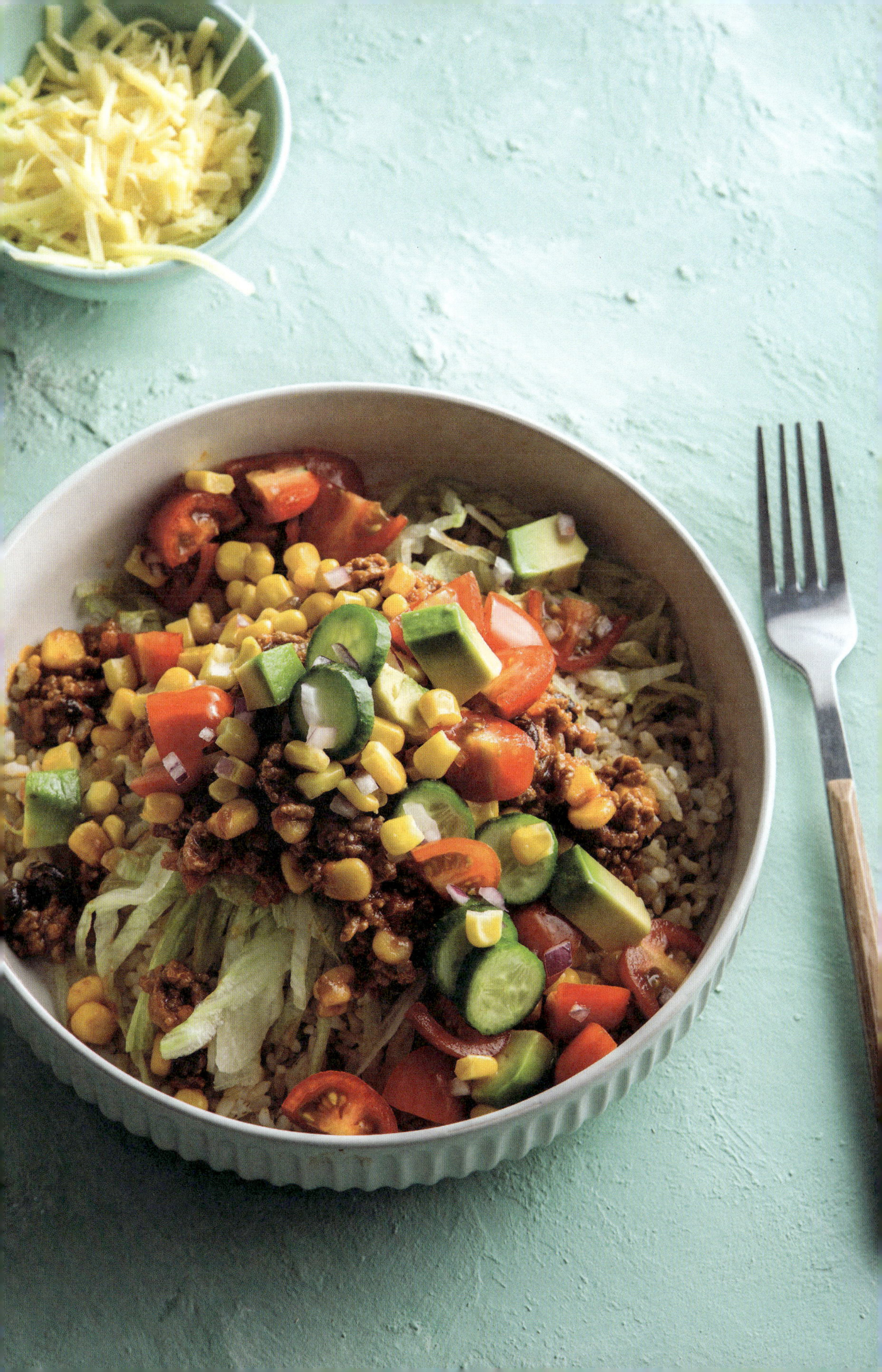

Serves 4

UPSIDE-DOWN NACHOS

It's the corn chip base that makes nachos not too healthy. So here we flip the dish upside down, topping the protein-packed and fibre-filled beans with a handful of crushed-up chips – still delicious but so much better for us.

Meat sauce

2 tablespoons extra-virgin olive oil
½ small red onion, finely chopped
500 g extra-lean beef mince (see Note on page 195)
1 x 400 g can black beans, drained and rinsed
1 x 400 g can corn kernels, drained
1 x 400 g can crushed or diced tomatoes
1 garlic clove, minced
1 teaspoon smoked or sweet paprika
1 tablespoon low-sugar barbecue sauce
sea salt and freshly ground black pepper

Quick guacamole

1 avocado
juice of 1 lime
sea salt

To serve

50 g (½ cup) grated tasty cheddar
plain Greek-style yoghurt
50 g (1 cup) good-quality plain corn chips
pickled jalapeños (optional)

For the meat sauce, heat the olive oil in a large heavy-based frying pan over medium–high heat. Add the onion and cook for a few minutes, or until soft and translucent.

Add the mince to the pan and use a spatula to break it up. Cook for a few minutes, stirring occasionally. Once the mince is nice and brown, add the beans, corn, tomatoes, garlic, paprika and barbecue sauce. Season with salt and pepper, stir together to combine everything and cook until the mixture starts to simmer. Turn the heat to low, place the lid on the pan and cook for 10–15 minutes. Remove the lid and continue cooking until any excess liquid has evaporated.

Meanwhile, to make the quick guacamole, use the back of a fork to mash the avocado with the lime juice and a good pinch of salt in a small bowl.

Divide the meat sauce among bowls and top with grated cheese, a dollop of yoghurt, a generous spoonful of guacamole and some jalapenos, if you like. Finish by crushing up a handful of corn chips over each serve for that upside-down nacho experience!

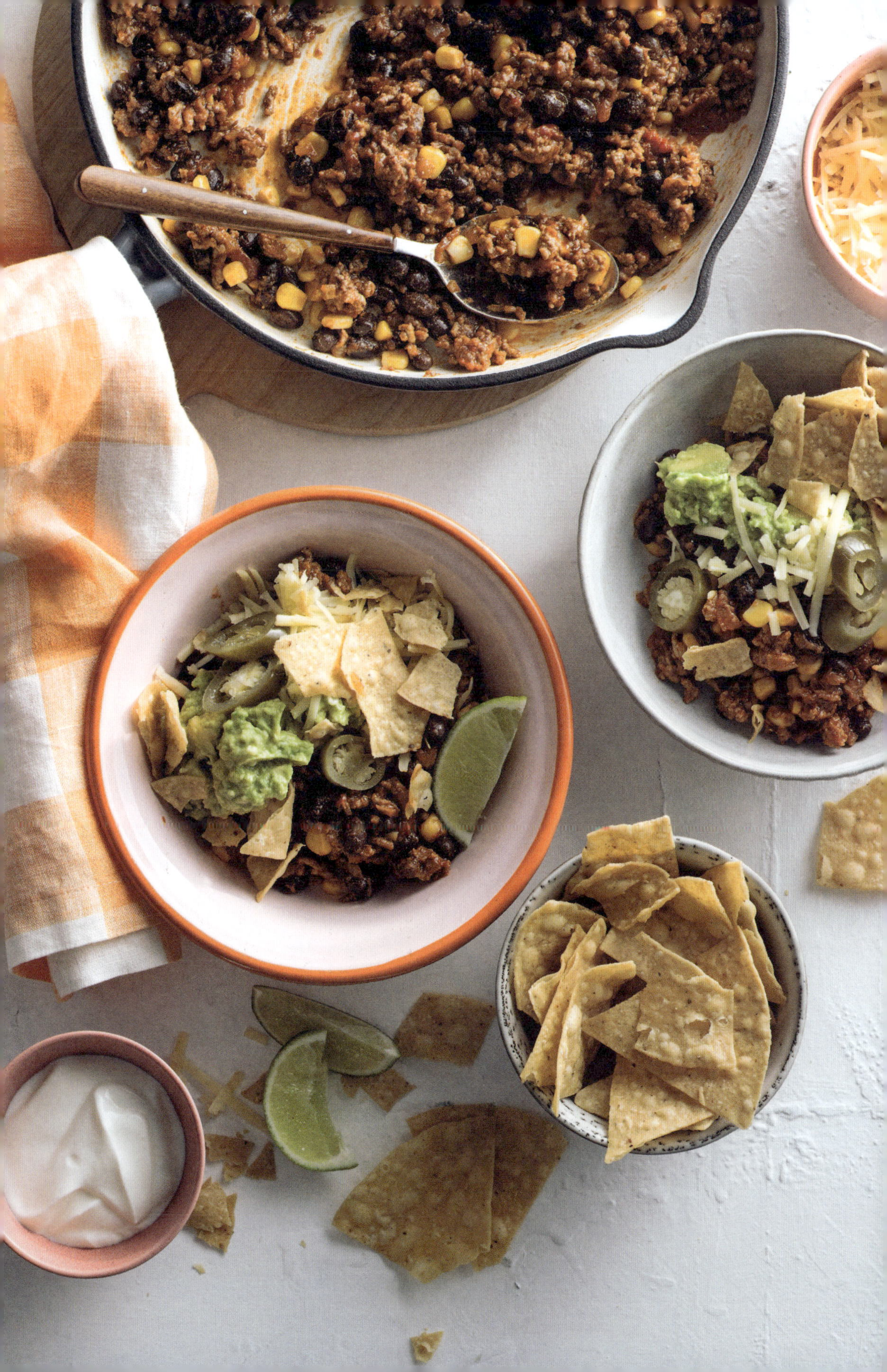

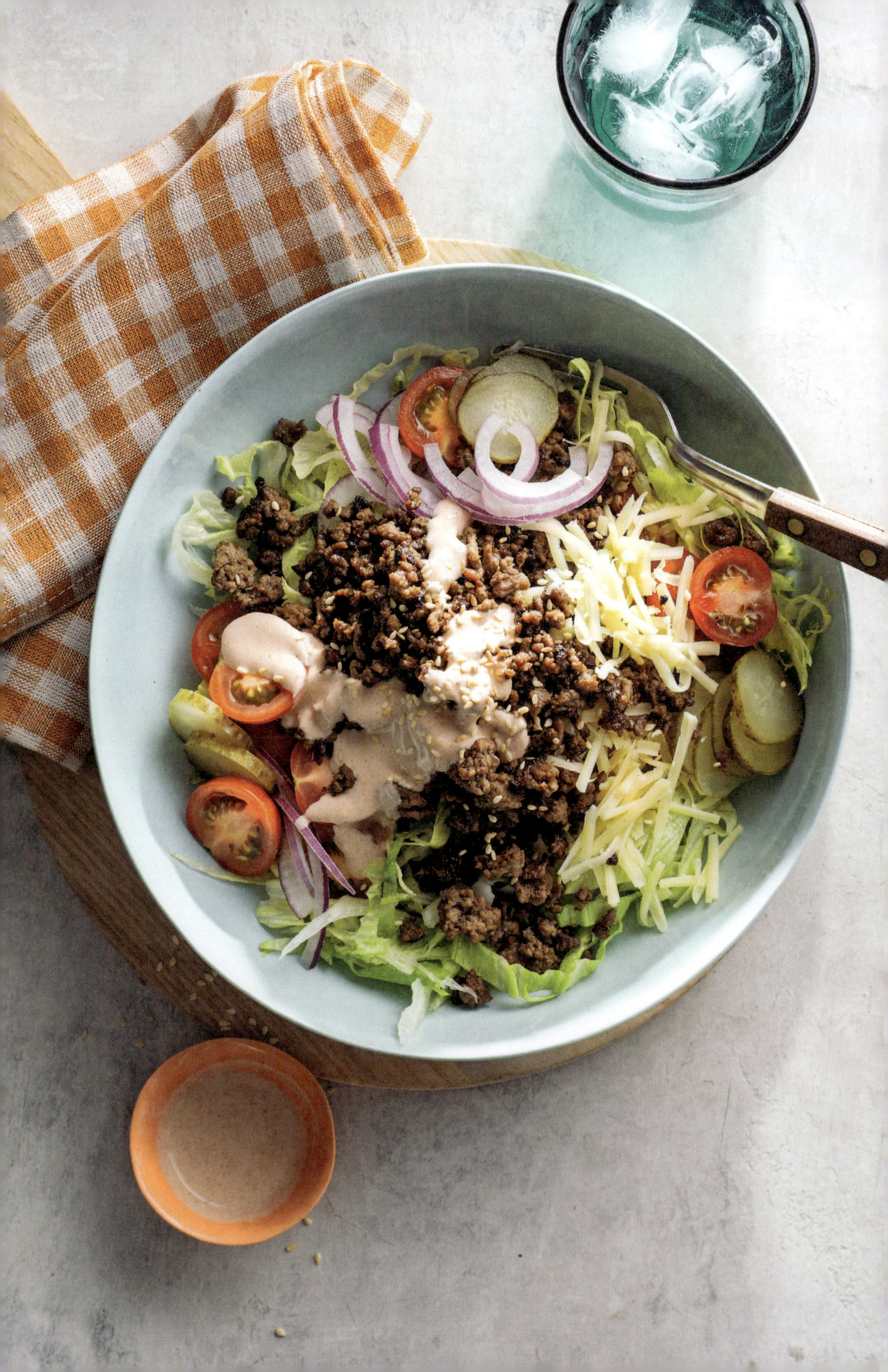

Serves 4

BIG MAC SALAD

Don't be fooled by the name. This salad may have the essence of a well-known burger but it is packed full of nutrition! It is a great way to enjoy a little good-quality red meat.

- 1 tablespoon extra-virgin olive oil
- 500 g extra-lean beef mince (see Note)
- 1 teaspoon garlic powder
- 1 teaspoon onion powder
- 1 teaspoon worcestershire sauce
- sea salt and freshly ground black pepper
- 1 small iceberg lettuce, finely sliced
- 100 g (1 cup) grated tasty cheddar
- 150 g (1 cup) cherry tomatoes, halved
- ½ red onion, finely diced
- 4 dill pickles, thinly sliced
- 2 tablespoons toasted sesame seeds

Dressing

- 125 g (½ cup) plain Greek-style yoghurt
- 2 teaspoons tomato sauce (try a reduced-sugar variety)
- 2 teaspoons dijon or American mustard
- ½ teaspoon smoked or sweet paprika
- 1 tablespoon red wine vinegar

Heat the olive oil in a large frying pan over medium–high heat. Add the mince, garlic and onion powder and worcestershire sauce, then season with salt and pepper. Break up the beef and cook until it has browned, stirring occasionally. This will take 6–8 minutes.

Mix all of the dressing ingredients in a jar with a lid and shake until well combined.

Divide the lettuce, cheddar, cherry tomatoes, onion and dill pickles among bowls. When ready to serve, top with the mince mixture, drizzle over the dressing and scatter with toasted sesame seeds.

NOTE

See the note about choosing beef mince on page 195. If you prefer, you can also swap beef for chicken or turkey mince.

04

SNACKS

Not everyone needs to snack, but if and when you do, it's best to have something nourishing as well as tasty to hand. This chapter is a selection of my favourite snacks. Some can even double as a light meal, such as the high-protein egg muffins on page 218. You'll notice they all make many serves so they can be stashed away to enjoy on those occasions you feel like something extra.

Serves 20

CARAMEL-PECAN CHOCOLATE BARK

I've taken inspiration from two sources for this snack. The first is a date dark chocolate bark making the rounds online at the moment. The second is one of my favourite treats ever, Turtles, which I used to enjoy on holiday in Hawaii long before having kids! Oh, boy, does this version bring back delicious memories. Along with being so tasty, these are also full of fibre and antioxidant goodness. Remember, though, each little portion is very energy-dense so stick to the serving recommendations of one at a time. These keep well in an airtight container for up to 2 weeks – if they last that long.

120 g pecans
500 g medjool dates, pitted
4 tablespoons smooth, runny peanut butter (or other runny natural nut spread)
200 g dark chocolate (70 per cent cocoa or higher)
sea salt

Gently toast the pecans in a frying pan over medium heat, tossing often for 5–7 minutes until they begin to turn golden. Set aside on a chopping board, then chop roughly with a large knife.

Line a baking tray with baking paper. Use a small knife to slice each date so it opens like a book. Arrange the dates on a tray so they slightly overlap and gently press down on them so they connect and create one big sheet of dates.

Drizzle the peanut butter over the dates and use the back of a spoon to smooth and spread it evenly over the dates. Sprinkle the crushed toasted pecans on top.

Break the chocolate into chunks and microwave in a heatproof bowl for 30 seconds at a time, stirring after each burst, until the chocolate has melted. (This takes about 1 minute and 30 seconds in my microwave.)

Pour the melted chocolate evenly over the bark, using a spoon to spread it if you need to. Place the tray in the fridge for at least an hour to set.

Sprinkle with a little sea salt before cutting into 20 pieces and storing in an airtight container.

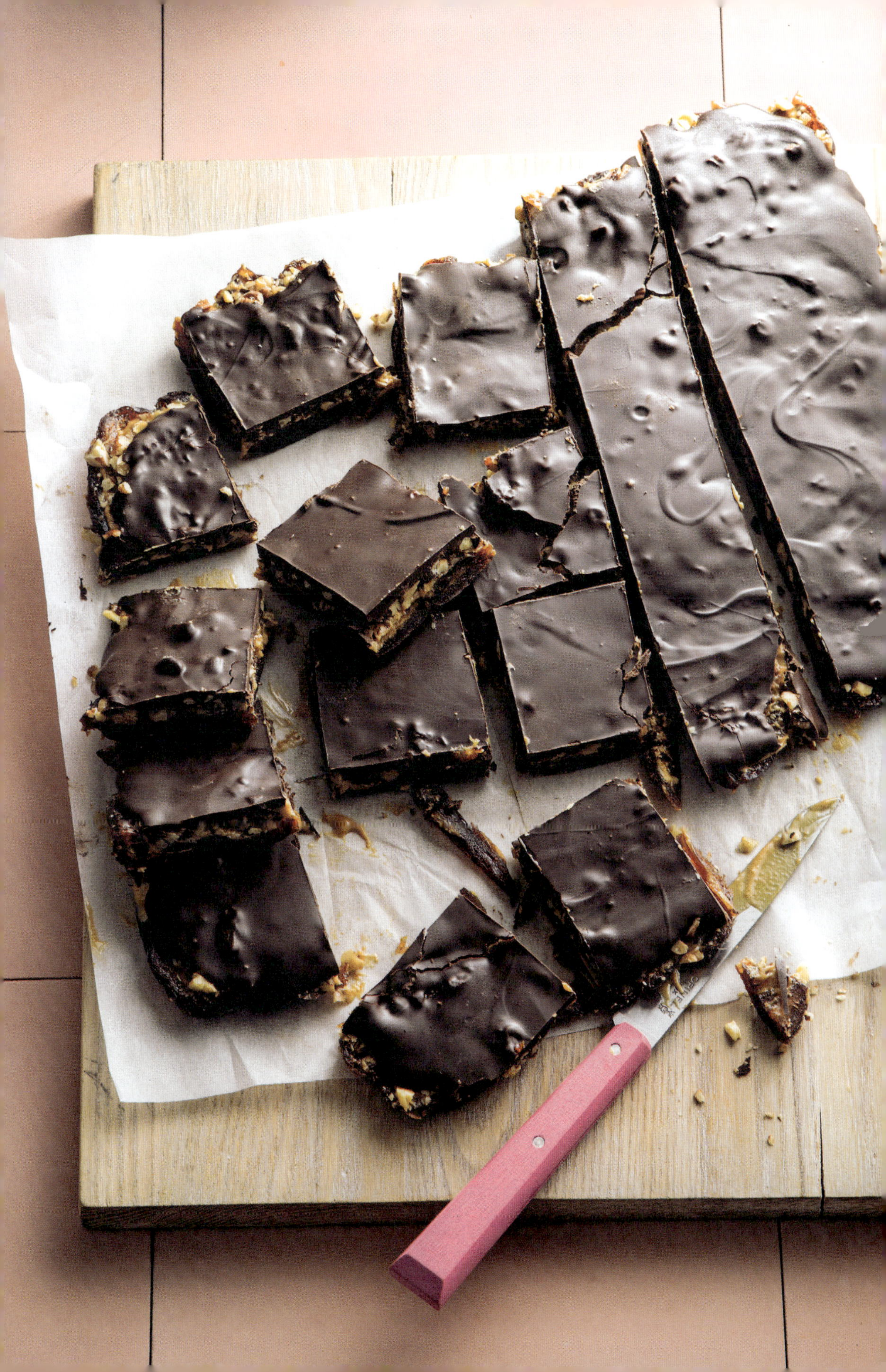

Makes 10–12

FROZEN YOGHURT CLUSTERS

This is such a sensational little snack, but beware! If you've got kids, no yoghurt cluster will be safe around them. This recipe is also very versatile as you can use a variety of different yoghurts, fruits and other favourite ingredients in the mixture. You can either keep the clusters plain or, for a more indulgent snack, dip or drizzle the frozen clusters in melted dark chocolate.

- 250 g mixed berries
- 200 g vanilla or berry probiotic yoghurt (or any yoghurt of your choice)
- 1 tablespoon honey or maple syrup
- 150 g good-quality dark chocolate (70 per cent cocoa or higher)

Line a tray with non-stick baking paper. If using raspberries and blueberries, halve them; cut strawberries into small pieces.

Mix the berries, yoghurt and honey or maple syrup in a bowl until well combined. Dollop heaped tablespoons of the mixture onto the lined tray. Place in the freezer for at least 4 hours so the clusters can set.

Break the chocolate into chunks and microwave in a heatproof bowl for 30 seconds at a time, stirring after each burst, until the chocolate has melted. Allow it to sit for 5 minutes to cool slightly.

Drizzle each cluster liberally with the melted chocolate, then return the tray to the freezer for at least 15 minutes to set before eating. Store any leftovers in an airtight container in the freezer for up to a month.

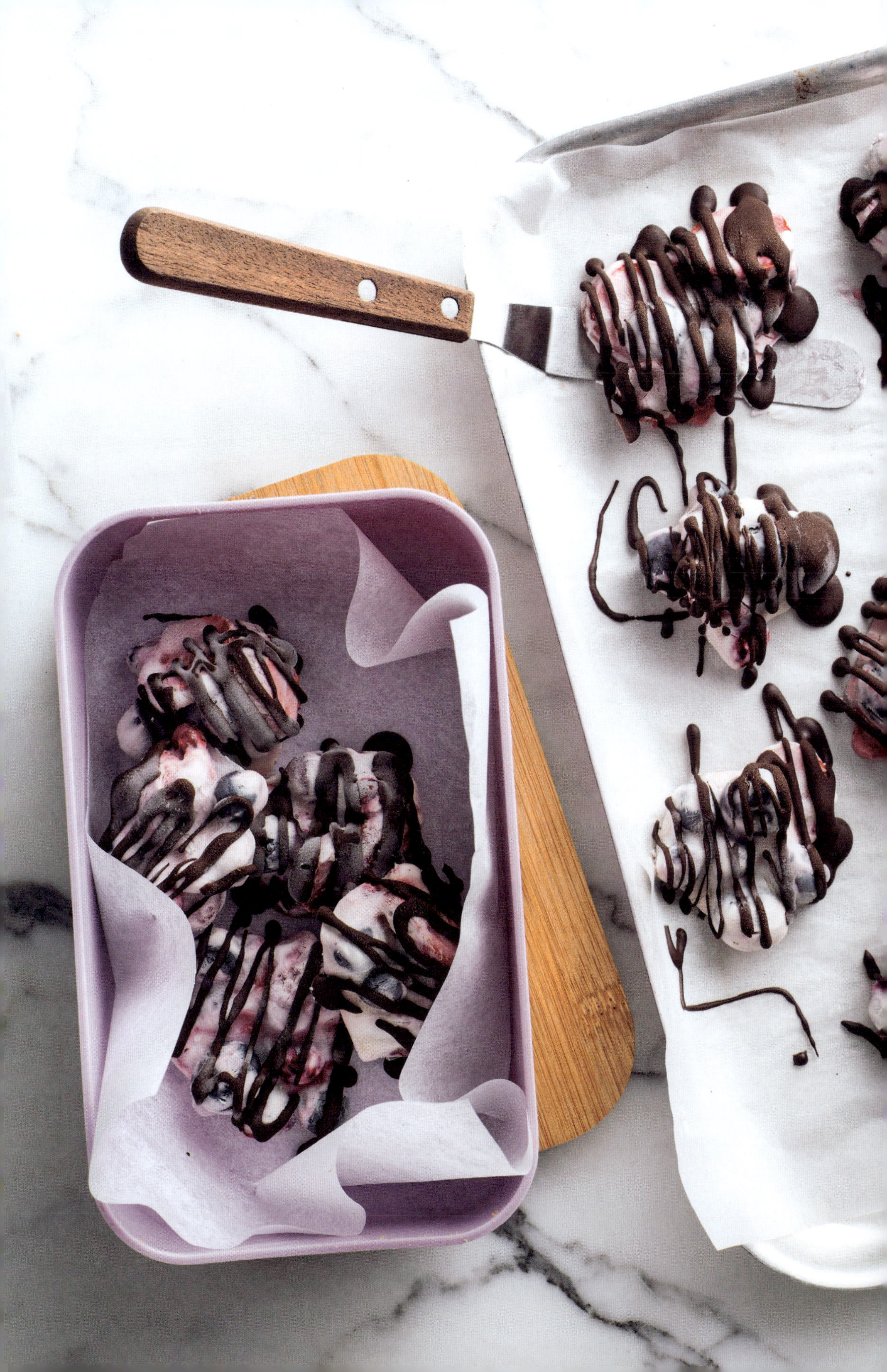

Serves 4

FOUR-INGREDIENT CHOCOLATE MOUSSE

If you're still on the fence about tofu, this might get you over the line. The silken variety is the perfect texture for this beautiful mousse and you'll honestly not even know you're eating tofu!

100 g good-quality dark chocolate (70 per cent cocoa or higher)
500 g silken tofu, drained
2 tablespoons maple syrup
1 teaspoon vanilla extract

To serve
plain Greek-style yoghurt
mixed berries

Break the chocolate into chunks and microwave in a heatproof bowl for 30 seconds at a time, stirring after each burst, until the chocolate has melted.

Combine the tofu, maple syrup and vanilla in a food processor and whizz until smooth. Add the melted chocolate and process again until smooth and combined.

Divide between serving bowls or glasses and place in the fridge to set for at least an hour.

Serve topped with a dollop of yoghurt and some mixed berries.

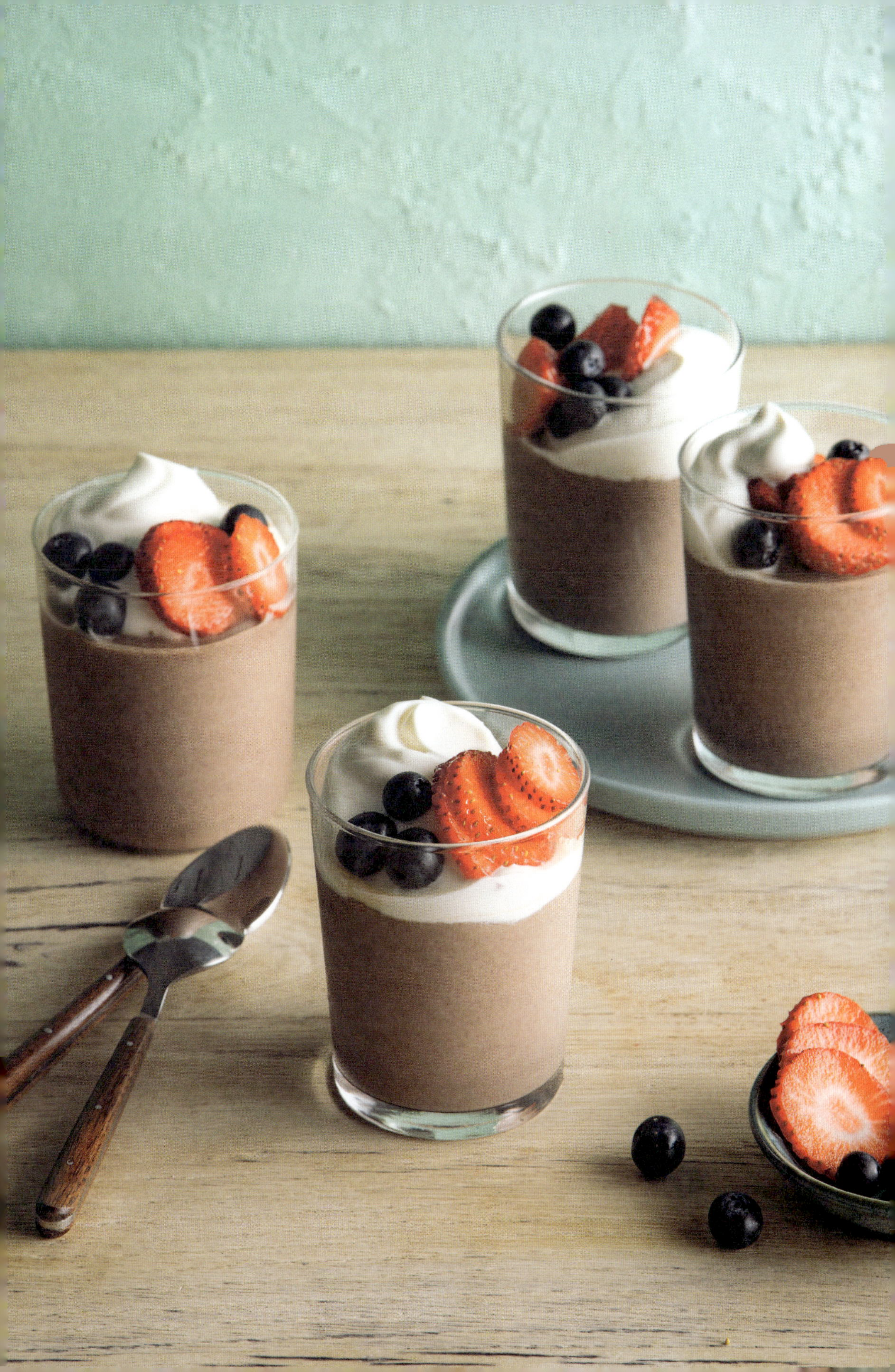

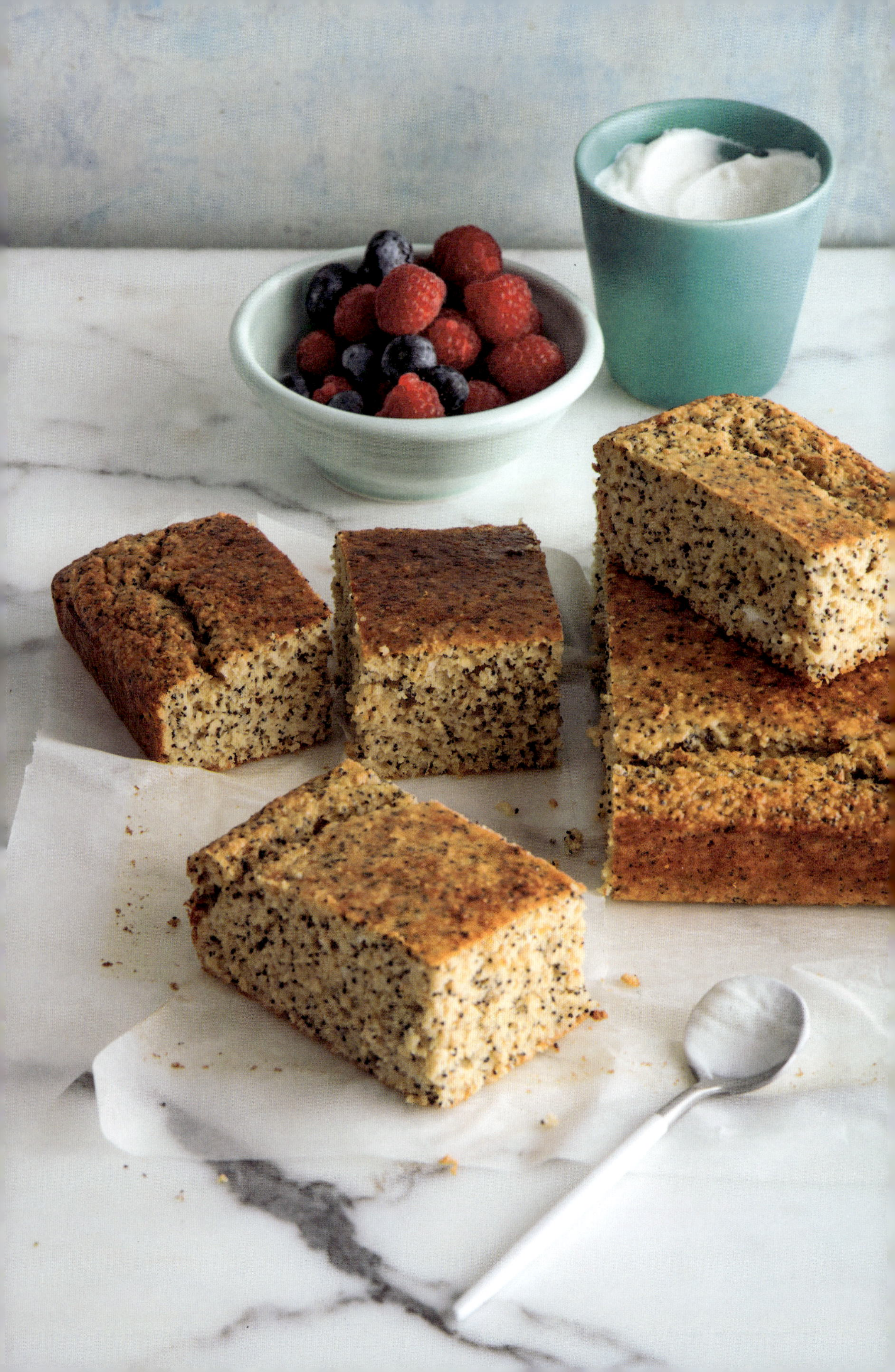

Makes 10

HIGH-PROTEIN LEMON AND POPPY SEED SLICE

I love a lemon and poppyseed muffin – the tang of lemon and the tiny little crunch of poppy seeds is so appealing. This recipe can be made into muffins too but I quite like it as a slice or loaf. As with my other recipes, it's had a healthy glow-up too. I keep this in the fridge and eat it over the course of a week. It's lovely eaten cold or reheated a little in the microwave.

250 g (2½ cups) rolled oats
4 eggs
250 g (1 cup) plain yoghurt
125 ml (½ cup) maple syrup
zest and juice of 1 large lemon
sea salt
3 tablespoons vanilla protein powder (optional)
3 teaspoons baking powder
3 tablespoons poppy seeds

To serve (optional)
plain Greek-style yoghurt
mixed berries

Preheat the oven to 180°C. Line a loaf tin with baking paper.

Blend the oats to a fine flour in a food processor.

Whisk the eggs and yoghurt in a large bowl, then add the maple syrup, lemon zest and juice, and whisk again. Add the oat flour, a pinch of salt, the protein powder (if using), baking powder and poppy seeds, then stir until combined. Pour the mixture into the tin.

Bake for 30–35 minutes, or until the slice is golden on top and a bamboo skewer inserted in the centre comes out clean.

Leave to cool for 10–20 minutes before slicing and serving. You can enjoy as is or serve warm with a dollop of yoghurt and some berries.

Makes around 15 servings (30 g each)

ROSEMARY-SPICED NUTS

According to the latest research, most of us should be eating a handful of mixed nuts a day. They're a great source of good fats, fibre and bioactive compounds – nutrients that also happen to reduce the risk of metabolic syndrome associated with perimenopause and menopause. Go for almonds, walnuts, hazelnuts, Brazil nuts, cashews, pecans and pistachios for these – grab a mixture or just choose your favourites.

- 560 g (4 cups) mixed nuts
- 2 tablespoons extra-virgin olive oil
- 1 teaspoon sea salt
- ½ teaspoon garlic powder
- ½ teaspoon onion powder
- 1 teaspoon dried rosemary

Preheat the oven to 150°C. Line a baking tray with baking paper.

Place all the ingredients in a bowl and toss together until the nuts are well coated. Spread out on the tray.

Bake for around 25 minutes, or until the nuts are golden. Take out of the oven and leave to cool for at least 20 minutes to allow the nuts to become crunchy.

Transfer the nuts to an airtight container and store in the fridge to stay crunchy and fresh.

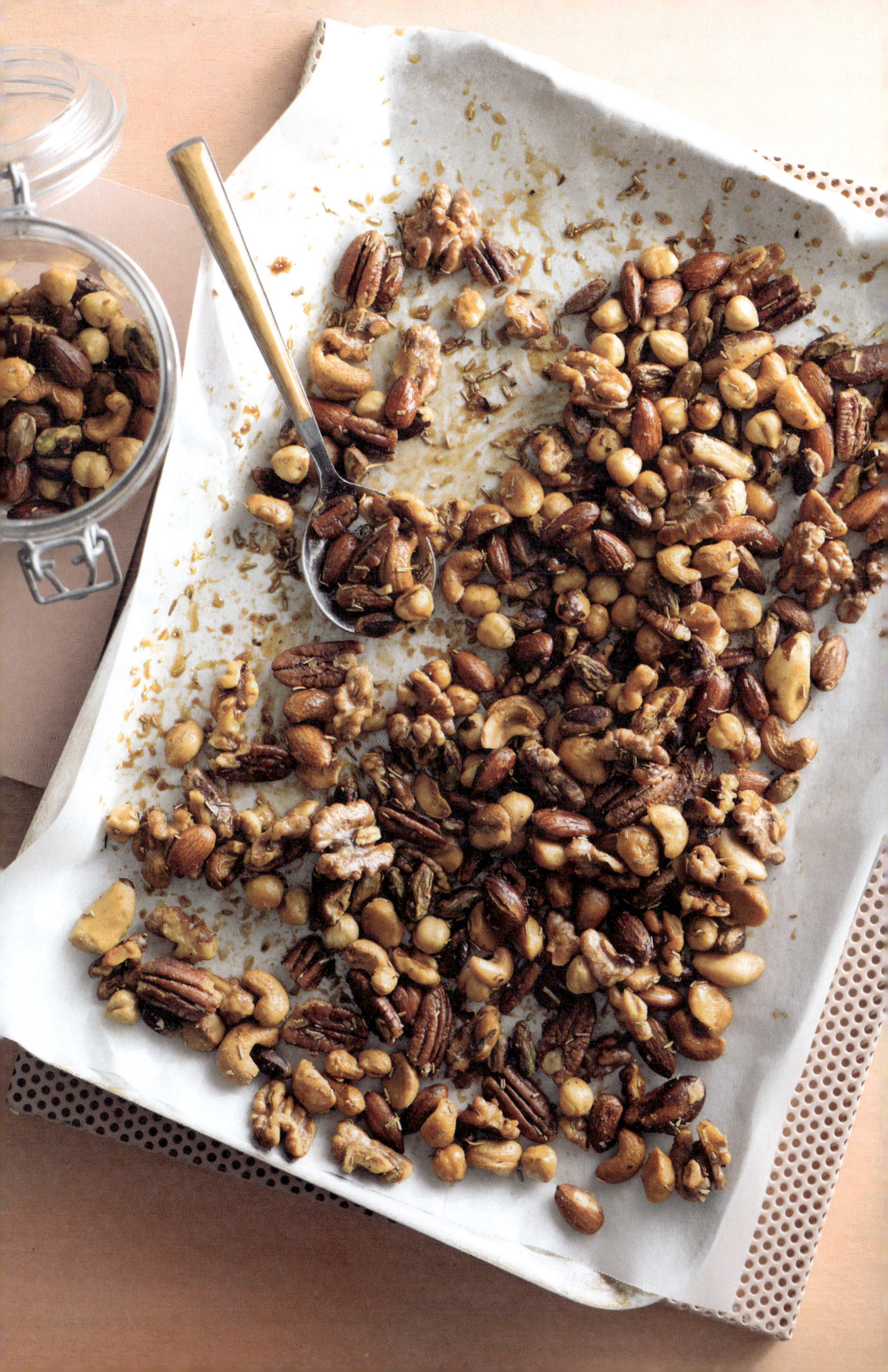

Serves 12

TURMERIC SEED CRACKERS

Packets of these gorgeous seed crackers can go for $10–15 at the grocery store, but making your own is so easy, it's almost silly. They're a great way to use up the odds and ends of packets of seeds in the pantry. A perfect crunchy snack by themselves, you can also serve them with your favourite dip.

- 60 g (½ cup) sunflower seeds
- 105 g (¾ cup) pumpkin seeds
- 115 g (¾ cup) sesame seeds
- 50 g (⅓ cup) flaxseeds
- 2 tablespoons psyllium husks
- ½ teaspoon ground turmeric
- 1 teaspoon sea salt
- freshly ground black pepper
- 560 ml (2¼ cups) filtered water

Preheat the oven to 150°C. Line two baking trays with baking paper.

Put all the dry ingredients in a large bowl with a good grind of pepper, then pour in the water and stir until well combined. Set aside to thicken for 30 minutes.

Spoon the mixture onto the trays and use the back of the spoon to spread it into an even layer around 5 mm thick.

Bake for around 1 hour, keeping an eye on it after 50 minutes to ensure it doesn't burn. Remove from the oven once it's golden.

Cool for 10 minutes, then peel from the paper before cutting or snapping into cracker-sized pieces.

Store any leftover crackers in an airtight container.

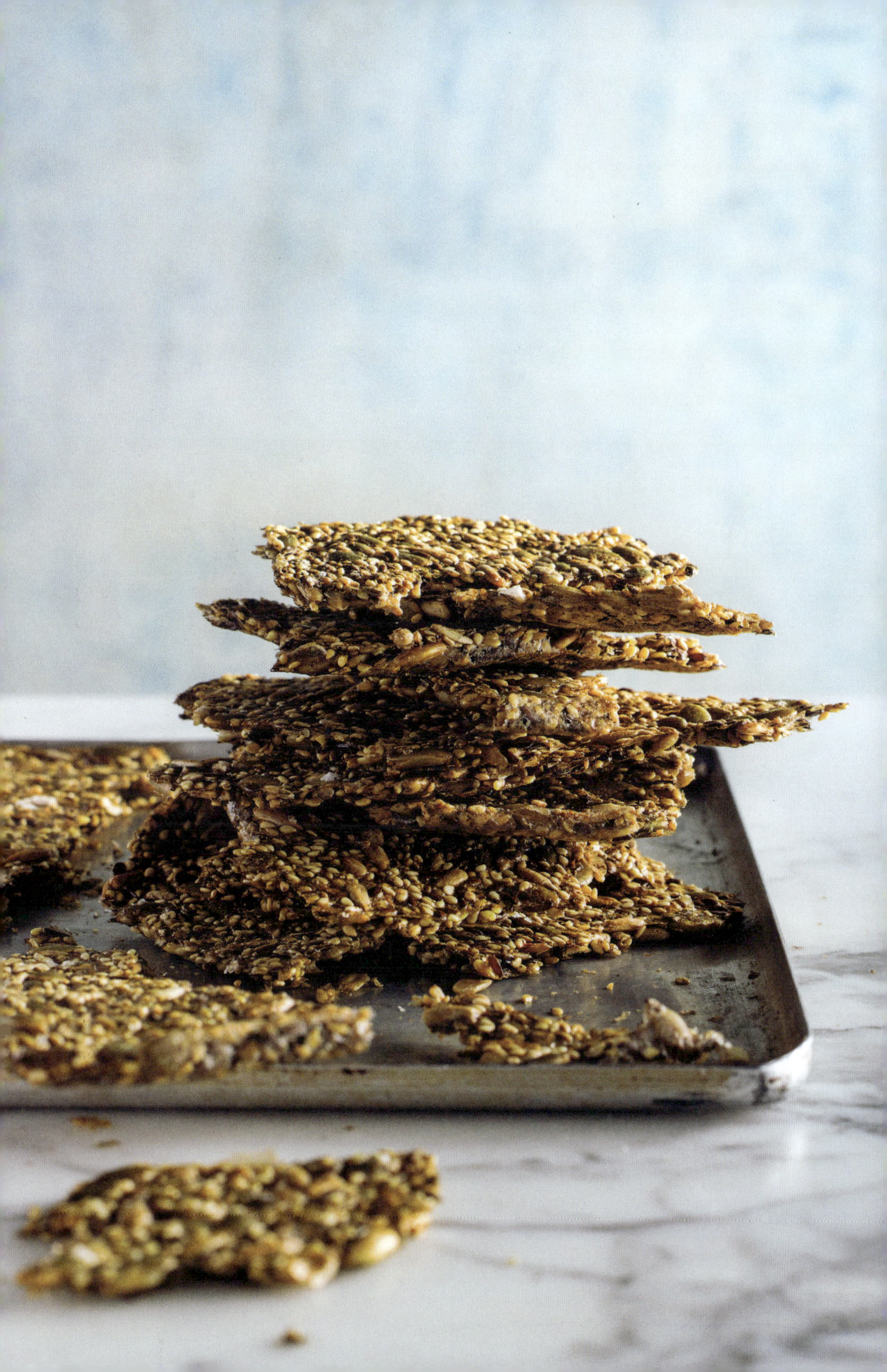

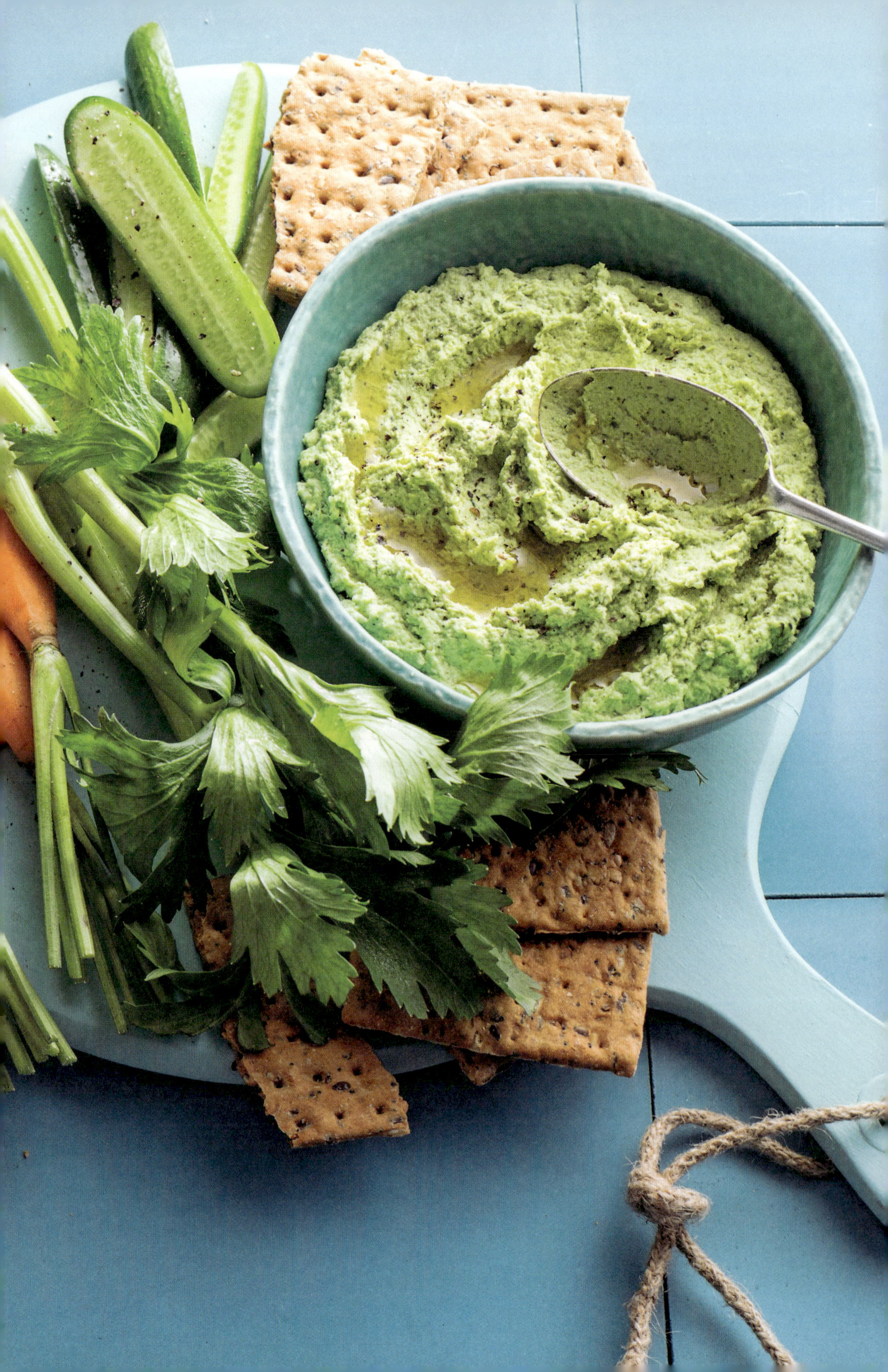

Serves 6

EDAMAME HUMMUS

This is a glow-up for a traditional hummus recipe – it's so good you'll want to eat it with everything. I love it as a snack with some veggie sticks or seed crackers (see page 214), but it would also be great in sandwiches or wraps, as part of a buddha bowl or tossed through a salad or pasta.

135 g (1½ cups) shelled edamame, thawed
2 garlic cloves
juice of 1 large lemon (around 3 tablespoons)
90 g (⅓ cup) tahini
¼ teaspoon ground cumin
small handful of coriander or flat-leaf parsley
sea salt and freshly ground black pepper
3 tablespoons extra-virgin olive oil
1 large ice cube

Combine the edamame, garlic, lemon juice, tahini, cumin and coriander or parsley in a food processor or blender, and season well with salt and pepper. Blend at a high speed until you have a rough paste, then start drizzling in the olive oil slowly as the blender is running. You may need to stop and scrape down the side as you go.

Continue adding the olive oil until the hummus reaches a creamy consistency (you may not need all the oil). Finally, add the ice cube to bring the mixture together.

Spoon some hummus onto a serving platter, top with a drizzle of olive oil, if you like, and add a pinch of sea salt.

Makes 12

HIGH-PROTEIN EGG MUFFINS

These egg muffins are like a mini hand-held omelette. They are so handy to grab on the go for a quick, high-protein snack or light meal. Play around with your fillings to suit you. As long as you get the base ingredients of egg, cottage cheese and cheese right, you can't really go wrong.

olive oil spray
8 eggs
265 g (1 cup) cottage cheese
50 g (½ cup) grated low-fat tasty cheddar, plus extra to sprinkle on top
sea salt and freshly ground black pepper
25 g (½ cup) baby spinach leaves, roughly chopped
150 g (1 cup) finely diced mixed vegetables (try mushrooms, onion, capsicum, zucchini, corn), finely diced

Preheat the oven to 180°C. Spray a 12-hole muffin tin with olive oil.

Put the eggs, cottage cheese, grated cheese and a good pinch of salt and pepper in a food processor and blend until smooth. Pour into a large jug or bowl with the spinach and vegetables.

Pour the mixture directly into the muffin holes, filling each nearly to the top. Sprinkle a pinch of extra cheddar over each muffin.

Bake for 20–25 minutes, or until the muffins are golden on top and a skewer inserted in the centre comes out clean.

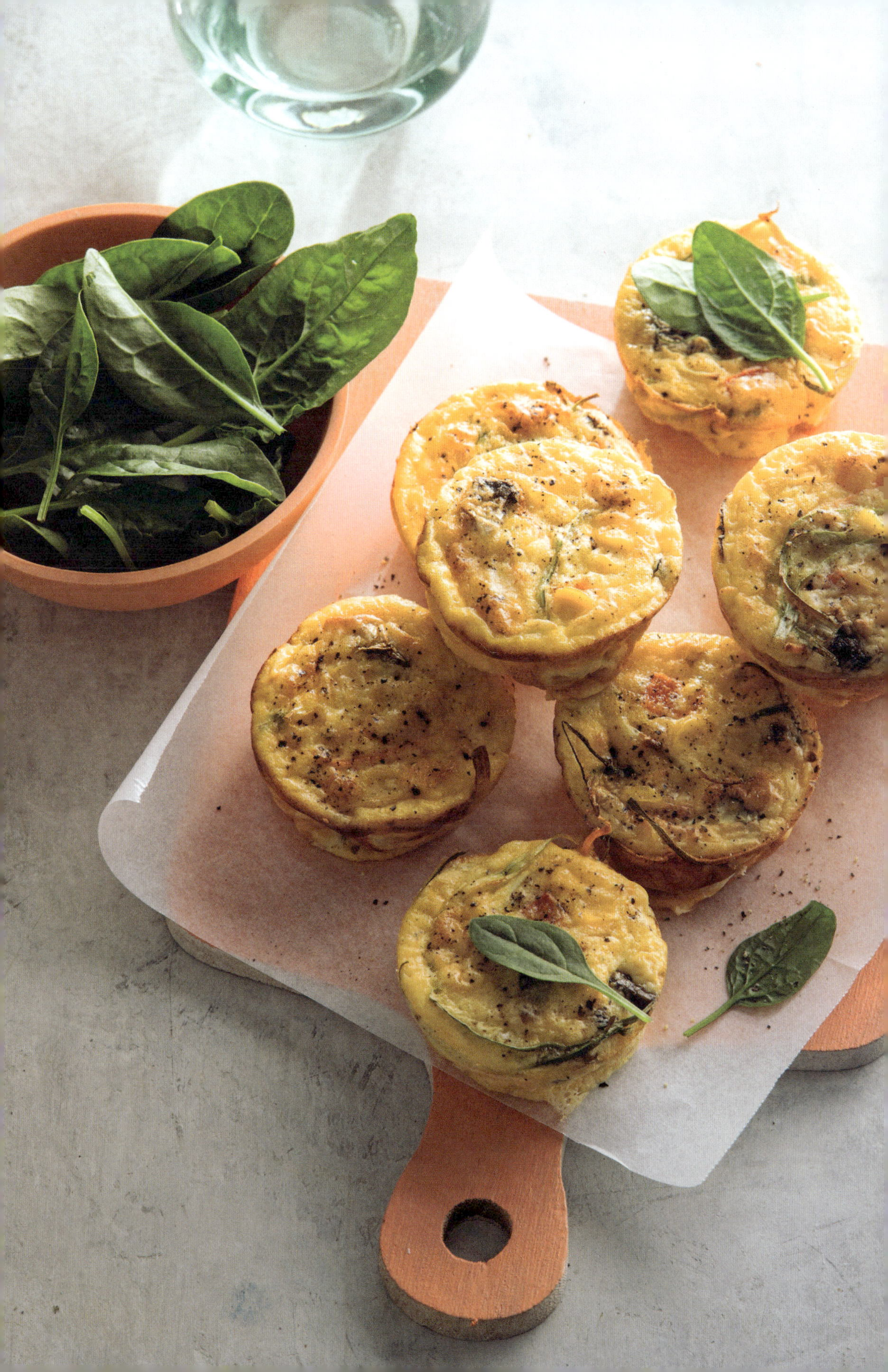

Conversion chart

Measuring cups and spoons may vary slightly from one country to another, but the difference is generally not enough to affect a recipe. All cup and spoon measures are level. One Australian metric measuring cup holds 250 ml (8 fl oz), one Australian tablespoon holds 20 ml (4 teaspoons) and one Australian metric teaspoon holds 5 ml. North America, New Zealand and the UK use a 15 ml (3-teaspoon) tablespoon.

LENGTH

METRIC	IMPERIAL
3 mm	⅛ inch
6 mm	¼ inch
1 cm	½ inch
2.5 cm	1 inch
5 cm	2 inches
18 cm	7 inches
20 cm	8 inches
23 cm	9 inches
25 cm	10 inches
30 cm	12 inches

LIQUID MEASURES

ONE AMERICAN PINT	ONE IMPERIAL PINT
500 ml (16 fl oz)	600 ml (20 fl oz)

CUP	METRIC	IMPERIAL
⅛ cup	30 ml	1 fl oz
¼ cup	60 ml	2 fl oz
⅓ cup	80 ml	2½ fl oz
½ cup	125 ml	4 fl oz
⅔ cup	160 ml	5 fl oz
¾ cup	180 ml	6 fl oz
1 cup	250 ml	8 fl oz
2 cups	500 ml	16 fl oz
2¼ cups	560 ml	20 fl oz
4 cups	1 litre	32 fl oz

DRY MEASURES

The most accurate way to measure dry ingredients is to weigh them. However, if using a cup, add the ingredient loosely to the cup and level with a knife; don't compact the ingredient unless the recipe states 'firmly packed'.

METRIC	IMPERIAL
15 g	½ oz
30 g	1 oz
60 g	2 oz
125 g	4 oz (¼ lb)
185 g	6 oz
250 g	8 oz (½ lb)
375 g	12 oz (¾ lb)
500 g	16 oz (1 lb)
1 kg	32 oz (2 lb)

OVEN TEMPERATURES

CELSIUS	FAHRENHEIT
100°C	200°F
120°C	250°F
150°C	300°F
160°C	325°F
180°C	350°F
200°C	400°F
220°C	425°F

CELSIUS	GAS MARK
110°C	¼
130°C	½
140°C	1
150°C	2
170°C	3
180°C	4
190°C	5
200°C	6
220°C	7
230°C	8
240°C	9
250°C	10

Acknowledgements

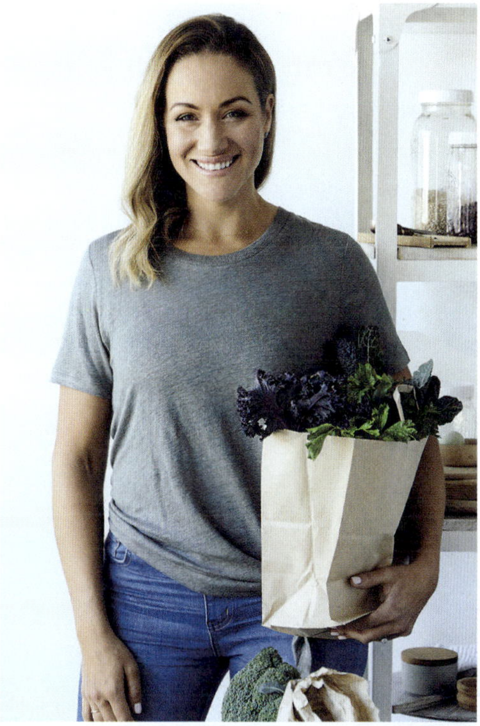

These books are a true honour to write but they take time: I often say it's like writing a university thesis, given the deep research and extensive writing that is involved! While the process is relatively short in duration, it is intense and it can take you away from your family and your kids for some time.

So my first big thank you is to my beautiful family: my husband Rob and my boys, Billy and Luis, for making space for me to do what I love and being patient while Mummy finished her book.

To my patients, who for nearly 20 years in clinical practice have trusted me with managing their health through their peri journey and taught me so much. Your stories and experiences have helped me to really understand how the perimenopause period can impact lives, and allowed me to learn and observe what works and how to tackle the specific complexities of this time.

To my publisher, Ingrid Ohlsson, who has been the most wonderful support for me for years now and always believed in me and trusted me to write these books – you have changed the entire course of my career and I'm forever grateful.

Also to my editors, Ariane Durkin and Katie Bosher, for making my research and my words into a carefully crafted book that flows and reads so beautifully!

And to the incredible designer Madeleine Kane, who has created the most beautiful, user-friendly resource.

Finally, thank you to Alan Benson, Vanessa Austin, Kerrie Ray, Lucinda Thompson, Sally Devenish and Jane Watkins.

Endnotes

page 9

Essentially, menopause is the ... Helen Paynter, 'Top Nutrition Tips for Menopause', *CSIRO*, 4 May, 2021, www.CSIRO.au

This mind-blowing fact ... 'Menopause', *Mount Sinai*, www.mountsinai.org

These immature eggs are in ... ibid.

By 37, we have roughly 25,000 ... ibid.

Our egg supply runs out ... Dr Louise Newson, *Preparing for the Perimenopause and Menopause*, Penguin Life, 2021

The average age Western women go ... 'Menopause', *Jean Hailes for Women's Health*, www.jeanhailes.org.au

Since the average life expectancy ... Mercedes Vélez Toral et al., 'Psychosocial interventions in perimenopausal and postmenopausal women: a systematic review of randomised and non-randomised trials and non-controlled studies', *Maturitas*, vol. 77, no. 2, 2013, pp 93–110.

We know that adopting healthy ... ibid.

Some women experience perimenopause ... David Steen Martin, 'Perimenopause can be more difficult than menopause for many', *Norton Healthcare*, December 15, 2021, www.nortonhealthcare.com

In fact, it's been suggested that ... Nanette Santoro, 'Perimenopause: From research to practice'; *Journal of Women's Health*, vol. 25, no. 4, 2016, pp332–339.

page 10

The age a woman goes into menopause ... Bauset et al., 2022.

Geographic location seems to ... ibid.

Bodily systems, including the cardiovascular ... Bauset et al., 'Nuts and Metabolic Syndrome: Reducing the Burden of Metabolic Syndrome in Menopause', *Nutrients*, vol. 14, no. 8, 2022, p1677.

This decline in hormones ... Dr Louise Newson, 2021; Jerilynn C. Prior, 'Progesterone for symptomatic perimenopause treatment: progesterone politics, physiology and potential for perimenopause', vol. 3, no. 2, 2011, pp109–120.

page 11

Women in peri are as likely to ... Jerilynn C Prior et al., 'Oral micronized progesterone for perimenopausal night sweats and hot flushes a Phase III Canada-Wide randomized placebo-controlled 4-month trial', *Scientific Reports*, vol. 13, no. 1, 2023, p9082.

As many as 85 per cent of women ... Bansal and Aggarwal, 2019.

Research indicates that these hot ... ibid.

Despite this, studies suggest that ... ibid.

When they happen, they usually last ... Dr Robert R Freedman, 'Menopausal hot flashes: Mechanisms, endocrinology, treatment'; *The Journal of Steroid Biochemistry Molecular Biology*, vol. 142, 2014, pp115–120.

Despite years of research, the exact ... Bansal and Aggarwal, 2019.

What is known is that a hot flush ... ibid.

What is known is that a hot flush ... ibid.

There's likely a genetic component ... ibid.

So far, the only consistent risk ... ibid.

page 12

When our blood pressure fluctuates ... Dr Louise Newson, 2021.

Night sweats come a close second ... Rebecca S.; 'Q&A: What are the differences between night sweats and hot flashes?'; *Menopause Now*, June 18, 2020, www.menopausenow.com

They're characterised by episodes ... ibid.

Much like hot flushes, night sweats ... Jerilynn C. Prior et al. 'Oral micronized progesterone for perimenopausal night sweats and hot flushes a Phase III Canada-wide randomized placebo-controlled 4-month trial', *Nature Portfolio: Scientific reports*, 2023, p9082.

Insomnia and night waking has ... Mengnan Zhao et al., 'Effects of exercise on sleep in perimenopausal women: a meta-analysis of randomized controlled trials', *Explore*, vol 19, no. 5, 2023, pp636-645.

Having disturbed sleep over ... ibid.

page 13

The decline in oestrogen during ... Kate M. Bermingham et al., 'Menopause is associated with postprandial metabolism, metabolic health and lifestyle: The ZOE PREDICT study'; *eBioMedicine*; vol. 85, 104303, 2022.

Peri can be a vulnerable period ... Jupil Ko and Young-Min Park; 'Menopause and the loss of skeletal muscles mass in women'; *Iranian Journal of Public Health*: vol 50, no. 2, 2021, pp413–414.

According to one study, women ... ibid.

Fat mass and waist circumference ... Hye Gyeong Jeong and Hyuntae Park; 'Metabolic disorders in menopause'; *Metabolites*, vol. 12, no. 10, 2022, p954.

Fat mass increases and there's ... ibid.

There's a rise in what is known ... Vasiliki Venetsanaki and Stergios A. Polyzos; 'Menopause and non-alcoholic fatty liver disease: a review focusing on therapeutic perspectives'; *Current Vascular Pharmacology*, vol. 17, no. 6, 2019, pp546–555.

page 14

This happens because the brain's ... Dr Louise Newson, 2021.

According to one study, 42 per cent ... Mary Infantino, 'The prevalence and pattern of gastroesophageal reflux symptoms in perimenopausal and menopausal women', *Journal of the American Association of Nurse Practitioners*, vol. 20, no. 5, 2008, pp266–272.

Not only does the drop in oestrogen ... Dr Louise Newson, 2021.

Causes include overeating ... Mary Infantino, 2008.

page 15

The most common psychological ... Alexandra M. Bodnaurc et al, 'Diet and depression during peri- and post-menopause: A Scoping Review Protocol', *Methods and Protocols*, vol. 5, no. 5, 2023, p91.

This makes a lot of sense given ... ibid.

Serotonin is our 'happy hormone' ... Stephanie Watson, 'Serotonin: The natural mood booster', *Harvard Health Publishing*, November 20, 2023, www.health.harvard.edu

By the time we've been through ... Bansal and Aggarwal, 2019.

Endorphins are associated with ... 'Endorphins: The brain's natural pain reliver, *Harvard Health Publishing*, July 20, 2021, www.health.harvard.edu

Many women report feeling cranky ... Alexandra M. Bodnaurc et al, 2023.

The cause, as always, is our hormones ... Kelly Bilodeau, 'Sleep, stress, or hormones? Brain fog during perimenopause', *Harvard Health Publishing*, April 9, 2021, www.health.harvard.edu

page 16

Some women find that the fluctuating ... Dr Louise Newson, 2021.

Vaginal dryness due to lowered oestrogen ... Bansal and Aggarwal, 2019.

It's widely accepted that sexual function ... Irene Scavello et al., 'Sexual health in menopause', *Medicina*, vol. 55, no. 9, 2019, p559.

This is a little-known symptom of peri ... Dr Louise Newson, 2021.

Peri (and particularly late peri) marks … Jo C. Lo et al., 'Bone and the Perimenopause', *Obstetrics and Gynecology Clinics of North America*, vol. 38, no. 3, 2011, pp503–517.

page 17

Hormones cause areas of the … Dr Louise Newson, 2021.

If breast tenderness is a concern … Cemile Idiz et al., 'The role of nutrition in women with benign cyclic mastalgia: a case-control study', *European Journal of Breast Health*, vol. 14, no. 3, 2018, pp156–159.

As oestrogen levels decline … Dr Louise Newson, 2021.

A GP who specialises … ibid.

Oestrogen helps to lubricate … ibid.

It tends to be at its worst … ibid.

page 21

The Mediterranean Diet has been … Dr Catherine Itsiopoulos and Vivienne Koutsis, *The Modern Mediterranean Diet: The world's most successful every diet for long-term health*, Macmillan Australia, 2023.

In one study, of a group of women … ibid.

page 22

Recently, I read that Japan is … Jennifer Chandler, 'Menopause around the world', *mindset health*, October 15, 2021; accessed Mar 5, 2024, www.mindsethealth.com

It's true that Japanese women … Takeshi Aso, 'Equol improves menopausal symptoms in Japanese women'; *The Journal of Nutrition*, vol. 140, no. 7, 2010, pp1386S–1389S.

This difference is believed to be … Y Somekawa et al., 'Soy intake related to menopausal symptoms, lipids, and bone mineral density in postmenopausal Japanese women', *Obstetrics and Gynaecology*, vol. 97, no. 1, 2001, pp109–15.

Like the Mediterranean diet … 'Menopause', *PCRM's Nutrition Guide for Clinicians*, 2024. Accessed March 5, 2024, www.nutritionguide.pcrm.org

Okinawa in Japan is one of the … 'The Okinawa Diet: Eating and living to 100', *Blue Zones*, 2024, accessed March 5, 2024, www.bluezones.com

Plant foods make up 90 per cent … ibid

DASH stands for … 'DASH Eating Plan', *National Heart, Lung, and Blood Institute*, December 29, 2021, accessed, March 5, 2024, nhlbi.nih.gov

In a 2022 study of perimenopausal … Shuping Hao et al., 'Dietary and exercise interventions for perimenopausal women: A health status impact study', *Frontiers in Nutrition*, vol. 8, 752500, 2022.

This way of eating provides … National Heart, Lung, and Blood Institute, 2021.

page 23

Overall, research shows that … Neal D. Barnard et al; 'The women's study for the alleviation of vasomotor symptoms (WAVS): a randomized controlled trial of a plant-based diet and whole soybeans for postmenopausal women'; *Menopause*, vol. 28, no. 10, 2021, pp1150–1156.

Whether you choose to follow … Bonnie Beezhold et al.,'Vegans report less bothersome vasomotor and physical menopausal symptoms than omnivores', *Maturitas*, 2018, pp12–17.

page 24

It is an essential nutrient … Meng-Xia Ji and Qi Yu, 'Primary osteoporosis in postmenopausal women', *Chronic Diseases and Translational Medicine*, vol. 1, no. 1, 2015, pp9–13.

page 25

The Cancer Council has safe sun … Zhaojun Mei et al. 'The role of vitamin D in menopausal women's health', *Frontiers in Physiology*, vol. 14: 2023, 1211896.

The glycaemic index (GI) is … Monique Tello, 'Menopause and insomnia: Could a low-GI diet help?' *Harvard Health Publishing*, January 17, 2020, www.health.harvard.edu

High-GI foods are rapidly … ibid.

Eating low-GI foods is also … ibid.

page 26

Magnesium essential for the … ibid.

Studies show that maintaining … ibid.

It's also been linked with … 'Alysha Owen, 'How to eat during perimenopause for your weight and health', *Zoe*, August 4, 2023. Accessed March 5, 2024, www.zoe.com

These fats can help with … 'How omega-3 can provide relief for menopausal symptoms' *Australian Menopause Centre*, February 11, 2016. Accessed March 5, 2024, www.menopausecentre.com.au

page 27

They bind to oestrogen receptors … 'Phytoestrogens', *Australian Menopause Centre*, October 24, 2022. Accessed March 5, 2024, www.menopausecentre.com.au

Because the decline of oestrogen … ibid.

There are two main types … ibid.

When iron levels are low … 'Iron: Are you deficient?'; *Australian Menopause Centre*, June 28, 2022. Accessed March 5, 2024, www.menopausecentre.com.au

Peri women, however, may … ibid.

page 29

Protein benefits: M. Drummen et al., 'Dietary protein and energy balance in relation to obesity and co-morbidities', *Frontiers in Endocrinology*, vol 9. 2018.

From around the age of 40 … 'The power of protein, more so during perimenopause and menopause'; *Australian Menopause Centre*, July 5, 2019. Accessed March 5, 2024, www.menopausecentre.com.au

page 30

When we describe a food … 'What are complete proteins?', *Cleveland Clinic*, December 5, 2022, accessed March 5, 2024, health.clevelandclinic.org

Incomplete protein describes … 'Incomplete Proteins', *Nibble Directory*, accessed March 5, 2024, umass.edu

If you're vegan, you can eat … Cleveland Clinic, Dec 5, 2022

page 31

So for example, if your current weight … Thais R. Silva et al., 'Nutrition in menopausal woman: A narrative review', *Nutrients*, vol. 13, no. 7, 2021, p2149.

1500 calories X 30 per cent … '4 Ways Protein Can Help you Shed Pounds', *Cleveland Clinic*, October 27, 2022, health.clevelandclinic.org

page 32

Protein counter: 'Protein counter factsheet', *Australian Nutrition 2011–2013 Food Nutrient Database*, February 2021, www.dieticianconnection.com

The amount we can absorb at … Cleveland Clinic, October 27, 2022.

However, protein powder … 'Information sheet: Soy & isoflavones', *Cancer Council*, accessed March 2024 www.cancer.org.au

page 35

Phytoestrogens interact with oestrogen … Desmawati Desmawati and Delmi Sulastri, 'Phytoestrogens and their health effect', *Open Access Macedonian Journal of Medical Sciences*, vol. 7, no. 3, 2019, pp 495–499.

There are four groups of phytoestrogens: 'Information sheet: Soy & isoflavones', *Cancer Council*.

page 36

The World Cancer Research Fund (WCRF) have … Information sheet: Soy & isoflavones', *Cancer Council*.

In fact, another study even … ibid.

page 37

The link between soy and reduced … 'Straight talk about soy', *Harvard T.H. Chan School of Public Health*, 2024, hsph.harvard.edu

A recent study on postmenopausal ... Neal D. Barnard et al., 'The women's study for the alleviation of vasomotor symptoms (WAVS): a randomized controlled trial of a plant-based diet and whole soybeans for postmenopausal women', *Menopause*, vol. 28, no. 10, 2021, pp1150–1156.

In Japan, where ... Y Somekawa et al., 2001.

In studies, the therapeutic ... Desmawati Desmawati and Delmi Sulastri, 2019.

page 39

Plant lignans, found in flaxseeds, were ... 'Flaxseed for menopause: What does the science say?', *Nature's Best*, 2024, naturesbest.co.uk

Eating flaxseeds every day ... Nuray Egelioglu Cetisli et al., 'The effects of flaxseed on menopausal symptoms and quality of life', *Holistic Nursing Practice*, vol. 29, no. 3, 2015, pp151–157.

40 g of flaxseeds per day for 2 months .... André Lemay et al. 'Flaxseed dietary supplement versus hormone replacement therapy in hypercholesterolemic menopausal women', *Obstetrics and Gynecology*, vol. 100, no. 3, 2002, pp495–504.

A study in 2004 suggested that ... Jennifer D. Brooks, et al., 'Supplementation with flaxseed alters estrogen metabolism in postmenopausal women to a greater extent than does supplementation with an equal amount of soy', *American Journal of Clinical Nutrition*, vol 79, no. 2, 2004, pp318–325.

page 40

Tree nuts are also low ... Bauset et al., 2022.

The bioactive components ... ibid.

Nuts are associated with a ... ibid.

They're an integral part of the ... Thais R. Silva et al., 2021.

They have been shown to have ... Bauset, et al., 2022.

Nuts may play a role ... ibid.

It's recommended that we eat ... 'Nut consumption, nutrients and better health', *Nuts For Life*, August 15, 2019, www.nutsforlife.com.au

Many people avoid nuts because ... ibid.

Interestingly, we don't absorb between ... 'Are all kilojoules in nuts absorbed?' *Nuts For Life*, August 8, 2022, www.nutsforlife.com.au

This is because the fats get trapped ... ibid

page 41

On average, people who eat more ... 'Berries are among the healthiest foods you can eat', *Harvard T.H. Chan*, 2021, www.hsph.harvard.edu

Blueberries, blackberries and raspberries ... 'Blueberries, the post menopause superfood', *Menopause Natural Solutions*, August 13, 2021, www.menopausenaturalsolutions.com

Blueberries have been shown to ... ibid.

Eating strawberries daily can ... Rafaela G. Feresin, et al., 'Impact of daily strawberry consumption on blood pressure and arterial stiffness in pre- and stage-1 hypertensive postmenopausal women: a randomized trial', *Food & Function*, vol. 8, no. 11, 2017, pp4139–4149

The greater the intake of blueberries ... 'Blueberries, the Post Menopause Superfood', 2021.

Blueberries may also improve ... ibid.

A large observational study ... ibid.

page 42

Olive oil is associated with ... Heidi Godman, 'Harvard study: high olive oil consumption associated with longevity', *Harvard Health Publishing*, April 1, 2022, health.harvard.edu

If it doesn't specify 'cold-pressed' ... 'FAQs: Everything you might want to know about Cobram Estate', 2024, www.combramestate.com.au

Hydroxytyrosol has several beneficial ... Lorena Martínez et al., 'Hydroxytyrosol: Health benefits and use as functional ingredient in meat, *Medicines*, vol. 5, no. 1, 2018, p13.

page 43

Extra-virgin olive oil has been shown ... Thanh Truong Giang Ly et al., 'Protective effects and benefits of olive oil and its extracts on women's health', *Nutrients*, vol. 13, no. 12, 2021, p4279.

The polyphenols in extra-virgin olive ... ibid.

Extra-virgin olive oil can protect ... ibid.

However, there is a lot of information on ...Juan José Hidalgo-Mora et al., 'Diet to reduce the metabolic syndrome associated with menopause. The logic for olive oil', *Nutrients*, vol. 12, no. 10, 2020, p3184.

The PREDIMED study showed a ... Nancy Babio, et al., 'Mediterranean diets and metabolic syndrome status in the PREDIMED randomized trial', *Canadian Medical Association Journal*, vol. 186, no. 17, 2014, ppE649–E657.

Consuming as little as .... Godman, 2022.

In fact, extra-virgin olive oil ... ibid.

page 44

Omega-3 fatty acids are a type ... National Heart Foundation of Australia, 'Omega-3 fatty acids and plant-based diets', *Factsheet 2015*, www.heartfoundation.org.au

If you don't eat oily fish ... 'How Omega-3 Can Provide Relief for Menopausal Symptoms', www.menopausecentre.com.au

If you are vegan ... National Heart Foundation of Australia, 2015.

A cross-sectional, nationwide health ... Minjeong Chae and Kyong Park, 'Association between dietary omega-3 fatty acid intake and depression in postmenopausal women', *Nutrition Research and Practice*, vol. 15, no. 4, 2021, pp468–478.

Three high level studies showed ... Mina Mohammady et al., 'Effect of omega-3 supplements on vasomotor symptoms in menopausal women: A systematic review and meta-analysis', *European Journal of Obstetrics and Gynecology and Reproductive Biology*, September 2018, 228, pp295–302.

Omega-3 fatty acid intake showed ... Davide Decandia, et al., 'n-3 PUFA improve emotion and cognition during menopause: A systemic review', *Nutrients*, vol. 14, no. 9, 2022. p1982.

The Heart Foundation ... The Australian Heart Foundation, 'Fish and omega-3: Questions and answers Factsheet', 2015, www.heartfoundation.org.au

page 46

Lower-GI foods have been shown to ... Top Nutrition Tips for Menopause', Paynter, 2021.

Researchers who looked at the ... Tello, 2020.

They believed the drops in blood ...ibid.

page 48

A random controlled trial ... Thais R. Silva et al., 2021.

Fibre improves cholesterol levels ... https://nutritionaustralia.org/fact-sheets/fibre-2/

page 50

Fibre counter: 'Fibre', *Nutrition Australia*, October 2014 (Revised July 2021), www.nutritionaustralia.org

page 51

Given their undeniable health benefits ... 'We're not getting any better at eating fruit and veg: we need a coordinated approach to nutrition now', media release, *Dieticians Australia*, Canberra, 17 June, 2022.

Eating a wide variety of different coloured ... Paynter, 2021.

A higher consumption of cruciferous ... Sarah JO Nomura et al., 'Dietary intake of soy and cruciferous vegetables and treatment-related symptoms in Chinese American and non-Hispanic White breast cancer survivors', *Breast Cancer Research and Treatment*, vol. 168, no. 2, 2018, pp467–479.

Higher intake of whole plant foods ... Zhao-Min Liu et al., 'Whole plant foods intake is associated with fewer menopausal symptoms in Chinese postmenopausal women with prehypertension or untreated hypertension', *Menopause*, vol. 22, no. 5, 2015, pp496–504.

One study found that ... Barnard, et al., 2021.

The risk of developing ... Tello, 2020.

Getting adequate magnesium ... Katey Davidson, 'Can magnesium help relieve menopause symptoms?', *Healthline*, 23 June, 2020, www.healthline.com

A study of postmenopausal women ... ibid.

Another study found that ... Nuria Rosique-Esteban et al., 'Dietary magnesium and cardiovascular disease: A review with emphasis in epidemiological studies', *Nutrients*, vol. 10, no. 2, 2018, p168.

How many do we need? Australian Government, 'What is a serve of vegetables?', *Eat for health*, www.eatforhealth.gov.au

page 52

They have many roles, such as ... Barrea, et al., 2023 https://www.ncbi.nlm.nih.gov/pmc/articles/PMC9974675/

Oestrogen has been shown to ...

Luigi Barrea, et al., 'Probiotics and prebiotics: Any role in menopause-related diseases?', *Current Nutrition Reports*, vol. 12, no. 1, 2023, pp83–97.

Oestrogen regulates the gut ... ibid.

Dysbiosis in the gut ... ibid

Beneficial bacterial strains ... ibid.

If this link is proven, tailoring ... ibid.

Studies have shown a positive effect ... ibid.

A study found postmenopausal women ... Mehrnaz Shafie et al., 'The effect of probiotics on mood and sleep quality in postmenopausal women: A triple-blind randomized controlled trial', *Clinical Nutrition ESPEN*, vol. 50, 2022, pp15–23.

The pH level in the vagina declines ... Barrea, et al., 2023.

page 54

There you should find the name of ... Andrew M. Taylor and Hannah D. Holscher, 'A review of dietary and microbial connections to depression, anxiety, and stress', *Nutritional Neuroscience*, vol. 23, no. 3, 2020, pp237–250.

page 61

Women lose around 10 per cent ... Joan C. Lo et al., 'Bone and the perimenopause', *Obstetrics and Gynecology Clinics of North America*, vol. 38, no. 3, 2011, pp503–517.

Fractures can become a greater ... ibid.

In a US study of 2,000 women ... ibid.

Research showed that the rate ... ibid.

However, the mechanisms of age-related ... Oddom Demontiero et al., 'Aging and bone loss: new insights for the clinician', *Therapeutic Advances in Musculoskeletal Disease*, vol. 4, no. 2, 2012, pp61–76.

As we age, this process shifts ...ibid.

page 63

Lactose content: 'What is the lactose content of different dairy products?', *Dairy Australia*, 7 March, 2024, www.dairy.com.au

page 64

Calcium counter: 'Calcium content of common foods', *Factsheet, International Osteoporosis Foundation*, 2022, www.healthybonesaustralia.org.au

page 65

One of vitamin D's primary functions ... 'Vitamin D and Bone Health', *Factsheet, Healthy Bones Australia*, 2020, .www.healthybonesaustralia.org.au

Unfortunately, this means they miss ... ibid

Vitamin D has been shown to have ... Zhaojun Mei et al., 'The role of vitamin D in menopausal women's health', *Frontiers in Physiology*, vol. 14, 2023, 1211896.

page 66

Vitamin K is most commonly known for ... P Weber, 'Vitamin K and bone health', *Nutrition*, vol. 17, no. 10, 2001, ppage 880-887.

Due to vitamin K's role in blood clotting ... Celia Rodríguez-Olleros Rodríguez and Manuel Díaz Curiel, 'Vitamin K and bone health: A review on the effects of vitamin K deficiency and supplementation and the effect of non-vitamin K antagonist oral anticoagulants on different bone parameters', *Journal of Osteoporosis*, 2019, 2069176.

The best sources of vitamin K ... 'Vitamin K: Fact sheet for health professionals', *National Institutes of Health*, updated 29 March 2021, www.ods.od.nih.gov

These exercises put pressure on the. ... Xinyu Chang et al., 'Regulation of bone health through physical exercise: Mechanisms and types', *Frontiers in Endocrinology*, vol. 13, 2022, 1029475.

page 67

Symptoms of iron deficiency: 'Iron deficiency anemia', *Mayo Clinic*, 2024, www.mayoclinic.org

If you're unable to build back your ... Jennifer Harrington, 'Iron deficiency anemia in peri-menopause', *Menopause Natural Solutions*, September 12, 2023, www.menopausenaturalsolutions.com

Generally speaking, women with regular periods ... Australian Government, 'Nutrient reference values: Iron', *Eat for health*, www.eatforhealth.gov.au

page 68

Iron Counter: ibid.

page 70

During peri, women can experience ... Laurel Kelly, 'Consumer health: Diabetes and menopause', *Mayo Clinic*, November 16, 2021, www.newsnetwork.mayoclinic.org

This means that sugar (or glucose) remains ... 'Blood sugar (glucose)', *Columbine Health Systems Center for Health Aging (Colorado State University)*, 2021, www.research.colostate.edu

Age is an independent risk factor ... Jennifer Rodgers et al., 'Cardiovascular risks associated with gender and aging', *Journal of Cardiovascular Development and Disease*, vol. 6, no. 2, 2019, p19.

The incidence of CVD in adults aged ... Maddalena Lettino et al., 'Cardiovascular disease in the elderly: proceedings of the European Society of Cardiology – Cardiovascular Round Table', *European Journal of Preventative Cardiology*, vol. 20, no. 10, 2022, pp1412–1424.

It's probably no great shock to ... Rodgers, et al., 2019.

Ageing can cause change in the heart... 'Heart health and aging', *National Institute on Aging*, Reviewed 1 June 2018, www.nia.nih.gov

Research also suggests that ... Seong-Hee Ko and Hyun-Sook Kim, 'Menopause-associated lipid metabolic disorders and foods beneficial for postmenopausal women', *Nutrients*, vol. 12, no. 1, 2020, p202.

Certain parts of the brain shrink ... 'How the aging brain affects thinking', *National Institute on Aging*, Reviewed 27 June 2023, www.nia.nih.gov

The neurons in the brain that ... ibid.

Additionally, the blood flow to the ... ibid.

Metabolic syndrome occurs when ... Hidalgo-Mora et al., 2020.

This cluster includes irregular blood ...ibid.

Excess abdominal weight is a trigger ... ibid.

In Chapter 4, we'll discuss how declining oestrogen ... Kexin Zhang et al., 'Metabolic diseases and healthy aging: identifying environmental and behavioural factors and promoting public health', *Frontiers in Public Health*, vol. 11, 2023, 1253506.

page 71

So, if you have a coffee with lunch ... Rob Newsom, 'How Long Does it Take for Caffeine to Wear Off?, *Sleep Foundation*, January 9, 2024, www.sleepfoundation.org

page 72

In one study, caffeine was associated ... Stephanie S. Faubion et al., 'Caffeine and menopausal symptoms: what is the association?', *Menopause*, vol. 22, no. 2, 2015, pp155–158.

Caffeine is known to enhance ... Ginger Plumbo, 'Study suggests caffeine intake may worsen menopausal hot flashes, night sweats', *Mayo Clinic*, July 22, 2014, www.newsnetwork.mayclinic.org

Caffeine counter, 'Caffeine', *Health Direct*, www.healthdirect.gov.au

page 73

A low-fat, vegetarian diet has been shown ... N. D. Barnard et al., 'Effectiveness of a low-fat vegetarian diet in altering serum lipids in healthy premenopausal women', *American Journal of Cardoiology*, vol. 85, no. 8, 2000, pp969–972.

Another trial following women ... Cara L. Carty et al., 'Low-fat dietary pattern and change in body-composition traits in the Women's Health Initiative Dietary Modification Trial', *The American Journal of Clinical Nutrition*, vol. 93, no. 3, 2011, pp516–524.

page 75

Interestingly, research shows that... Lacey M. Gould, et al., 'Metabolic effects of menopause: a cross-sectional characterization of body composition and exercise metabolism', *Menopause*, vol. 29, no. 4, 2022 pp377–389.

Almost 39 per cent of women enter... Sakshi Chopra, et al., 'Weight management module for perimenopausal women: A practical guide for gynecologists', *Journal of Mid-Life Health*, vol. 10, no. 4, 2019, pp165–172.

This weight gain along with a ... ibid.

The great news, however, is that ... ibid.

page 76

However, if we actively include more protein ... Stephen J. Simpson, 'Weight gain during the menopause transition: Evidence for a mechanism dependent on protein leverage', *BJOG: An International Journal of Obstetrics and Gynaecology*, vol. 130, no. 1, 2022, pp4–10.

Supporting this theory is the ... ibid.

Skeletal muscle is the biggest organ in ... Muthu Periasamy et al., 'Skeletal muscle thermogenesis and its role in whole body energy metabolism', *Diabetes and Metabolism Journal*, vol. 41, no. 5, 2017, pp327–336.

As we lose lean muscle tissue ... Chopra et al., 2019.

Lowered oestrogen and increased ... ibid.

Oestrogen decline is believed to ... ibid.

Peri and menopausal women ... ibid.

page 77

In addition liver disease ... ibid.

Higher fat mass, particularly ... ibid.

Studies have shown an association ... Bauset et al., 2022.

This fat accumulation tends to focus ... Chopra, et al., 2019.

Joint pain, particularly in weight-bearing ... ibid.

Higher weight or body mass index ... ibid.

page 83

Not only do you deeply deserve ... Sophie Yelland et al., 'The role of diet in Managing menopausal symptoms: A narrative review', *Nutrition Bulletin*, vol. 48, no. 1, 2023, pp43–65.

Given how challenging losing and ... Kaitlin Vogel, 'Menopausal women may benefit from weight loss drugs like Ozempic, Wegovy', *Health*, December 14, 2023, www.health.com

Since weight gain during peri ... ibid.

The most common ones are ... 'Ozempic helps weight loss by making you feel full. But certain foods can do the same thing – without the side-effects,' *Hunter Medical Research Institute*, March 21, 2023, www.hmri.org.au

Ozempic is taken as a weekly ... 'Brand name: Ozempic™', *Health Direct*, 2024, www.healthdirect.gov.au

However, Ozempic has surged in ... ibid.

Research has shown an average ... W. Timothy Garvey et al., 'Two-year effects of semaglutide in adults with overweight or obesity: the STEP 5 trial', *Nature Medicine*, vol. 28, 2022, pp2083–2091.

page 84

Like Ozempic, Saxenda is also injected ... 'How Saxenda® works', *Saxenda®*, July 2023, www.saxenda.com

Research subjects taking Saxenda ...: 'Saxenda (liraglutide) for the treatment of obesity, US', *Clinical Trials Arena*, August 4, 2023, www.clinicaltrialsarena.com

It works on the brain to decrease appetite ... 'Phentermine and Topiramate', *MedlinePlus*, 2024, www.medlineplus.gov

Research has shown a greater than ... Kim et al., 'Postmarketing Surveillance Study of the Efficacy and Safety of Phentermine in Patients with Obesity', *Korean Journal of Family Medicine*, vol. 34, no. 5, 2013, pp298–306.

One study showed that one year ... John PAGE H. Wilding, et al., 'Weight regain and cardiometabolic effects after withdrawal of semaglutide: The STEP 1 trial extension', *Diabetes, Obesity & Metabolism*, vol. 24, no. 8, 2022, pp1553–1564.

page 86

'Body mass index (BMI) and waist measurement', *Australian Government: Department of Health and Aged Care*, July 29, 2021, www.health.gov.au

page 91

And the more frequent the exercise ... Zhao et al., 2023.

Strength training also helps to ... Ana Mariá Capel-Alcaraz et al., 'The efficacy of strength exercises for reducing the symptoms of menopause: A Systematic Review', *Journal of Clinical Medicine*, vol. 12, no. 2, 2023, p548.

In fact, this has been confirmed ... bid.

page 92

Aerobic exercise (aka cardio)... Zhao et al., 2023.

Resistance training (aka strength training) ... Capel-Alcaraz et al., 2023.

Shuping Hao et al., 'Dietary and exercise interventions for perimenopausal women: A health status impact study', *Frontiers in Nutrition*, vol. 8. 2022, 752500.

Exercise interventions showed that ... Zhao et al., 2023.

In the research, it seems lighter ... ibid.

page 93

Exercise, particularly high-intensity aerobic ... Zhao et al., 2023.

Exercise has been shown to play ... Carol Hamilton Zehnacker and Anita Bemis-Dougherty, 'Effect of weighted exercises on bone mineral density in post-menopausal women. A systematic review', *Journal of Geriatric Physical Therapy*, vol. 30, no. 2, 2007, pp79–88.

Weight-bearing exercise like walking ... Ma et al., 'Effects of walking on the preservation of bone mineral density in perimenopausal and postmenopausal women: a systematic review and meta-analysis', 2013.

Index

Pan Macmillan acknowledges the Traditional Custodians of Country throughout Australia and their connections to lands, waters and communities. We pay our respect to Elders past and present and extend that respect to all Aboriginal and Torres Strait Islander peoples today. We honour more than sixty thousand years of storytelling, art and culture.

First published 2024 in Australia
by Pan Macmillan Australia Pty Limited
Level 25, 1 Market Street, Sydney, New South Wales
Australia 2000

A catalogue record for this book is available from the National Library of Australia

Design by Madeleine Kane
Edited by Katie Bosher
Index by Helena Holmgren
Prop and food styling by Vanessa Austin
Food preparation by Kerrie Ray
Colour + reproduction by Splitting Image Colour Studio
Printed in China by Imago Printing International Limited

10 9 8 7 6 5 4 3 2 1